DEVELOPMENTAL TRAUMA

Developmental Trauma offers a comprehensive introduction to the research findings that help us understand the effects on human development of early childhood trauma and adaptation to stress. It explains how developmental trauma disorder (DTD) differs from posttraumatic stress disorder (PTSD) and emerges from a toxic seed planted at the beginning of an individual's lifespan development. This important volume examines relational traumas and adverse childhood experiences, such as exposure to family and community violence, polyvictimization (multiple repeated childhood traumas), and disruptions to parent-child bonds, which lay the foundation for future relationships. The volume considers how DTD affects self-regulation capacities, identity development, self-esteem, and faith in oneself and others as well as increases the likelihood of comorbidities, including ADHD and autism spectrum disorders. Individuals with indications of developmental trauma face lifelong challenges in their ability to develop and maintain trusting relationships, to build and utilize healthy coping strategies, and to adjust to school and, eventually, the workplace. Uniquely, Daniel Cruz goes beyond individual levels of analysis that focus almost exclusively on patients and explores toxic stress embedded in social systems and institutional policies and procedures that cause individuals to suffer, experience psychiatric and medical problems, and that lead to social and economic adversities, such as poverty, homelessness, and involvement in criminal activity. Key topics explored include institutional betrayal, such as sexual assaults and workplace bullying, and judicial betrayal, when failures from the legal system do not adequately protect victims of trauma, for example in cases of domestic violence.

Developmental Trauma is for students of child and adolescent psychology, developmental psychology, clinical psychology, primary care and health psychology, education, social work, and urban studies. It is relevant for graduate students in applied fields, such as clinical and counseling psychology, and those working with diverse children as well as public health and policy.

Daniel Cruz is a psychologist, researcher, educator, and consultant and has provided psychotherapy and psychological evaluations to children and families in diverse settings. He served as a behavioral scientist in the family medicine training program at Mountainside Medical Center in Verona, New Jersey. Daniel has worked with individuals facing considerable adversity, including addiction, violence, human trafficking, discrimination, and suicide, who often distrust the social systems and institutions designed to protect them, such as child welfare and law enforcement agencies. He is past president of the Latino Mental Health Association of New Jersey.

DEVELOPMENTAL TRAUMA

Theory, Research, and Practice

Daniel Cruz

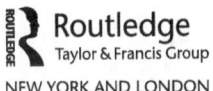 Routledge
Taylor & Francis Group

NEW YORK AND LONDON

Designed cover image: Elva Etienne/Moment via Getty Images

First published 2023
by Routledge
605 Third Avenue, New York, NY 10158

and by Routledge
4 Park Square, Milton Park, Abingdon, Oxon OX14 4RN

Routledge is an imprint of the Taylor & Francis Group, an informa business

© 2023 Daniel Cruz

ISBN: 978-1-032-30363-5 (hbk)
ISBN: 978-1-032-30346-8 (pbk)
ISBN: 978-1-003-30471-5 (ebk)

DOI: 10.4324/9781003304715

Typeset in Bembo
by Taylor & Francis Books

CONTENTS

ACKNOWLEDGEMENTS

My work as a psychologist, researcher, and writer would not have been possible without the love and support of my family and friends. I want to thank my mother, Milagros, or "miracle" in Spanish, who raised my sister and me as a strong and resilient single mother. We are grateful to you for always being such a kind, spiritual, and loving mother who taught us to value respect, humility, faith, forgiveness, and kindness. I also thank my sister, Wanda, for her strength, perseverance, and love and for blessing our family with my nieces and nephews, Wanda Jr., Desteny, Damaryse, Cristina, and Luis. To my cousin, Carmen, my late aunt, Julia, and my late cousin, Ernesto, thank you for always being there for our family. We are forever grateful to you for your years of love and support.

A special thank you to Matthew Lichten for his support, wisdom, compassion, and unwavering commitment to helping others and making this world a better place. You are indeed an inspiration to us all! Likewise, thanks to Hassey, Michael, and family for their kindness and support. To Grandma B and Aunt Roberta, thank you for your love, encouragement, sacrifice, and dedication to family. Your warmth, laughter, and words of wisdom are indelibly ingrained in my memories.

I want to acknowledge several friends and colleagues who have positively influenced my thinking over the years, provided feedback on chapters, and encouraged me throughout this process: Tamara Altman, Beata Beaudoin, Natasha Manning, John Gabriel, Gianni Pirelli, and all the staff and faculty at Mountainside Medical Center's Family Medicine Residency Training program.

Thank you to Helen Pritt, Shreya Bajpai, Shivranjani Singh, and the entire team at Routledge Psychology for their guidance and support and for making this process enjoyable.

1

EFFECTS OF EARLY CHILDHOOD STRESS AND TRAUMA

How do you define stress? What is stressful for you personally? How do you handle stress? Do you become overwhelmed and "shut down" emotionally – do you become silent, avoid others, and bottle up your feelings? Or, do you express your frustrations for the outside world to see? Do you think your approaches to dealing with stress are generally healthy? Or, do you sometimes regret the things you say or do when you experience heightened levels of stress?

Stress is something we all experience daily to varying degrees. Stress can lead us to experience fear and anxiety. It can also manifest as anger and/or sadness and depression in some individuals. In 1981, Kanner and colleagues coined the phrase "daily hassles" to reflect the fact that we routinely experience stress at school, work, or home (e.g., financial stress, stress from managing multiple personal and family responsibilities; Kanner et al., 1981). For children, stress is often associated with peer relationships and conflicts, tests and quizzes, and trying to manage school responsibilities and assignments with social and extra-curricular activities. Stress from daily hassles, which are presumably minor and reasonably predictable but arguably common, is linked to a variety of psycho-logical problems, including anxiety, insomnia, opioid abuse, and medical pro-blems such as asthma, obesity, and high blood pressure (Asselmann et al., 2017; Mize & Kliewer, 2017; Moss et al., 2020, 2021; Preston et al., 2018; Tinajero et al., 2020; Wirtz & von Känel, 2017).

But what exactly is stress?

Many of us intuitively understand stress to be a subjective (and hopefully relatively brief) emotional response to circumstances that challenge our sense of perceived control and leave us feeling overwhelmed and emotionally vulnerable. We may

DOI: 10.4324/9781003304715-1

also experience multiple stressors at any given point, making it challenging for us to stay present for ourselves and our loved ones. However, researchers' and practitioners' in-depth examinations of stress, including its meaning and objective measurement, reveal that stress is remarkably complex (e.g., Epel et al., 2018; McEwen & McEwen, 2017; O'Connor et al., 2021). Consider, for example, that stress can be acute (with a sudden onset and short duration) or chronic (longstanding and pervasive); caused by internal (physiological disturbances, such as vitamin deficiencies, and medical problems, such as thyroid dysfunction) or external (social stressors, such as those linked to gender norms, as well as poverty or being the victim of bullying); and correspond to discrete, isolated events or to long-term, repeated episodes that give rise to extreme fear, helplessness, and anxiety (Agnafors et al., 2017; Jung et al., 2019; Messerli-Bürgy et al., 2018; Muentner et al., 2021; Shaw & Starr, 2019; Watters & Martin, 2021; Zhang et al., 2020). I want to devote space here to discussing stress more carefully because it is critical to establishing a good understanding of trauma in general and developmental trauma specifically, which will be discussed in detail in the next chapter.

Stress and the General Adaptation Syndrome (GAS)

In his now classical studies of stress, Hans Selye included a detailed account of an individual's response to physiological stress – the general adaptation syndrome (GAS) – in which he argued that challenges to our state of homeostasis predictably give rise to a collection of sequenced reactions that involve three stages (Cunanan et al., 2018; Lu et al., 2021; O'Connor et al., 2021). In the earliest stage, which he referred to as the alarm reaction, the body assembles its energy resources (e.g., increases in blood oxygenation, heart rate, and blood pressure and, in turn, physical strength and energy) to deal with an immediate threat or an aversive event. In the alarm phase, the individual is alerted to something dangerous in their surroundings, and they experience distress as a consequence. The alarm reaction is followed by the resistance stage, where the body continuously mobilizes its energy reserves and attempts to return to a state of equanimity (the term *allostasis* is often used in the scientific literature to describe this process). In this state, the individual will remain on high alert (i.e., they maintain focus on the source or sources of danger), but, at the same time, they will use whatever strategies they have available to them to cope. In the final stage – the exhaustion stage – the body experiences fatigue (i.e., depletion of resources) from repeated attempts to cope with the stressor, eventually recovers from the initial alarm reaction, and re-enters a state of homeostasis.

Scholars have described this physiological stress response process in a number of different ways. For example, you may have heard of Walter Cannon's now mainstream phrase, "the fight, flight, and freeze" response, or more recently, the fight-flight-freeze-fawn adaptation (Öztürk et al., 2021; Zingela et al., 2022). The process has also been referred to as the sympathetic and parasympathetic response, or you might be familiar with the hypothalamic-pituitary-adrenal (HPA) axis, the sympathetic-adreno-medullar (SAM) axis, and the microbiota-gut-brain (MGB), which refer to the brain regions involved in the release of hormones, neurotransmitters, and the immune stress response process (Kim & Shin, 2018; Kothgassner et al., 2021; Roos et al., 2017).

Chronic Stress

One of the mysteries of our stress response system is that while it prepares us for immediate action, and, from an evolutionary framework, it improves our chances of survival, these same responses can make us physically sick, feel emotionally vulnerable, and place us at risk for several mental health problems. The physiological stress response described earlier in this chapter (i.e., the immediate and elevated release of glucocorticoids and neurotransmitters) is indeed linked to poor psychological and physical health, especially for experiences of prolonged stress and for children who are dependent on safe, predictable, and supportive environments to develop foundational cognitive, physiological, and emotion-regulation capacities (Agorastos & Chrousos, 2022; Kim et al., 2022; Lupien et al., 2018; McEwen, 2017)

Children are particularly susceptible to the adverse effects of stress because they lack the life experience that provides guidance regarding how to cope effectively in these situations. In addition, children often do not have a broad range of response options to deal with stress. For example, children usually cannot decide to leave school because they are frustrated with their academic performance or worried about bullying by peers. Consequently, children are far more vulnerable than adults are to mental health problems because early stress leads to psychological and physical health consequences (Koss & Gunnar, 2018; Monk et al., 2019; Nelson & Gabard-Durnam, 2020). These mental health problems can vary considerably from one child to another, depending, in part, on stress-mediated biological and epigenetic vulnerabilities (e.g., disturbances in neurotransmitter genes that regulate mood and cognition, such as catechol-O-methyltransferase and monoamine oxidase, as well as changes in heart-rate variability, which is an objective measure of physiological stress and cardiovascular-disease risk influenced, in part, by stress and stress appraisals, self-regulation, the prefrontal cortex, norepinephrine activity, and personality; Golds et al., 2020; Kim et al., 2018; McLaughlin & Lambert, 2017; Mulcahy et al., 2019; Rowell & Neal-Barnett, 2021; Schiweck et al., 2019). However, some children are naturally more sensitive than others.

Fear

Empirically supported models of trauma and the broader neuroscience literature on stress, cognition, and learning have now collectively established that fear conditioning mediates the types of pathogenic reactions seen in victims of trauma (Deslauriers et al., 2018; Jovanovic et al., 2020; Marusak et al., 2021; Stenson et al., 2021). Fear conditioning refers to the implicit or unconscious learning that takes place in situations that prompt an alarm reaction and that give rise to persistent, stereotyped, and often global fear-mediated reactions immediately following such events. Widespread worry, restlessness, and mental distraction, including flashback memories that yield graphic recollections of the first alarming event, illustrate conditioned fear responses. Fear expedites learning to prepare us to anticipate and respond to future threats quickly and effectively. This inclination, however, can seriously impede our sense of coherence and lead to, for example, high rates of "false alarms."

Pause and Reflect: Fear and Scary Movies

What was the scariest movie you ever saw growing up as a child or adolescent? Think back to the film that scared you the most and ask yourself what made that movie so scary for you? How did you learn to cope with the fear you experienced? How did you overcome it?

For me, it was *The Exorcist* (1973) and Wes Craven's *A Nightmare on Elm Street* (1999). The first film is about a 12-year-old girl who is possessed by a demonic entity. Her family, with the help of two priests, attempts to save her through prayer and, later in the film, an exorcism. I saw that movie when I was young, but it feels like I just saw it yesterday because the images of the movie and the memories of me watching the film in my living room are striking. It wasn't the movie alone, however, that scared me. It was the fact that, immediately following the film, there was a news report of a real-life exorcism, which complicated my ability to separate what I just saw in the movie at the time from real life. Understanding the movie's plot and the story's favorable resolution – that *good will always overcome evil* – helped me to manage the intensity of my fear. For some people, the horror film(s) that caused them to experience this intense level of fear and anxiety will also cause them to experience and re-experience these feelings for the rest of their lives.

Stress and Anxiety

Anxiety often arises from chronic stress and is characterized by pervasive fear, restlessness, loss of perceived control, cognitive rumination, and a tendency to expect the worst possible outcomes regardless of the circumstances. Research suggests that individuals who experience anxiety often report high levels of insomnia; cardiac problems; physiological responses, such as sweating and palpitations; depression; gastrointestinal problems; and disruptions in attention, concentration, and memory (Asselmann et al., 2017; Caporino et al., 2017; Lathren et al., 2019; Marques de Miranda et al., 2020; Panchal et al., 2021).

Children may develop characteristics of separation anxiety, for example, where they experience psychological distress when separated from caregivers because they fear something bad will happen during their parents' absence. Likewise, some children warrant treatment for social anxiety disorder (SAD), a psychiatric condition marked by pervasive fear and avoidance of social situations, often due to fear of rejection, embarrassment, and being judged negatively by others (Lawrence et al., 2019). Children with separation anxiety and SAD often warrant evaluation and treatment from healthcare providers. Studies have demonstrated that they often have a broad range of co-morbid psychiatric disorders, such as generalized anxiety, selective mutism, trichotillomania (compulsive hairpulling), anorexia, depression, and experiences of traumatic stress (Dogan et al., 2019; Matthies et al., 2018; Menzies et al., 2021). They tend to experience bullying, concentration problems, and mood disturbances, including panic attacks, angry outbursts, and school avoidance and refusal.

Cognitive Appraisals

Although physiological stress is mediated by the autonomic system (automatic and outside of our conscious awareness), researchers have confirmed that the way we perceive stressful events can worsen or enhance our responses to them. In their seminal work on stress, Lazarus and Folkman (1984) proposed a transactional model, which illuminates the differences between stress, or the events that happen to us in life, and our corresponding cognitive appraisals, or the ways in which we interpret and then later respond to such stressors. What the theory conveys is that, in the strictest sense, stress doesn't necessarily happen *to* us, it happens *with* us – with our active involvement; our unique temperaments, personalities, and coping resources; and, as I hope to convey in later chapters, the patterned responses and memory traces of our (and our families' and ancestors') strengths, adaptations, and resiliencies.

Carl Rogers, and his now well-respected model of humanistic psychology, believed that we are all born with the capacity to grow and develop to reach a point of unimaginable potential, despite life stressors and adversities. According to Rogers (1980), "Individuals have within themselves vast resources for self-understanding and for altering their self-concepts, basic attitudes, and self-directed behavior; these resources can be tapped if a definable climate of facilitative psychological attitudes can be provided" (pp. 115–117).

The point here is that we tend to cope with stress by evaluating (and re-evaluating) stressors and considering/carrying out both immediate and delayed responses (i.e., our immediate fight or flight reactions versus our careful reflection about possible strategic responses to these same stressors). Stress is an objective event that may lead to expected responses in some people (e.g., fear, depression, anxiety, stress-mediated health problems) and unexpected reactions in others (i.e., grit and determination, goal-directed behaviors, spirituality). In other words, stress is best viewed from the standpoint of a highly fluid and reciprocal (person-environment) interaction that gives rise to both challenges (helplessness, panic, behavioral dysregulation) as well as strengths.

Case in Point

Are you familiar with the concept of *hardiness*? Hardiness is a personality trait that describes individuals who are highly resistant to stress (Khosravi & Namani, 2021; Vagni et al., 2020). These individuals appear to have a natural propensity to cope with stress in adaptive ways, and as such, they tend to have better health. Hardiness is positively correlated with optimism, emotional intelligence, improved immunity, life satisfaction, mental flexibility, resilience, and problem-focused coping, and it is negatively correlated with anger, depression, neuroticism, avoidance coping, cognitive rumination, and anxiety (Bartone & Homish, 2020; Pandey & Shrivastava, 2017; Thomassen et al., 2018, 2022). Research suggests that hardy individuals not only cope well with stress, but they also develop strengths from it (i.e., the concept of stress-related growth, which refers to individuals' experiences of personal growth in response to stressful life experiences). Scholars have increasingly referred to hardiness and to the strengths that develop from positive adaptations to stress as *transformational coping* (LaRocca et al., 2018). Transformational coping refers to an individual's ability to re-evaluate stressful events so that they are neutral (a more mindful or peaceful state), positive, and personally meaningful (Mohr & Rosén, 2017). How does one develop hardiness? Feldman and Christensen (2008) offer the following description, and recommendations, which they refer to as the four Cs of hardiness:

> a strong *commitment* to self, work, family, and other important values; a sense of *control* over one's life; ... the ability to see change as a *challenge*, rather than a threat ... [and] *coherence*, a belief that one's internal and external environments are predictable and that things will work out as well as can be expected.
>
> *(p. 333)*

The idea that stress causes us to react in predetermined ways could instead be reframed to reflect the fact that stress appraisals mediate our responses to stress. As a number of scholars have observed: (1) more stress does not necessarily equate to more severe psychological problems; (2) some people thrive under stress and pressure; (3) what one person deems to be stressful, another may view as benign; and (4) an individual's cognitive appraisals and behavioral responses to stress vary considerably as a result of personal, social, and cultural differences. There is a substantial body of research evidence to suggest, for example, that stress, stress appraisals, and stress-related coping behaviors depend on, among other things, age, gender, socioeconomic status, personality, and attachment styles (Cristóbal-Narváez, 2017; Ebner & Singewald, 2017; Edman et al., 2017; Lathren et al., 2019; Malesza, 2019; Roos et al., 2017; Sommerfeldt et al., 2019). Thus, a critical aspect of stress is that our appraisals of it become automatic and reflexive "knee-jerk" reactions that are inextricably linked to automatic physiological processes (fight or flight response), especially if our automatic assumptions (described below) are not challenged.

In therapy, providers working with individuals under stress often attempt to help them distinguish between their automatic physiological reactions to stress (fight or flight) and their interpretations of those events (cognitive appraisals and reappraisals). This is a central goal, for example, in cognitive behavioral therapy and rational emotive behavior therapy, both of which often provide didactic training on distinguishing automatic (and often maladaptive) thoughts from those that are logical and reality based. Cognitive scholars have identified several maladaptive thinking patterns, which they refer to as cognitive errors and distortions, that underlie psychological disorders such as anxiety, depression, and trauma. If we don't challenge our automatic assumptions, we may develop automatic negative thoughts that become habitual and problematic. From the perspective of cognitive therapy, stress and anxiety predictably give rise to maladaptive automatic thoughts or schemas that are irrational, negatively skewed, and fear driven. Individuals in therapy learn skills to challenge such assumptions, including the tendency to make arbitrary inferences without measurable evidence, to assume the worst possible outcome in any given scenario (i.e., catastrophizing), and to discount positive events or positive aspects of events. In therapy, patients carefully examine and challenge statements such as: "I can't trust anyone because everyone really has bad intentions, some just hide it better than others," "Why should I try, I know I'm going to fail," "God doesn't love me; otherwise, I wouldn't have experienced the things I did so why should I care anymore," and "This is all my fault, I should have known better." Decades of systematic research suggest notable gains to social, emotional, and physical wellness for individuals who learn to reappraise stressful events using rational, evidence-based, and solution-focused ideas (e.g., Benbow & Anderson, 2019; Carpenter et al., 2018; Crowe & McKay, 2017; David et al., 2018; Kodal et al., 2018; Silk et al., 2018; Villabø et al., 2018). But, before we continue with this discussion, consider the following reflection exercise:

> Look at this fish in a bowl and ask yourself the following questions: Is this fish happy? Sad? Frustrated? Does it feel isolated? Is it aware that it is in a bowl and that there is a larger outside world? Is it aware that the world has many rewards, but also many potential dangers?

These were some of the questions posed by primatologist Dr. Jane Goodall in a documentary called *Inside Animal Minds* (NOVA, 2014). In this video, Dr. Goodall challenges us to consider the inferences we make to other species and to question whether such inferences are warranted. She uses the term

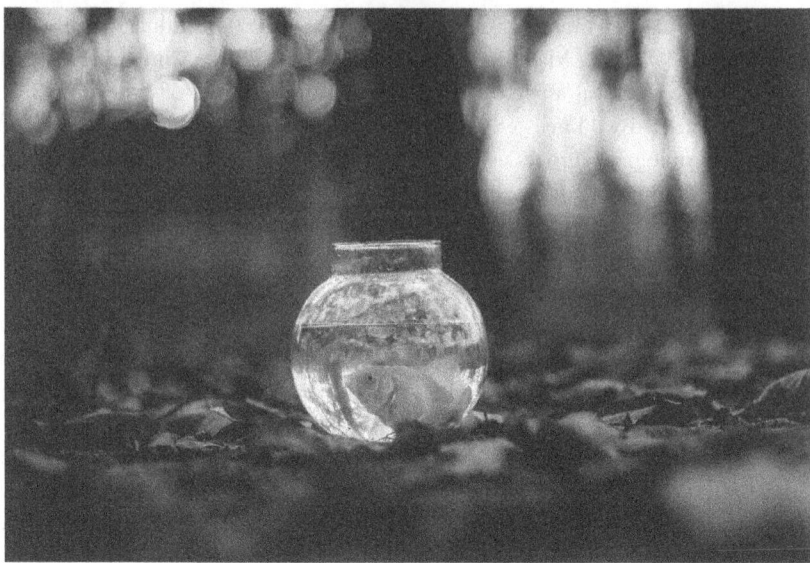

FIGURE 1.1 Goldfish in fish tank. Photograph by A. Zayan (2018).

anthropomorphism to refer to the attributions we make (sometimes erroneously) to describe the attributes of others (including other species, like the goldfish in this example). Researchers have used this concept to better understand our ideas and assumptions about life, death, suffering, meaning in life, self-identity and values, interpersonal attachments, stereotypes, and our ideas about normal and abnormal behavior (Wan & Chen, 2021; Williams et al., 2020; Yue et al., 2021). I raise this analogy because sometimes it is helpful for us to think about children (and even other adults for that matter) as anthropomorphic – to the extent that it orients us to question what we observe (and often don't observe), assume, and expect from people exposed to stress and trauma. More specifically, one might question whether a "happy" child is indeed happy, or whether they are masking deep-seated emotional pain. The point being – some children develop "normal" reactions to traumatic stress, some appear to have no symptoms at all, and still others may not show any classical symptoms of trauma that would typically warrant a diagnostic evaluation. We know that children respond to stress differently from other children, adolescents, or adults depending on their biological vulnerability and resiliency, social and emotional support from family and friends, and their age and stage of development.

Early Stress and Coping in Children

There are several stressors that we commonly see in children and that we generally expect children to resolve as they become adolescents and young adults.

A common worry was the subject of a recent study by Cheetham-Blake and colleagues (2019), who interviewed children as part of their qualitative investigation. Children reported experiencing psychological distress and rumination from their experiences of bullying and intimidation. These children often struggled to understand why they were being bullied in the first place and how they could differentiate friends from enemies effectively. Some children, however, recognized that they were targeted because of their physical appearance. In my own clinical practice, I have seen children who are targeted because of their height or weight, acne, inability to buy the latest fashions, lack of athletic ability, autistic characteristics, sexual orientation, and limited English-language proficiency. Respondents in the Cheetham-Blake et al. (2019) study also experienced fear of failure, getting into trouble at home or school, concerns about possibly changing schools if their parents transitioned to new jobs, and differing views about the importance of learning life lessons, such as bullying. More specifically, some parents felt that bullying is a rite of passage with important lessons to be learned, whereas others disagreed and addressed the problem differently. Indeed, these findings are consistent with several studies reporting on children's experiences of stress and anxiety and their natural concerns about the well-being of their family and friends, achieving in school, eating well, making friends, and feeling safe and secure (Mendoza et al., 2017; Taylor & Ruiz, 2017; Tudor et al., 2019).

How children cope with stress has been the subject of many studies (Caporino et al., 2017; Chishima et al., 2018; Eschenbeck et al., 2018; Nijhof et al., 2018; Schneider et al., 2018). Scholars have postulated that supportive caregivers and consistent habits and routines help children regulate their emotions and behaviors and manage psychological distress. In other words, when children experience stress, they look to their caregivers to model how to cope with stress effectively so they can regulate their own emotions (the alarm phase of GAS). Children often attempt to cope by crying, throwing tantrums, seeking support from caregivers, or by trying to escape until they either get the help they need from others or exhaust their ability to express discomfort (the resistance and exhaustion phases of GAS). Children also cope with stress by trying to avoid memories of the upsetting events, distracting themselves with displays of maladaptive behaviors at home or school, or by using more adaptive tactics, such as prayer, seeking social and emotional support, or engaging in play. Children may also use fantasy and imagination to help regulate their emotions in response to a stressful event. For example, some children will immerse themselves in cartoons, comic books, superhero movies, social media, or video games to assert age-appropriate power and control in stressful situations (e.g., Lim & Nam, 2020; Milani et al., 2018; Plante et al., 2019; Wartberg et al., 2021).

Children may also tend to become disconnected from others during play or in other situations during or after experiencing a stressful event. They may be using this time to self-regulate, problem solve, or substitute memories of their life with images that are less stressful and radically different. Perhaps they are thinking about existential issues, such as formulating ideas about why "bad" things happen to "good" people and vice-versa. Alternatively, it could be that they are afraid to confront the memories of their trauma, and they use disconnection as a strategy to help keep them detached. Other children may be unable to express their thoughts and feelings related to trauma either because of cultural norms or because they lack the presence of adults who can appropriately listen and respond to their concerns.

Concluding Thoughts

Stress is a complex concept, and reactions to stress and trauma vary widely from person to person. When we experience stress, we attempt to cope through whatever means we have available to us at the time. Circumstances linked to the experience of extreme fear or terror, marked by the real and immediate possibility of death, cause a significant but purposeful disruption to our physiological state of homeostasis. Experiences of trauma cause a shift to the way an individual evaluates and reacts to danger in general, but this eventually generalizes to all situations, including those that may be reasonably safe. For children with trauma who go on to develop clinical signs and symptoms of trauma, such as posttraumatic stress disorder, the level of fear and anxiety they experience will likely disrupt their social, emotional, and behavioral control. These children experience intrusive thoughts and reminders of the original trauma, which may cause them to act in ways that may frustrate others.

In the next chapter, I expand on stress and trauma in children from a more clinical perspective and discuss developmental trauma disorder. I introduce the concept of toxic stress to allude to the types of stress reactions that cause severe and often less recognizable trauma symptoms in children. Toxic stress occurs when a child experiences longstanding abuse or neglect, most often at the hands of their caregivers. But many of these children do not display typical signs of trauma. I also describe the concept of developmental trauma, which refers to early trauma that takes multiple forms (e.g., neglect and maltreatment), is severe and ongoing, and involves the caregiving system (parents and other caregivers). The combination of repeated childhood trauma and the absence of parental nurturing, support, and protection can be particularly devastating. The next chapter describes developmental trauma in detail, including its history and theoretical tenets as well as clinical evaluation procedures.

References

Agnafors, S., Svedin, C. G., Oreland, L., Bladh, M., Comasco, E., & Sydsjö, G. (2017). A Biopsychosocial Approach to Risk and Resilience on Behavior in Children Followed from Birth to Age 12. *Child Psychiatry and Human Development*, 48(4), 584–596. https://doi.org/10.1007/s10578-016-0684-x.

Agorastos, A., & Chrousos, G. P. (2022). The neuroendocrinology of stress: The stress-related continuum of chronic disease development. *Molecular Psychiatry*, 27(1), 502–513. https://doi.org/10.1038/s41380-021-01224-9.

Asselmann, E., Wittchen, H.-U., Lieb, R., & Beesdo-Baum, K. (2017). A 10-year prospective-longitudinal study of daily hassles and incident psychopathology among adolescents and young adults: Interactions with gender, perceived coping efficacy, and negative life events. *Social Psychiatry and Psychiatric Epidemiology*, 52(11), 1353–1362. https://doi.org/10.1007/s00127-017-1436-3.

Bartone, P. T., & Homish, G. G. (2020). Influence of hardiness, avoidance coping, and combat exposure on depression in returning war veterans: A moderated-mediation study. *Journal Of Affective Disorders*, 265, 511–518. https://doi.org/10.1016/j.jad.2020.01.127.

Benbow, A. A., & Anderson, P. L. (2019). Long-term improvements in probability and cost biases following brief cognitive behavioral therapy for social anxiety disorder. *Cognitive Therapy and Research*, 43(2), 412–418. https://doi.org/10.1007/s10608-018-9947-0.

Caporino, N. E., Read, K. L., Shiffrin, N., Settipani, C., Kendall, P. C., Compton, S. N., Sherrill, J., Piacentini, J., Walkup, J., Ginsburg, G., Keeton, C., Birmaher, B., Sakolsky, D., Gosch, E., & Albano, A. M. (2017). Sleep-related problems and the effects of anxiety treatment in children and adolescents. *Journal of Clinical Child And Adolescent Psychology*, 46(5), 675–685. https://doi.org/10.1080/15374416.2015.1063429.

Carpenter, J. K., Andrews, L. A., Witcraft, S. M., Powers, M. B., Smits, J., & Hofmann, S. G. (2018). Cognitive behavioral therapy for anxiety and related disorders: A meta-analysis of randomized placebo-controlled trials. *Depression and Anxiety*, 35(6), 502–514. https://doi.org/10.1002/da.22728.

Cheetham-Blake, T. J., Family, H. E., & Turner-Cobb, J. M. (2019). 'Every day I worry about something': A qualitative exploration of children's experiences of stress and coping. *British Journal of Health Psychology*, 24(4), 931–952. https://doi.org/10.1111/bjhp.12387.

Chishima, Y., Mizuno, M., Sugawara, D., & Miyagawa, Y. (2018). The influence of self-compassion on cognitive appraisals and coping with stressful events. *Mindfulness*, 9(6), 1907–1915. https://doi.org/10.1007/s12671-018-0933-0.

Craven, W., Depp, J., Saxon, J., Blakley, R., & Langenkamp, H. (1999). *A Nightmare on Elm Street 1–4*. New York: New Line Home Entertainment.

Cristóbal-Narváez, P., Sheinbaum, T., Myin-Germeys, I., Kwapil, T. R., de Castro-Catala, M., Domínguez-Martínez, T., Racioppi, A., Monsonet, M., Hinojosa-Marqués, L., van Winkel, R., Rosa, A., & Barrantes-Vidal, N. (2017). The role of stress-regulation genes in moderating the association of stress and daily-life psychotic experiences. *Acta Psychiatrica Scandinavica*, 136(4), 389–399. https://doi.org/10.1111/acps.12789.

Crowe, K., & McKay, D. (2017). Efficacy of cognitive-behavioral therapy for childhood anxiety and depression. *Journal of Anxiety Disorders*, 49, 76–87. https://doi.org/10.1016/j.janxdis.2017.04.001.

Cunanan, A. J., DeWeese, B. H., Wagle, J. P., Carroll, K. M., Sausaman, R., Hornsby, W. G., 3rd, Haff, G. G., Triplett, N. T., Pierce, K. C., & Stone, M. H. (2018). The general adaptation syndrome: A foundation for the concept of periodization. *Sports Medicine*, 48(4), 787–797. https://doi.org/10.1007/s40279-017-0855-3.

David, D., Cotet, C., Matu, S., Mogoase, C., & Stefan, S. (2018). 50 years of rational-emotive and cognitive-behavioral therapy: A systematic review and meta-analysis. *Journal of Clinical Psychology*, 74(3), 304–318. https://doi.org/10.1002/jclp.22514.

Deslauriers, J., Acheson, D. T., Maihofer, A. X., Nievergelt, C. M., Baker, D. G., Geyer, M. A., Risbrough, V. B., & Marine Resiliency Study Team (2018). COMT val158met polymorphism links to altered fear conditioning and extinction are modulated by PTSD and childhood trauma. *Depression and Anxiety*, 35(1), 32–42. https://doi.org/10.1002/da.22678.

Dogan, B., Yoldas, C., Kocabas, O., Memis, C. O., Sevincok, D., & Sevincok, L. (2019). The characteristics of the comorbidity between social anxiety and separation anxiety disorders in adult patients. *Nordic Journal of Psychiatry*, 73(6), 380–386. https://doi.org/10.1080/08039488.2019.1642381.

Ebner, K., & Singewald, N. (2017). Individual differences in stress susceptibility and stress inhibitory mechanisms. *Current Opinion in Behavioral Sciences*, 14, 54–64. https://doi.org/10.1016/j.cobeha.2016.11.016.

Edman, J. S., Greeson, J. M., Roberts, R. S., Kaufman, A. B., Abrams, D. I., Dolor, R. J., & Wolever, R. Q. (2017). Perceived stress in patients with common gastrointestinal disorders: Associations with quality of life, symptoms, and disease management. *Explore*, 13(2), 124–128. https://doi.org/10.1016/j.explore.2016.12.005.

Epel, E. S., Crosswell, A. D., Mayer, S. E., Prather, A. A., Slavich, G. M., Puterman, E., & Mendes, W. B. (2018). More than a feeling: A unified view of stress measurement for population science. *Frontiers in Neuroendocrinology*, 49, 146–169. https://doi.org/10.1016/j.yfrne.2018.03.001.

Eschenbeck, H., Schmid, S., Schröder, I., Wasserfall, N., & Kohlmann, C.-W. (2018). Development of coping strategies from childhood to adolescence: Cross-sectional and longitudinal trends. *European Journal of Health Psychology*, 25(1), 18–30. https://doi.org/10.1027/2512-8442/a000005.

Feldman, M. D., & Christensen, J. F. (2008). *Behavioral medicine: A guide for clinical practice*. New York: McGraw-Hill Medical.

Friedkin, W., & Blatty, W. P. (1973). *The Exorcist*. Los Angeles: Warner Bros.

Golds, L., de Kruiff, K., & MacBeth, A. (2020). Disentangling genes, attachment, and environment: A systematic review of the developmental psychopathology literature on gene-environment interactions and attachment. *Development and Psychopathology*, 32(1), 357–381. https://doi.org/10.1017/S0954579419000142.

Jovanovic, T., Stenson, A. F., Thompson, N., Clifford, A., Compton, A., Minton, S., van Rooij, S. J. F., Stevens, J. S., Lori, A., Nugent, N., Gillespie, C. F., Bradley, B., & Ressler, K. J. (2020). Impact of ADCYAP1R1 genotype on longitudinal fear conditioning in children: Interaction with trauma and sex. *Neuropsychopharmacology*, 45(10), 1603–1608. https://doi.org/10.1038/s41386-020-0748-2.

Jung, S. J., Kang, J. H., Roberts, A. L., Nishimi, K., Chen, Q., Sumner, J. A., Kubzansky, L., & Koenen, K. C. (2019). Posttraumatic stress disorder and incidence of thyroid dysfunction in women. *Psychological Medicine*, 49(15), 2551–2560. https://doi.org/10.1017/S0033291718003495.

Kanner, A. D., Coyne, J. C., Schaefer, C., & Lazarus, R. S. (1981). Comparison of two modes of stress measurement: Daily hassles and uplifts versus major life events. *Journal of Behavioral Medicine*, 4(1), 1–39. http://dx.doi.org/10.1007/BF00844845.

Khosravi, A., & Namani, E. (2021). Investigating the structural model of the relationship between self-compassion and psychological hardiness with family cohesion in women with war-affected spouses: The mediating role of self-worth. *Contemporary Family Therapy*, 44, 1–8. https://doi.org/10.1007/s10591-021-09579-5.

Kim, H. G., Cheon, E. J., Bai, D. S., Lee, Y. H., & Koo, B. H. (2018). Stress and heart rate variability: A meta-analysis and review of the literature. *Psychiatry Investigation*, 15 (3), 235–245. https://doi.org/10.30773/pi.2017.08.17.

Kim, J., Li, L., Korous, K. M., Valiente, C., & Tsethlikai, M. (2022). Chronic stress predicts post-traumatic stress disorder symptoms via executive function deficits among urban American Indian children. *Stress*, 25(1), 97–104. https://doi.org/10.1080/10253890.2021.2024164.

Kim, Y. K., & Shin, C. (2018). The microbiota-gut-brain axis in neuropsychiatric disorders: Pathophysiological mechanisms and novel treatments. *Current Neuropharmacology*, 16(5), 559–573. https://doi.org/10.2174/1570159X15666170915141036.

Kodal, A., Fjermestad, K., Bjelland, I., Gjestad, R., Öst, L. G., Bjaastad, J. F., Haugland, B., Havik, O. E., Heiervang, E., & Wergeland, G. J. (2018). Long-term effectiveness of cognitive behavioral therapy for youth with anxiety disorders. *Journal of Anxiety Disorders*, 53, 58–67. https://doi.org/10.1016/j.janxdis.2017.11.003.

Koss, K. J., & Gunnar, M. R. (2018). Annual Research Review: Early adversity, the hypothalamic-pituitary-adrenocortical axis, and child psychopathology. *Journal Of Child Psychology and Psychiatry, and Allied Disciplines*, 59(4), 327–346. https://doi.org/10.1111/jcpp.12784.

Kothgassner, O. D., Goreis, A., Glenk, L. M., Kafka, J. X., Pfeffer, B., Beutl, L., Kryspin-Exner, I., Hlavacs, H., Palme, R., & Felnhofer, A. (2021). Habituation of salivary cortisol and cardiovascular reactivity to a repeated real-life and virtual reality Trier Social Stress Test. *Physiology & Behavior*, 242, 113618. https://doi.org/10.1016/j.physbeh.2021.113618.

LaRocca, M. A., Scogin, F. R., Hilgeman, M. M., Smith, A. J., & Chaplin, W. F. (2018). The impact of posttraumatic growth, transformational leadership, and self-efficacy on PTSD and depression symptom severity among combat Veterans. *Military Psychology*, 30(2), 162–173. https://doi.org/10.1080/08995605.2018.1425073.

Lathren, C., Bluth, K., & Park, J. (2019). Adolescent self-compassion moderates the relationship between perceived stress and internalizing symptoms. *Personality and Individual Differences*, 143, 36–41. https://doi.org/10.1016/j.paid.2019.02.008.

Lawrence, P. J., Murayama, K., & Creswell, C. (2019). Systematic review and meta-analysis: anxiety and depressive disorders in offspring of parents with anxiety disorders. *Journal of the American Academy of Child and Adolescent Psychiatry*, 58(1), 46–60. https://doi.org/10.1016/j.jaac.2018.07.898.

Lazarus, R. S., & Folkman, S. (1984). Coping and Adaptation. In W. D. Gentry (Ed.), *The Handbook of Behavioral Medicine* (pp. 282–325.). New York: Guilford.

Lim, Y., & Nam, S. J. (2020). Exploring factors related to problematic internet use in childhood and adolescence. *International Journal of Mental Health and Addiction*, 18, 891–903. https://doi.org/10.1007/s11469-018-9990-9.

Lu, S., Wei, F., & Li, G. (2021). The evolution of the concept of stress and the framework of the stress system. *Cell Stress*, 5(6), 76–85. https://doi.org/10.15698/cst2021.06.250.

Lupien, S. J., Juster, R. P., Raymond, C., & Marin, M. F. (2018). The effects of chronic stress on the human brain: From neurotoxicity, to vulnerability, to opportunity. *Frontiers in Neuroendocrinology*, 49, 91–105. https://doi.org/10.1016/j.yfrne.2018.02.001.

Malesza, M. (2019). Stress and delay discounting: The mediating role of difficulties in emotion regulation. *Personality and Individual Differences*, 144, 56–60. https://doi.org/10.1016/j.paid.2019.02.035.

Marques de Miranda, D., da Silva Athanasio, B., Sena Oliveira, A. C., & Simoes-E-Silva, A. C. (2020). How is COVID-19 pandemic impacting mental health of children and adolescents? *International Journal of Disaster Risk Reduction*, 51, 101845. https://doi.org/10.1016/j.ijdrr.2020.101845.

Marusak, H. A., Hehr, A., Bhogal, A., Peters, C., Iadipaolo, A., & Rabinak, C. A. (2021). Alterations in fear extinction neural circuitry and fear-related behavior linked to trauma exposure in children. *Behavioural Brain Research*, 398, 112958. https://doi.org/10.1016/j.bbr.2020.112958.

Matthies, S., Schiele, M. A., Koentges, C., Pini, S., Schmahl, C., & Domschke, K. (2018). Please don't leave me: Separation anxiety and related traits in borderline personality disorder. *Current Psychiatry Reports*, 20(10), 83. https://doi.org/10.1007/s11920-018-0951-6.

McEwen, B. S. (2017). Neurobiological and systemic effects of chronic stress. *Chronic Stress*, 1, 2470547017692328. https://doi.org/10.1177/2470547017692328.

McEwen, C. A., & McEwen, B. S. (2017). Social structure, adversity, toxic stress, and intergenerational poverty: An early childhood model. *Annual Review of Sociology*, 43, 445–472. https://doi.org/10.1146/annurev-soc-060116-053252.

McLaughlin, K. A., & Lambert, H. K. (2017). Child trauma exposure and psychopathology: Mechanisms of risk and resilience. *Current Opinion in Psychology*, 14, 29–34. https://doi.org/10.1016/j.copsyc.2016.10.004.

Mendoza, M. M., Dmitrieva, J., Perreira, K. M., Hurwich-Reiss, E., & Watamura, S. E. (2017). The effects of economic and sociocultural stressors on the well-being of children of Latino immigrants living in poverty. *Cultural Diversity and Ethnic Minority Psychology*, 23(1), 15–26. https://doi.org/10.1037/cdp0000111.

Menzies, R. E., Zuccala, M., Sharpe, L., & Dar-Nimrod, I. (2021). Are anxiety disorders a pathway to obsessive-compulsive disorder?: Different trajectories of OCD and the role of death anxiety. *Nordic Journal of Psychiatry*, 75(3), 170–175. https://doi.org/10.1080/08039488.2020.1817554.

Messerli-Bürgy, N., Arhab, A., Stülb, K., Kakebeeke, T. H., Zysset, A. E., Leeger-Aschmann, C. S., Schmutz, E. A., Ehlert, U., Kriemler, S., Jenni, O. G., Munsch, S., & Puder, J. J. (2018). Physiological stress measures in preschool children and their relationship with body composition and behavioral problems. *Developmental Psychobiology*, 60(8), 1009–1022. https://doi.org/10.1002/dev.21782.

Milani, L., La Torre, G., Fiore, M., Grumi, S., Gentile, D. A., Ferrante, M., Miccoli, S., & De Blasio, P. (2018). Internet gaming addiction in adolescence: Risk factors and maladjustment correlates. *International Journal of Mental Health and Addiction*, 16, 888–904. https://doi.org/10.1007/s11469-017-9750-2.

Mize, J. L., & Kliewer, W. (2017). Domain-specific daily hassles, anxiety, and delinquent behaviors among low-income, urban youth. *Journal of Applied Developmental Psychology*, 53, 31–39. https://doi.org/10.1016/j.appdev.2017.09.003.

Mohr, D., & Rosén, L. A. (2017). The impact of protective factors on posttraumatic growth for college student survivors of childhood maltreatment. *Journal of Aggression, Maltreatment & Trauma*, 26(7), 756–771. https://doi.org/10.1080/10926771.2017.1304478.

Monk, D., Mackay, D. J. G., Eggermann, T., Maher, E. R., & Riccio, A. (2019). Genomic imprinting disorders: Lessons on how genome, epigenome and environment interact. *Nature Reviews Genetics*, 20(4), 235–248. https://doi.org/10.1038/s41576-018-0092-0.

Moss, R. H., Conner, M., & O'Connor, D. B. (2020). Exploring the effects of daily hassles on eating behaviour in children: The role of cortisol reactivity. *Psychoneuroendocrinology*, 117, 104692. https://doi.org/10.1016/j.psyneuen.2020.104692.

Moss, R. H., Conner, M., & O'Connor, D. B. (2021). Exploring the effects of daily hassles and uplifts on eating behaviour in young adults: The role of daily cortisol levels. *Psychoneuroendocrinology*, 129, 105231. https://doi.org/10.1016/j.psyneuen.2021.105231.

Muentner, L., Kapoor, A., Weymouth, L., & Poehlmann-Tynan, J. (2021). Getting under the skin: Physiological stress and witnessing paternal arrest in young children with incarcerated fathers. *Developmental Psychobiology*, 63(5), 1568–1582. https://doi.org/10.1002/dev.22113.

Mulcahy, J. S., Larsson, D. E., Garfinkel, S. N., & Critchley, H. D. (2019). Heart rate variability as a biomarker in health and affective disorders: A perspective on neuroimaging studies. *Neuroimage*, 202, 116072. https://doi.org/10.1016/j.neuroimage.2019.116072.

Nelson, C. A., 3rd, & Gabard-Durnam, L. J. (2020). Early adversity and critical periods: Neurodevelopmental consequences of violating the expectable environment. *Trends in Neurosciences*, 43(3), 133–143. https://doi.org/10.1016/j.tins.2020.01.002.

Nijhof, S. L., Vinkers, C. H., van Geelen, S. M., Duijff, S. N., Achterberg, E., van der Net, J., Veltkamp, R. C., Grootenhuis, M. A., van de Putte, E. M., Hillegers, M., van der Brug, A. W., Wierenga, C. J., Benders, M., Engels, R., van der Ent, C. K., Vanderschuren, L., & Lesscher, H. (2018). Healthy play, better coping: The importance of play for the development of children in health and disease. *Neuroscience and Biobehavioral Reviews*, 95, 421–429. https://doi.org/10.1016/j.neubiorev.2018.09.024.

NOVA. (2014). *NOVA: Inside Animal Minds* [video]. BBC Productions; NOVA Productions. https://www.pbs.org/wgbh/nova/series/inside-animal-minds.

O'Connor, D. B., Thayer, J. F., & Vedhara, K. (2021). Stress and health: A review of psychobiological processes. *Annual Review of Psychology*, 72, 663–688. https://doi.org/10.1146/annurev-psych-062520-122331.

Öztürk, E., Erdoğan, B., & Derin, G. (2021). Psychotraumatology and dissociation: A theoretical and clinical approach. *Medicine-Science*, 10(1), 246–254. http://dx.doi.org/10.5455/medscience.2021.02.041.

Panchal, U., Salazar de Pablo, G., Franco, M., Moreno, C., Parellada, M., Arango, C., & Fusar-Poli, P. (2021). The impact of COVID-19 lockdown on child and adolescent mental health: Systematic review. *European Child & Adolescent Psychiatry*, 1–27. https://doi.org/10.1007/s00787-021-01856-w.

Pandey, D., & Shrivastava, P. (2017). Mediation effect of social support on the association between hardiness and immune response. *Asian Journal of Psychiatry*, 26, 52–55. https://doi.org/10.1016/j.ajp.2017.01.022.

Plante, C. N., Gentile, D. A., Groves, C. L., Modlin, A., & Blanco-Herrera, J. (2019). Video games as coping mechanisms in the etiology of video game addiction. *Psychology of Popular Media Culture*, 8(4), 385–394. https://doi.org/10.1037/ppm0000186.

Preston, K. L., Schroeder, J. R., Kowalczyk, W. J., Phillips, K. A., Jobes, M. L., Dwyer, M., Vahabzadeh, M., Lin, J. L., Mezghanni, M., & Epstein, D. H. (2018). End-of-day reports of daily hassles and stress in men and women with opioid-use disorder: Relationship to momentary reports of opioid and cocaine use and stress. *Drug and Alcohol Dependence*, 193, 21–28. https://doi.org/10.1016/j.drugalcdep.2018.08.023.

Rogers, C. R. (1980). *Way of being*. Boston, MA: Houghton Mifflin.

Roos, L. E., Knight, E. L., Beauchamp, K. G., Berkman, E. T., Faraday, K., Hyslop, K., & Fisher, P. A. (2017). Acute stress impairs inhibitory control based on individual differences in parasympathetic nervous system activity. *Biological Psychology*, 125, 58–63. https://doi.org/10.1016/j.biopsycho.2017.03.004.

Rowell, T., & Neal-Barnett, A. (2021). A systematic review of the effect of parental adverse childhood experiences on parenting and child psychopathology. *Journal of Child & Adolescent Trauma*, 15(1), 167–180. https://doi.org/10.1007/s40653-021-00400-x.

Schiweck, C., Piette, D., Berckmans, D., Claes, S., & Vrieze, E. (2019). Heart rate and high frequency heart rate variability during stress as biomarker for clinical depression: A systematic review. *Psychological Medicine*, 49(2), 200–211. https://doi.org/10.1017/S0033291718001988.

Schneider, R. L., Arch, J. J., Landy, L. N., & Hankin, B. L. (2018). The longitudinal effect of emotion regulation strategies on anxiety levels in children and adolescents. *Journal of Clinical Child and Adolescent Psychology*, 47(6), 978–991. https://doi.org/10.1080/15374416.2016.1157757.

Shaw, Z. A., & Starr, L. R. (2019). Intergenerational transmission of emotion dysregulation: The role of authoritarian parenting style and family chronic stress. *Journal of Child and Family Studies*, 28(12), 3508–3518. https://doi.org/10.1007/s10826-019-01534-1.

Silk, J. S., Tan, P. Z., Ladouceur, C. D., Meller, S., Siegle, G. J., McMakin, D. L., Forbes, E. E., Dahl, R. E., Kendall, P. C., Mannarino, A., & Ryan, N. D. (2018). A randomized clinical trial comparing individual cognitive behavioral therapy and child-centered therapy for child anxiety disorders. *Journal of Clinical Child and Adolescent Psychology*, 47(4), 542–554. https://doi.org/10.1080/15374416.2016.1138408.

Sommerfeldt, S. L., Schaefer, S. M., Brauer, M., Ryff, C. D., & Davidson, R. J. (2019). Individual differences in the association between subjective stress and heart rate are related to psychological and physical well-being. *Psychological Science*, 30(7), 1016–1029. https://doi.org/10.1177/09567976bell9555.

Stenson, A. F., van Rooij, S. J., Carter, S. E., Powers, A., & Jovanovic, T. (2021). A legacy of fear: Physiological evidence for intergenerational effects of trauma exposure on fear and safety signal learning among African Americans. *Behavioural Brain Research*, 402, 113017. https://doi.org/10.1016/j.bbr.2020.113017.

Taylor, Z. E., & Ruiz, Y. (2017). Contextual stressors and the mental health outcomes of Latino children in rural migrant-farmworker families in the Midwest. *Journal of Rural Mental Health*, 41(4), 284–298. https://doi.org/10.1037/rmh0000082.

Thomassen, Å. G., Hystad, S. W., Johnsen, B. H., Johnsen, G. E., & Bartone, P. T. (2018). The effect of hardiness on PTSD symptoms: A prospective mediational approach. *Military Psychology*, 30(2), 142–151. https://doi.org/10.1080/08995605.2018.1425065.

Thomassen, Å. G., Johnsen, B. H., Hystad, S. W., & Johnsen, G. E. (2022). Avoidance coping mediates the effect of hardiness on mental distress symptoms for both male and female subjects. *Scandinavian Journal of Psychology*, 63(1), 39–46. https://doi.org/10.1111/sjop.12782.

Tinajero, R., Tudos, P. G., Cribbet, M. R., Rau, H. K., Silver, M. A., Bride, D. L., & Suchy, Y. (2020). Reported history of childhood trauma and stress-related vulnerability: Associations with emotion regulation, executive functioning, daily hassles, and pre-sleep arousal. *Stress and Health: Journal of the International Society for the Investigation of Stress*, 36(4), 405–418. https://doi.org/10.1002/smi.2938.

Tudor, K., Sarkar, M., & Spray, C. (2019). Exploring common stressors in physical education: A qualitative study. *European Physical Education Review*, 25(3), 675–690. https://doi.org/10.1177/1356336X18761586.

Vagni, M., Giostra, V., Maiorano, T., Santaniello, G., & Pajardi, D. (2020). Personal accomplishment and hardiness in reducing emergency stress and burnout among COVID-19 emergency workers. *Sustainability*, 12(21), 9071. https://doi.org/10.3390/su12219071.

Villabø, M. A., Narayanan, M., Compton, S. N., Kendall, P. C., & Neumer, S.-P. (2018). Cognitive–behavioral therapy for youth anxiety: An effectiveness evaluation in community practice. *Journal of Consulting and Clinical Psychology*, 86(9), 751–764. https://doi.org/10.1037/ccp0000326.

Wan, E. W., & Chen, R. P. (2021). Anthropomorphism and object attachment. *Current Opinion in Psychology*, 39, 88–93. https://doi.org/10.1016/j.copsyc.2020.08.009.

Wartberg, L., Thomasius, R., & Paschke, K. (2021). The relevance of emotion regulation, procrastination, and perceived stress for problematic social media use in a representative sample of children and adolescents. *Computers in Human Behavior*, 121, 106788. https://doi.org/10.1016/j.chb.2021.106788.

Watters, E. R., & Martin, G. (2021). Health outcomes following childhood maltreatment: An examination of the biopsychosocial model. *Journal of Aging and Health*, 33 (7–8),596–606. https://doi.org/10.1177/08982643211003783.

Williams, L. A., Brosnan, S. F., & Clay, Z. (2020). Anthropomorphism in comparative affective science: Advocating a mindful approach. *Neuroscience & Biobehavioral Reviews*, 115, 299–307. https://doi.org/10.1016/j.neubiorev.2020.05.014.

Wirtz, P. H., & von Känel, R. (2017). Psychological stress, inflammation, and coronary heart disease. *Current Cardiology Reports*, 19(11), 111. https://doi.org/10.1007/s11886-017-0919-x.

Yue, D., Tong, Z., Tian, J., Li, Y., Zhang, L., & Sun, Y. (2021). Anthropomorphic strategies promote wildlife conservation through empathy: The moderation role of the public epidemic situation. *International Journal of Environmental Research and Public Health*, 18(7), 3565. https://doi.org/10.3390/ijerph18073565.

Zayan, A. [photographer]. (2018, March 6). *Goldfish in fish tank* [digital image]. Retrieved from https://unsplash.com/photos/URaZrRvKQqM.

Zhang, J., Shuai, L., Yu, H., Wang, Z., Qiu, M., Lu, L., Cao, X., Xia, W., Wang, Y., & Chen, R. (2020). Acute stress, behavioural symptoms, and mood states among school-age children with attention-deficit/hyperactive disorder during the COVID-19 outbreak. *Asian Journal of Psychiatry*, 51, 102077. https://doi.org/10.1016/j.ajp.2020.102077.

Zingela, Z., Stroud, L., Cronje, J., Fink, M., & van Wyk, S. (2022). The psychological and subjective experience of catatonia: A qualitative study. *BMC Psychology*, 10, 173. https://doi.org/10.1186/s40359-022-00885-7.

2

INTRODUCTION TO DEVELOPMENTAL TRAUMA DISORDER

> Developmental Trauma compromises an individual's identity, self-worth, and personality; emotional regulation and self-regulation; and ability to relate to others and engage in intimacy. In many, it leads to ongoing despair, lack of meaning, and a crisis of spirituality.
>
> *(Lingiardi & McWilliams, 2017, p.190)*

Trauma is likely to be familiar to most readers. If someone told you they were traumatized, you would likely conclude that something terrible happened to them (some life-changing event) and perhaps they likely experienced fear, anxiety, depression, concentration problems, and memory disturbances as a result. Trauma that occurs during early, formative years may give rise to complex and often unrecognizable symptoms. These symptoms are highly consequential to our understanding and treatment of these children.

Childhood Trauma and PTSD

Early childhood trauma occurs when a child experiences an event that causes actual or perceived harm that poses a threat to their survival. This may include events such as surviving a house fire, direct physical or sexual abuse, witnessing domestic violence, prolonged separation from parents, bodily injury, parental substance abuse, assault, or, more recently, school violence such as a mass shooting. Trauma often leads to a heightened state of physiological arousal, which fundamentally alters the child's felt sense of safety, security, and homeostasis (Dunn et al., 2020; Iffland et al., 2020; Magwai & Xulu, 2022; Motsan et al., 2021)

Trauma also often causes children to have poor self-regulation, which refers to the ability to monitor and direct our thoughts, feelings, and actions in ways

DOI: 10.4324/9781003304715-2

that are socially acceptable (Gruhn & Compas, 2020; Jenness et al., 2021). For example, whereas we usually suppress or at least try to contain thoughts about death and dying, individuals with trauma may have more difficulty doing so. Since traumatic events are often unpredictable, children who have experienced such events may begin to view the world as unpredictable, and they may start to ask themselves troubling questions, such as *Am I safe? If this happened to me, what else could happen to me? Why didn't my parents protect me? Why didn't God protect me?* You can see how this line of thinking can devastatingly change someone's beliefs about life, safety, and security. This is especially likely for young children, who understand the world in ways that vastly differ from how adults see the world. For traumatized children, feelings may become dysregulated, and they will be at higher risk of emotional numbing, anger and irritability, and anxiety. These reactions likely developed to protect children from any further traumas, but these same adaptations actually create heightened risk for repeated traumas (the diathesis-stress theory holds that stress and trauma are cumulative or dose-dependent, meaning that previous traumas, in addition to genetic risks, temperament, and socioeconomic stressors, interact in such a way that they become additive and, in turn, more damaging; Dye, 2018; Popovic et al., 2019; Scheeringa, 2021; Stoltz et al., 2017; Zhu et al., 2020).

Some children who have experienced stress and trauma will develop symptoms that correspond to posttraumatic stress disorder (PTSD) (Uppendahl et al., 2020; Woolgar et al., 2022). PTSD is a psychiatric disorder brought on by exposure to a highly stressful and potentially life-threatening event, such as witnessing a school shooting, experiencing sexual or physical abuse, or surviving an accident or a natural disaster. PTSD is associated with intrusive images, reactions, and memories connected to the original trauma, which interfere with social, behavioral, and emotional capacities. Children who experience traumatic stress often display several concerning behaviors, such as recurrent nightmares, sadness and lability, anger and aggression, bed wetting (i.e., enuresis and encopresis; Castillo & Pham, 2022; Hébert et al., 2018; Secrist et al., 2019; Sousa et al., 2018), and anxiety (Gardner et al., 2019; Ulmer-Yaniv et al., 2018). These symptoms are considered in detail in the fifth edition of the DSM (American Psychiatric Association, 2013). The DSM-5 is widely used by healthcare providers to determine whether a child's symptoms are severe enough to warrant a diagnosis of PTSD.

Children who have experienced trauma and developed measurable mental health symptoms associated with the trauma may present with indications of PTSD that warrant a careful diagnostic evaluation. The symptoms of PTSD, as defined by DSM-5 criteria, are characterized by persistent and intrusive thoughts, hyperarousal (i.e., heightened startle in response to unexpected sounds or movements), deliberate avoidance of trauma reminders, and alterations to conscious awareness (i.e., dissociation, derealization, and depersonalization; Cheng et al., 2020; Hoeboer et al., 2021; Jin et al., 2019). Trauma symptoms that are persistent (i.e., that last longer than a month after the traumatic event(s)) and are accompanied by social, behavioral, and academic impairments indicate the presence of PTSD and differentiate it from other psychiatric disturbances (e.g., acute stress disorder, which is similar to PTSD but symptoms last from three days to a month; American Psychiatric Association, 2013).

Children who experience intrusive thoughts that are accompanied by heightened states of arousal as a result of their trauma often have difficulty sleeping because they experience distressing nightmares (Brindle et al., 2018; Mysliwiec et al., 2018; Secrist et al., 2019; Wamser-Nanney & Chesher, 2018). They may wake up in the middle of the night screaming from night terrors that force them to relive the trauma. Other children may resort to avoiding sleep altogether rather than having to live through another night of terror. Avoidance symptoms for traumatized children with PTSD become noticeable when children shut down emotionally, meaning that they become emotionally numb. These children may appear "robotic" in that adults may view them to be emotionally disconnected or even cold towards others. Children may become emotionally numb to avoid having to experience or re-experience additional emotional injury and to prevent the possibility of additional traumas.

Children who undergo a shift in their worldview after trauma are marked by a tendency to view life as cold, harsh, cruel, and dangerous. These children also tend to disconnect from others. It is important to realize, however, that some seemingly aloof children experience profound emotional pain, rumination, self-blame, and recurrent thoughts of suicide and are desperately in need of social support and connection (Cervin et al., 2021; Degnan et al., 2022; Tsur et al., 2021). Children who have undergone trauma are also more likely to experience anger, irritability, a heightened startle reaction, and concentration problems. All of these directly correspond to hyperarousal symptoms of PTSD, which may give some insight into a child's state of mind and level of emotional suffering.

Children and Trauma: Diagnostic Issues

Although children with PTSD share many symptoms with adults who suffer from the same disorder, several scholars, relying on decades of rigorous scholarship in the developmental sciences, have recently urged the American Psychiatric Association (APA) to formerly differentiate PTSD between children and adults in the DSM-5 (Foa et al., 2018; Sachser et al., 2018). This initiative has only recently gained recognition within the clinical and scientific communities, and studies are being done to better understand how PTSD differs between children and adults. One of the main arguments in favor of differentiating between the two groups is that the criteria for PTSD were developed almost exclusively with adults in mind. Several scholars contend that young children cannot develop PTSD (as we have come to understand it with adults) because they have undeveloped and inconsistent cognitive, emotional, and behavioral capacities as well as immature nervous systems (e.g., Cross et al., 2017; Dye, 2018). Children have not reached full maturation of the limbic system, which is an implicit memory system activated by the fight-flight-freeze response (Campbell, 2022; Keding et al., 2021; Mercurio et al., 2022). Because traumatic memories are often mediated by the limbic system, children are more likely than adults to forget the details of their trauma when asked by an adult and to instead show trauma through play (Dimitrova et al., 2021; Fung et al., 2022; McRae et al., 2021; Wolf et al., 2022). We now know that children can develop PTSD, that PTSD can and should be treated by providers differently, and that we should assess how a child's age and developmental competencies influence their expressions of trauma.

One approach to diagnosing children with trauma, especially for those who fail to meet the criteria for PTSD, is to revise the requirements of the DSM so that it is more developmentally sensitive to children (Bartels et al., 2021; Hitchcock et al., 2022; Moner et al., 2022). In other words, we might use different vocabulary to talk to children about their trauma and emphasize the areas of trauma that are unique to them (e.g., traumatic re-enactments in their interactions with peers during playtime). We might also focus more on trauma that is particularly relevant for children, such as any harm to the well-being of caregivers or disruptions to the quality of the parent-child relationship (e.g., having a caregiver who is medically ill and unable to care for the child, foster care placement, loss of a primary caregiver). In turn, we could then use this information to slightly shift, but not completely do away with, PTSD as we have come to understand it. Using this revised method, we would be better able to identify and treat traumatized children more effectively.

In their highly influential work with traumatized children, Sheeringa and colleagues (2003, 2005, 2011) proposed a developmental model of trauma, which conferred a preschool subtype of PTSD for children between the ages of 0 and 6. The preschool PTSD subtype provides more insight into the ways in which young children experience trauma and, at the same time, the ways in which they may show those symptoms in clinical circumstances. The alternative set of criteria used for the preschool PTSD subtype includes several changes to the standard DSM-PTSD criteria, ranging from adjustments to clinical thresholds (e.g., lowered from three to one avoidance symptom) to the removal of items deemed inappropriate for children (e.g., expression of immediate distress following the trauma; nightmares that necessarily include traumatic content; sense of a foreshortened future, which requires complex cognitive skills; McKinnon et al., 2019; Meiser-Stedman et al., 2017; Moner et al., 2022; Scheeringa, 2019; Woolgar et al., 2022). DSM-5 criteria for the preschool PTSD subtype require that the "duration of the disturbance [referring to trauma symptoms] is more than one month" (American Psychiatric Association, 2013, p. 273). These revised criteria were designed with both assessment and treatment in mind, underscoring the recognition that symptoms of PTSD may naturally present themselves in children's play behaviors and not necessarily in their verbal responses to the myriad of questions posed by assessors in standard clinical interviews.

Developmental Trauma Disorder (DTD)

In 2009, Bessel van der Kolk and colleagues published the first comprehensive proposal on a new diagnostic syndrome referred to as developmental trauma disorder (DTD) (DePierro et al., 2022; Spinazzola et al., 2021; van der Kolk et al., 2009). At that time, van der Kolk et al. (2009) recognized significant limitations in the DSM-IV-TR PTSD classification (American Psychiatric Association, 2000). They noticed that people who experienced significant trauma during their childhoods often receive inaccurate or incomplete diagnoses later in life. They also reported on a number of studies suggesting that although childhood trauma is present among 40% to 70% of psychiatric populations, the differing presentations of trauma-related disorders span a wide range, frequently go unnoticed and, therefore, are often underreported.

In their proposal, van der Kolk et al. (2009) focused on repeatedly traumatized children and adolescents who presented with overlapping symptoms of PTSD and a variety of mental health conditions, such as attention deficit hyperactive disorder (ADHD), conduct disorder, and bipolar disorder. High comorbidities between PTSD and other disorders have also been found in other studies, including Kessler et al.'s 1995 National Comorbidity Study (Kessler et al., 1995). In that study, 79% of all individuals diagnosed with PTSD met criteria for at least one other disorder, and 44% met criteria for three or more additional disorders. Both Kessler et al. (1995) and van der Kolk et al. (2009) surmised from these findings that the diagnosis of PTSD only accounts for a limited portion of the symptoms experienced by individuals who have experienced childhood trauma. As such, DTD was introduced as a new type of trauma that included many of these symptoms and comorbidities as primary, rather than secondary, characteristics.

Children who have experienced interpersonal trauma and are at risk of DTD have more severe and pervasive problems than are common in children with PTSD. Consider the fact that before children can be diagnosed with PTSD, we must carefully consider several other possible alternative diagnoses that either co-occur with PTSD or better explain the traumatic stress reaction. For example, we must rule out or distinguish PTSD from a broad range of disorders, including acute stress, depression, anxiety, dissociative identity disorder, psychosis, and medical problems.

DTD, on the other hand, conceptualizes these comorbidities as associated (and reasonably expected) *dimensions* of trauma rather than differentiated diagnostic entities. In other words, proponents of DTD claim that the diagnosis accounts for these comorbidities while, at the same time, maintaining enough distinction to qualify as a discrete diagnostic entity. The DTD diagnosis is conceptualized as capturing the full spectrum of "lasting personality changes following catastrophic stress" that go "well beyond the classic PTSD criteria" (Luxenberg et al., 2001, p. 376). Interestingly, van der Kolk et al. (2009), using large-scale data from the Child and Adolescent Needs and Strengths (CANS) Survey and the National Child Traumatic Stress Network, found that 24% to 46% of children with trauma histories characteristic of DTD failed to meet the criteria for PTSD.

The DTD diagnosis is intended to classify the complex and pervasive exposure to life-threatening events that (1) occur during sensitive periods of infant and child development; (2) disrupt interpersonal attachments; (3) compromise an individual's safety and security; and (4) alter cognitive, behavioral, and emotional control (Ford, 2017, 2021; Spinazzola et al., 2018). The diagnosis directly pertains to complex neurobehavioral disturbances, referring to the broad range of changes to the nervous system that occur in children who have been exposed to recurrent episodes of life-threatening events, such as violence in the home or prolonged separation from primary caregivers. These experiences fundamentally alter children's cognitive, emotional, physiological, and relational capacities (Beal et al., 2019; Kira, 2022; Kisiel et al., 2017; Van Nieuwenhove & Meganck, 2019).

DTD is set apart from PTSD in that the former necessarily results from a toxic seed planted at the beginning of an individual's lifespan development (sometimes preceding a child's birth during pregnancy), whereas the causal events that lead to PTSD can occur at any point (or points) in one's life cycle. More specifically, DTD emerges from *prolonged and cumulative interpersonal trauma that disrupts the development of secure attachments to caregivers*, or what scholars have increasingly referred to as adverse childhood experiences, or ACEs (Grady et al., 2017; Ihme et al., 2022; Karatzias et al., 2022; Malvaso et al., 2022). Interpersonal trauma has been conceptualized as trauma that primarily involves the disruption of interpersonal relationships (Mekawi et al., 2021; Mikolajewski & Scheeringa, 2022).

Children with DTD live in persistent states of fear and terror, especially those who have experienced recurring (and inescapable) trauma. These experiences become transformative developmental experiences that alter children's global appraisals and future responses to stress (Deuter et al., 2020; Fitzgerald, 2021; Mętel et al., 2020). These children become dysregulated because their bodies are consistently mobilizing the high levels of stress hormones, metabolic resources (e.g., glucose), and neurotransmitters necessary to prepare for imminent danger (Danese & Baldwin, 2017). This heightened fear propensity disrupts self-awareness, interpersonal communication, and mastery of age-appropriate developmental competencies (e.g., establishing healthy relationship parameters, identifying and expressing feelings, tolerating ambiguity, and distrusting others; Garon-Bissonnette et al., 2022; Toof et al., 2020).

Individuals who have endured significant stress in their lives, especially during early childhood or adolescence, are at increased risk of experiencing avoidance, anger, frustration, and anxiety as primary ways of being in the world, regardless of their circumstances (Hagan et al., 2018). These types of responses can be damaging to an individual's development and ability to function. Because DTD develops in early childhood (sometimes before the child has expressive language), DTD symptoms may remain latent until interpersonal interactions later in life give rise to traumatic memories (Gander et al., 2020; Zhu et al., 2020). Consequently, the symptoms may be elusive to most adults who interact with them, and these children may not be recognized as having trauma, and, critically, they may fail to get the types of support they need to recover.

Scholars are increasingly finding that when they compare children with DTD and PTSD, children with DTD are differentiated by (1) poorer self-identity development; (2) more consistent problems in relationships, including with primary caregivers; (3) higher rates of exposure to family and community violence; and (4) more comorbidities with panic, disruptive behavior, separation anxiety, and ADHD disorders (Copeland et al., 2018; Ford 2017, 2021; Spinazzola et al., 2018). Moreover, DTD causes more longstanding alterations in conscious awareness (e.g., dissociation, traumatic amnesia) and personality development, which, in turn, place DTD children at risk for psychological problems, chronic and debilitating medical conditions, and personality disorders in adulthood (Cyr et al., 2022; Jankovic et al., 2021; Rüfenacht et al., 2021; Tschoeke et al., 2021; Zdankiewicz-Ścigała & Ścigała, 2018).

Because children with DTD rely on dissociation as a primary coping strategy in response to psychological distress, they develop limited, and often incomplete, individual identities. In working with DTD individuals, I have been struck by the degree of loneliness and emotional disconnect these individuals experience, but often suppress, around others. For example, a depressed and suicidal individual may pretend to be happy and outgoing around others to avoid social rejection, bullying, and re-victimization. These children may continue to use these strategies as adolescents and adults, meaning that they could go their entire life virtually unknown to others.

Case in Point

Developmental Trauma and Self-Identity Development

In the late nineteenth century, William James (1890), one of psychology's most influential thinkers, advanced a theory of identity that reflects what he referred to as *self-consciousness*. James's theory holds that an individual's identity, which he referred to as the *self*, is both a physical entity and that entity's intersubjective experience. In other words, the self is both "an object of experience ... and a subject of experience" (Wozniak, 2018, p. 1656). The physical (e.g., body, clothing), social (e.g., the ways we relate to others at home, in school, or at work), and spiritual (e.g., personality, insight) selves, together with one's conscious awareness and emotional experience, mediate the objective–subjective identity continuum that defines who we are and how we present ourselves to others.

Who we are and how we present ourselves to others can sometimes be markedly different, and this is especially true for individuals affected by early childhood stress and trauma. Individuals with trauma often have significant disruptions to their identity development. They experience identity confusion that is intimately tied to their traumas, and this, in turn, often gives rise to problematic behaviors, dysfunctional relational styles, maladaptive coping responses, and a general distrust for themselves and others.

Given the critical role that loss of identity holds in understanding children with DTD, I invite readers to consider the loss of one's identity in more detail by using the movie *Invasion of the Body Snatchers*.

Invasion of the Body Snatchers as Metaphor for Loss of Identity in Developmental Trauma

Breaking News

Run! Hide! Protect Yourselves from the Alien Imposters! No one is Trustworthy!
… Not Even Our Selves

Invasion of the Body Snatchers (1956) is a science-fiction horror film adapted from a novel, *The Body Snatchers*, authored by Jack Finney in 1955. The premise of the film is that people are slowly being replaced by alien imposters, who create exact replicas of individual people. The extraterrestrial species, referred to as pod people in the story (i.e., toxic seeds that eventually mature into a human form in a plot to take over our world to save their own), also steal people's thoughts and memories, but they are unable to replicate human emotion.

> Your new bodies are growing in there. They're taking you over cell for cell, atom for atom. There is no pain. Suddenly, while you're asleep, they'll absorb your minds, your memories, and you're reborn.
>
> Dr. Kauffman, Invasion of the Body Snatchers *(Siegel, 1956)*

In the end, people lose their identities. They lose parts of themselves in the aftermath of the traumatic invasion, and they must fight with all their power to regain their original personas.

I use the *Invasion of the Body Snatchers* as an allegory for developmental trauma because children with trauma often have difficulty forming a cohesive identity, show emotional numbing, and experience ongoing conflicts about whom they can trust (including whether they can trust themselves). They feel like strangers in their bodies and like strangers in the world. In addition, early childhood abuse and neglect have been systematically linked to alexithymia (i.e., lack of expressed words or feelings; Zdankiewicz-Ścigała & Ścigała, 2020), and both childhood trauma and alexithymia heighten children's risk for chronic migraines, alcohol abuse, and dissociation (Bottiroli et al., 2018; Zdankiewicz-Ścigała & Ścigała, 2018).

The DTD diagnosis has failed to gain formal recognition by the APA. The APA cites several problems with the diagnosis of DTD, including limitations with the research on the topic, which has tended to rely on retrospective rather than prospective studies. These reasons, in part, have ultimately contributed to the APA's decision to not include the DTD diagnosis in the DSM-5.

Categorical and Dimensional Models of Trauma

When we work with children and evaluate them for trauma, we do so with the highest standards of evidence in mind. The DSM provides us with detailed descriptions of the kinds of behaviors we may come to see in children with trauma. The DSM and its diagnoses underscore the scientific evidence, advances in research, and data-driven decision-making that go into the development of these classifications. Thus far, I have emphasized, from a clinical point of view, the diagnostic categories linked to children's responses to trauma. In the next and final section of this chapter, I aim to elucidate their scientific underpinnings.

The *empirical approach* to understanding children with trauma chiefly relies on observable and measurable evidence to justify our theories so that we can, in turn, apply these theories to explain and predict behaviors. This approach requires us to study DTD through carefully designed experiments, much like those we use to test the effectiveness of new medications (i.e., an experimental group is compared with a placebo group). If we maintain objectivity, which is a requirement of the empirical model, we can assess the validity of our claims through experiments and assess their reliability through replication studies by other researchers to confirm the accuracy of our conclusions. Because there is power in numbers when it comes to the scientific method, empirical scholars want to recruit as many children as possible so that we can generalize our findings to the larger population (i.e., to all children with characteristics of DTD).

This now mainstream view has been primarily influenced by decades of research in psychiatry and medicine, which has traditionally emphasized biological causes (e.g., family history and genetic risks, abnormal brain development), systematic evaluation procedures, and objective measurement standards (e.g., symptom count and intensity, degree of functional impairment, standardized parent- and teacher-report questionnaires). In the same vein, advances in modern science and technology, such as those seen in neuroimaging (e.g., fMRI, EEG, PET scans), now allow us to measure and record brain activity and to use data from these findings to advance policies.

PTSD conceptualized as a distinct diagnosis confers many advantages to researchers, practitioners, and policymakers. For example, epidemiologists who study the prevalence of trauma in children can use the information that they glean to raise public awareness, work to prevent or reduce health disparities, and advocate for social and economic resources (e.g., parity of healthcare insurance reimbursement for mental health disorders such as DTD, and testing large-scale studies on DTD and its sequalae). A clear diagnosis of PTSD promotes interdisciplinary collaborations in research and practice, and it facilitates local, national, and international communications.

At the same time, reliance on the scientific approach has given rise to several unresolved and, in some cases, highly controversial issues. For example, numerous scholars have disputed the validity of categorical taxonomies of trauma, citing the reductionist, symptom-specific models of trauma as being inextricably linked to unyielding reimbursement policies from health maintenance organizations as well as pressures from pharmaceutical companies to maintain distinct groups so that they can develop lucrative new treatments (Hawn et al., 2022; Kaçar-Başaran & Arkar, 2022; Lynch et al., 2021; Stanton et al., 2020; Williams & Levinson, 2022). In other words, when providers evaluate a child for trauma and when they have worked through their evidence-based guidelines to confirm it, they must justify the diagnosis and the need for treatment to insurance companies for reimbursement. Insurance companies evaluate the necessity of treatment based on a specific diagnosis, and they, in turn, specify the kinds of available services and projected length of treatment available.

Health maintenance organizations also define the quality of evidence needed to justify treatment, and this can be challenging for children with DTD, who often require long-term care. These organizations tend to prioritize brief self-report assessments and interventions, generally allocate 8–12 sessions of treatment, and emphasize symptom reduction as the primary indicator of successful treatment. A number of scholars have expressed concerns with this practice on several grounds, including that it undermines the kinds of complex adaptations that we see in DTD children (Alegría et al., 2021; Dickson-Gomez et al., 2022; Ghosh, 2021; Heboyan et al., 2021). The fact that these children dissociate from reality, and thus have limited awareness of their symptoms, calls into question the validity of their self-reports. Research indeed suggests that individuals with DTD either underestimate their trauma symptoms on self-report or they provide highly inconsistent responses, which limits the diagnostic and predictive validity of such measures (Boyer et al., 2022; Cogan et al., 2021; Hall, 2022).

One of the most significant controversies surrounding the diagnosis of trauma is whether trauma should be conceptualized as a single, symptom-specific categorical diagnosis or whether it should be reconceptualized as a dimension of symptoms across a continuum. If we emphasize the identifiable aspects of trauma (e.g., distinct causes, numbers of symptoms on self-report in line with the APA's definition of trauma), then we may be regretfully dismissing any given child's intersubjective experience, expressed mental health problems (or lack thereof), and unique stress adaptations used to cope with the original trauma.

There has been a gradual change in the field of mental health to diversify the scientific methods we use to study DTD in children and to study mental health disorders more broadly. Although we have traditionally emphasized categorical views of mental illness, often characterized by clearly delineated signs, symptoms, and criteria, we are beginning to recognize that dimensional approaches provide us with distinctive and equally relevant insights. As definitions and conceptualizations of trauma have changed over the years and across the versions of the DSM, researchers and practitioners must contend with mounting empirical evidence advancing spectrum diagnoses and hybrid models that encompass both categorical taxonomies and symptom dimensions. The differing views of trauma, including whether we should emphasize categorical taxonomies or dimensions on a spectrum from normal to pathogenic to resilient, are underscored by the PTSD and DTD frameworks.

Concluding Thoughts

In this chapter, I have discussed several approaches to the diagnosis of trauma, ranging from traditional models of PTSD to more contemporary frameworks explicitly designed for children. The fact that much of our understanding of trauma is derived from adult models is a limitation we are now beginning to address in contemporary practice. We know that traumatic events predictably give rise to PTSD, but we are beginning to appreciate the kinds of adaptations in children who developed their foundations in a context of ongoing trauma. Children with developmental trauma demonstrate a broad range of symptoms, which may or may not mirror those of PTSD. The loss of a caregiver, in physical or symbolic terms, causes lifelong disturbances because it shatters our fundamental ideas about the world as a safe, secure, and predictable place. A critical distinction between PTSD and DTD, therefore, is that DTD is influenced by attachment, which serves as the primary template for all future relationships. In the next chapter, I describe attachment theory in detail, including its biological and conceptual underpinnings as well as its implications for assessment and intervention.

References

Alegría, M., Frank, R. G., Hansen, H. B., Sharfstein, J. M., Shim, R. S., & Tierney, M. (2021). Transforming mental health and addiction services. *Health Affairs (Project Hope)*, 40(2), 226–234. https://doi.org/10.1377/hlthaff.2020.01472.

American Psychiatric Association. (2000). *Diagnostic and statistical manual of mental disorders* (4th ed., text rev.). Washington, DC: American Psychiatric Association.

American Psychiatric Association. (2013). *Diagnostic and statistical manual of mental disorders* (5th ed.). Washington, DC: American Psychiatric Association.

Bartels, L., Sachser, C., & Landolt, M. A. (2021). Age-related similarities and differences in networks of acute trauma-related stress symptoms in younger and older preschool children. *European Journal of Psychotraumatology*, 12(1), 1948788. https://doi.org/10.1080/20008198.2021.1948788.

Beal, S. J., Wingrove, T., Mara, C. A., Lutz, N., Noll, J. G., & Greiner, M. V. (2019). Childhood adversity and associated psychosocial function in adolescents with complex trauma. *Child & Youth Care Forum*, 48(3), 305–322. https://doi.org/10.1007/s10566-018-9479-5.

Bottiroli, S., Galli, F., Viana, M., Sances, G., & Tassorelli, C. (2018). Traumatic experiences, stressful events, and alexithymia in chronic migraine with medication overuse. *Frontiers in Psychology, 9*, 704. https://doi.org/10.3389/fpsyg.2018.00704.

Boyer, S. M., Caplan, J. E., & Edwards, L. K. (2022). Trauma-related dissociation and the dissociative disorders: Neglected symptoms with severe public health consequences. *Delaware Journal of Public Health*, 8(2), 78–84. https://doi.org/10.32481/djph.2022.05.010.

Brindle, R. C., Cribbet, M. R., Samuelsson, L. B., Gao, C., Frank, E., Krafty, R. T., Thayer, J. F., Buysse, D. J., & Hall, M. H. (2018). The relationship between childhood trauma and poor sleep health in adulthood. *Psychosomatic Medicine*, 80(2), 200–207. https://doi.org/10.1097/PSY.0000000000000542.

Campbell, K. A. (2022). The neurobiology of childhood trauma, from early physical pain onwards: As relevant as ever in today's fractured world. *European Journal of Psychotraumatology*, 13(2), 2131969. https://doi.org/10.1080/20008066.2022.2131969.

Castillo, J., & Pham, S. (2022). Enuresis and psychological concerns in a foster care population. *Psychological Trauma: Theory, Research, Practice, and Policy*. Advance online publication. https://doi.org/10.1037/tra0001192.

Cervin, M., Salloum, A., Ruth, L. J., & Storch, E. A. (2021). Posttraumatic symptoms in 3–7 year old trauma-exposed children: Links to impairment, other mental health symptoms, caregiver PTSD, and caregiver stress. *Child Psychiatry and Human Development*, 52(6), 1173–1183. https://doi.org/10.1007/s10578-020-01093-3.

Cheng, J., Liang, Y., Fu, L., & Liu, Z. (2020). The relationship between PTSD and depressive symptoms among children after a natural disaster: A 2-year longitudinal study. *Psychiatry Research*, 292, 113296. https://doi.org/10.1016/j.psychres.2020.113296.

Cogan, C. M., Paquet, C. B., Lee, J. Y., Miller, K. E., Crowley, M. D., & Davis, J. L. (2021). Differentiating the symptoms of posttraumatic stress disorder and bipolar disorders in adults: Utilizing a trauma-informed assessment approach. *Clinical Psychology & Psychotherapy*, 28(1), 251–260. https://doi.org/10.1002/cpp.2504.

Copeland, W. E., Shanahan, L., Hinesley, J., Chan, R. F., Aberg, K. A., Fairbank, J. A., van den Oord, E. J. C. G., & Costello, E. J. (2018). Association of childhood trauma exposure with adult psychiatric disorders and functional outcomes. *JAMA Network Open*, 1(7), e184493. https://doi.org/10.1001/jamanetworkopen.2018.4493.

Cross, D., Fani, N., Powers, A., & Bradley, B. (2017). Neurobiological development in the context of childhood trauma. *Clinical Psychology: Science and Practice*, 24(2), 111–124. https://doi.org/10.1111/cpsp.12198.

Cyr, G., Godbout, N., Cloitre, M., & Bélanger, C. (2022). Distinguishing among symptoms of posttraumatic stress disorder, complex posttraumatic stress disorder, and borderline personality disorder in a community sample of women. *Journal of Traumatic Stress*, 35(1), 186–196. https://doi.org/10.1002/jts.22719.

Danese, A., & Baldwin, J. R. (2017). Hidden wounds?: Inflammatory links between childhood trauma and psychopathology. *Annual Review of Psychology*, 68, 517–544. https://doi.org/10.1146/annurev-psych-010416-044208.

Degnan, A., Berry, K., Humphrey, C., & Bucci, S. (2022). The role of attachment and dissociation in the relationship between childhood interpersonal trauma and negative symptoms in psychosis. *Clinical Psychology & Psychotherapy*, 29(5), 1692–1706. https://doi.org/10.1002/cpp.2731.

DePierro, J., D'Andrea, W., Spinazzola, J., Stafford, E., van Der Kolk, B., Saxe, G., Stolbach, B., McKernan, S., & Ford, J. D. (2022). Beyond PTSD: Client presentations of developmental trauma disorder from a national survey of clinicians. *Psychological Trauma: Theory, Research, Practice and Policy*, 14(7), 1167–1174. https://doi.org/10.1037/tra0000532.

Deuter, C. E., Wingenfeld, K., Otte, C., Bustami, J., Kaczmarczyk, M., & Kuehl, L. K. (2020). Noradrenergic system and cognitive flexibility: Disentangling the effects of depression and childhood trauma. *Journal of Psychiatric Research*, 125, 136–143. https://doi.org/10.1016/j.jpsychires.2020.03.017.

Dickson-Gomez, J., Weeks, M., Green, D., Boutouis, S., Galletly, C., & Christenson, E. (2022). Insurance barriers to substance use disorder treatment after passage of mental health and addiction parity laws and the affordable care act: A qualitative analysis. *Drug and Alcohol Dependence Reports*, 3, 100051. https://doi.org/10.1016/j.dadr.2022.100051.

Dimitrova, L. I., Dean, S. L., Schlumpf, Y. R., Vissia, E. M., Nijenhuis, E. R. S., Chatzi, V., Jäncke, L., Veltman, D. J., Chalavi, S., & Reinders, A. A. T. S. (2021). A neurostructural biomarker of dissociative amnesia: A hippocampal study in dissociative identity disorder. *Psychological Medicine*, 1–9. https://doi.org/10.1017/S0033291721002154.

Dunn, E. C., Nishimi, K., Neumann, A., Renaud, A., Cecil, C. A. M., Susser, E. S., & Tiemeier, H. (2020). Time-dependent effects of exposure to physical and sexual violence on psychopathology symptoms in late childhood: In search of sensitive periods in development. *Journal of the American Academy of Child and Adolescent Psychiatry*, 59(2), 283–295.e4. https://doi.org/10.1016/j.jaac.2019.02.022.

Dye, H. (2018). The impact and long-term effects of childhood trauma. *Journal of Human Behavior in the Social Environment*, 28(3), 381–392. https://doi.org/10.1080/10911359.2018.1435328.

Finney, J. (1955). *The body snatchers*. New York: Dell Publishing.

Fitzgerald, M. (2021). Developmental pathways from childhood maltreatment to young adult romantic relationship functioning. *Journal of Trauma & Dissociation*, 22(5), 581–597. https://doi.org/10.1080/15299732.2020.1869653.

Foa, E. B., Asnaani, A., Zang, Y., Capaldi, S., & Yeh, R. (2018). Psychometrics of the Child PTSD Symptom Scale for DSM-5 for trauma-exposed children and adolescents. *Journal of Clinical Child and Adolescent Psychology*, 47(1), 38–46. https://doi.org/10.1080/15374416.2017.1350962.

Ford, J. D. (2017). Complex trauma and developmental trauma disorder in adolescence. *Adolescent Psychiatry*, 7(4), 220–235. https://doi.org/10.2174/2210676608666180112160419.

Ford, J. D. (2021). Progress and limitations in the treatment of complex PTSD and developmental trauma disorder. *Current Treatment Options in Psychiatry*, 8(1), 1–17. https://doi.org/10.1007/s40501-020-00236-6.

Fung, H. W., Chien, W. T., Chan, C., & Ross, C. A. (2022). A cross-cultural investigation of the association between betrayal trauma and dissociative features. *Journal of Interpersonal Violence*, 38(1–2), 1630–1653. https://doi.org/10.1177/08862605221090568.

Gander, M., Buchheim, A., Bock, A., Steppan, M., Sevecke, K., & Goth, K. (2020). Unresolved attachment mediates the relationship between childhood trauma and impaired personality functioning in adolescence. *Journal of Personality Disorders*, 34 (Supplement B), 84–103. https://doi.org/10.1521/pedi_2020_34_468.

Gardner, M. J., Thomas, H. J., & Erskine, H. E. (2019). The association between five forms of child maltreatment and depressive and anxiety disorders: A systematic review and meta-analysis. *Child Abuse & Neglect*, 96, 104082. https://doi.org/10.1016/j.chiabu.2019.104082.

Garon-Bissonnette, J., Duguay, G., Lemieux, R., Dubois-Comtois, K., & Berthelot, N. (2022). Maternal childhood abuse and neglect predicts offspring development in early childhood: The roles of reflective functioning and child sex. *Child Abuse & Neglect*, 128, 105030. https://doi.org/10.1016/j.chiabu.2021.105030.

Ghosh, M. (2021). Mental health insurance in India: Lack of parity. *The lancet: Psychiatry*, 8(10), 860. https://doi.org/10.1016/S2215-0366(21)00287-X.

Grady, M. D., Levenson, J. S., & Bolder, T. (2017). Linking adverse childhood effects and attachment: A theory of etiology for sexual offending. *Trauma, Violence, & Abuse*, 18(4), 433–444. https://doi.org/10.1177/1524838015627147.

Gruhn, M. A., & Compas, B. E. (2020). Effects of maltreatment on coping and emotion regulation in childhood and adolescence: A meta-analytic review. *Child Abuse & Neglect*, 103, 104446. https://doi.org/10.1016/j.chiabu.2020.104446.

Hagan, M. J., Gentry, M., Ippen, C. G., & Lieberman, A. F. (2018). PTSD with and without dissociation in young children exposed to interpersonal trauma. *Journal of Affective Disorders*, 227, 536–541. https://doi.org/10.1016/j.jad.2017.11.070.

Hall, H. (2022). Dissociation and misdiagnosis of schizophrenia in populations experiencing chronic discrimination and social defeat. *Journal of Trauma & Dissociation*, 1–15. Advance online publication. https://doi.org/10.1080/15299732.2022.2120154.

Hawn, S. E., Wolf, E. J., Neale, Z., & Miller, M. W. (2022). Conceptualizing traumatic stress and the structure of posttraumatic psychopathology through the lenses of RDoC and HiTOP. *Clinical Psychology Review*, 95, 102177. https://doi.org/10.1016/j.cpr.2022.102177.

Hébert, M., Langevin, R., & Oussaïd, E. (2018). Cumulative childhood trauma, emotion regulation, dissociation, and behavior problems in school-aged sexual abuse victims. *Journal of Affective Disorders*, 225, 306–312. https://doi.org/10.1016/j.jad.2017.08.044.

Heboyan, V., Douglas, M. D., McGregor, B., & Benevides, T. W. (2021). Impact of mental health insurance legislation on mental health treatment in a longitudinal sample of adolescents. *Medical Care*, 59(10), 939–946. https://doi.org/10.1097/MLR.0000000000001619.

Hitchcock, C., Goodall, B., Wright, I. M., Boyle, A., Johnston, D., Dunning, D., Gillard, J., Griffiths, K., Humphrey, A., McKinnon, A., Panesar, I. K., Werner-Seidler, A., Watson, P., Smith, P., Meiser-Stedman, R., & Dalgleish, T. (2022). The early course and treatment of posttraumatic stress disorder in very young children: Diagnostic prevalence and predictors in hospital-attending children and a randomized controlled proof-of-concept trial of trauma-focused cognitive therapy, for 3- to 8-year-olds. *Journal of Child Psychology and Psychiatry, and Allied Disciplines*, 63(1), 58–67. https://doi.org/10.1111/jcpp.13460.

Hoeboer, C., de Roos, C., van Son, G. E., Spinhoven, P., & Elzinga, B. (2021). The effect of parental emotional abuse on the severity and treatment of PTSD symptoms in children and adolescents. *Child Abuse & Neglect*, 111, 104775. https://doi.org/10.1016/j.chiabu.2020.104775.

Iffland, B., Klein, F., Rosner, R., Renneberg, B., Steil, R., & Neuner, F. (2020). Cardiac reactions to emotional words in adolescents and young adults with PTSD after child abuse. *Psychophysiology*, 57(1), e13470. https://doi.org/10.1111/psyp.13470.

Ihme, H., Olié, E., Courtet, P., El-Hage, W., Zendjidjian, X., Mazzola-Pomietto, P., Consoloni, J. L., Deruelle, C., & Belzeaux, R. (2022). Childhood trauma increases vulnerability to attempt suicide in adulthood through avoidant attachment. *Comprehensive Psychiatry*, 117, 152333. Advance online publication. https://doi.org/10.1016/j.comppsych.2022.152333.

James, W. (1890). *The principles of psychology*. New York: H. Holt and Company.

Jankovic, M., Bogaerts, S., Klein Tuente, S., Garofalo, C., Veling, W., & van Boxtel, G. (2021). The complex associations between early childhood adversity, heart rate variability, cluster b personality disorders, and aggression. *International Journal of Offender Therapy and Comparative Criminology*, 65(8), 899–915. https://doi.org/10.1177/0306624X20986537.

Jenness, J. L., Peverill, M., Miller, A. B., Heleniak, C., Robertson, M. M., Sambrook, K. A., Sheridan, M. A., & McLaughlin, K. A. (2021). Alterations in neural circuits underlying emotion regulation following child maltreatment: A mechanism underlying trauma-related psychopathology. *Psychological Medicine*, 51(11), 1880–1889. https://doi.org/10.1017/S0033291720000641.

Jin, Y., Deng, H., An, J., & Xu, J. (2019). The Prevalence of PTSD Symptoms and Depressive Symptoms and Related Predictors in Children and Adolescents 3 Years After the Ya'an Earthquake. *Child Psychiatry and Human Development*, 50(2), 300–307. https://doi.org/10.1007/s10578-018-0840-6.

Kaçar-Başaran, S., & Arkar, H. (2022). Common vulnerability factors in obsessive-compulsive and major depressive disorders: A transdiagnostic hierarchical model. *Current Psychology: A Journal for Diverse Perspectives on Diverse Psychological Issues*. https://doi.org/10.1007/s12144-021-02599-2.

Karatzias, T., Shevlin, M., Ford, J. D., Fyvie, C., Grandison, G., Hyland, P., & Cloitre, M. (2022). Childhood trauma, attachment orientation, and complex PTSD (CPTSD) symptoms in a clinical sample: Implications for treatment. *Development and Psychopathology*, 34(3), 1192–1197. https://doi.org/10.1017/S0954579420001509.

Keding, T. J., Heyn, S. A., Russell, J. D., Zhu, X., Cisler, J., McLaughlin, K. A., & Herringa, R. J. (2021). Differential patterns of delayed emotion circuit maturation in abused girls with and without internalizing psychopathology. *American Journal of Psychiatry*, 178(11), 1026–1036. https://doi.org/10.1176/appi.ajp.2021.20081192.

Kessler, R. C., Sonnega, A., Bromet, E., Hughes, M., & Nelson, C. B. (1995). Posttraumatic stress disorder in the national comorbidity study. *Archives of General Psychiatry*, 52(12), 1048–1060. https://doi.org/10.1001/archpsyc.1995.03950240066012.

Kira, I. A. (2022). Taxonomy of stressors and traumas: An update of the development-based trauma framework (DBTF): A life-course perspective on stress and trauma. *Traumatology*, 28(1), 84–97. https://doi.org/10.1037/trm0000305.

Kisiel, C., Summersett-Ringgold, F., Weil, L. E. G., & McClelland, G. (2017). Understanding strengths in relation to complex trauma and mental health symptoms within child welfare. *Journal of Child and Family Studies*, 26(2), 437–451. https://doi.org/10.1007/s10826-016-0569-4.

Lingiardi, V., & McWilliams, N. (Eds.). (2017). *Psychodynamic diagnostic manual: PDM-2* (2nd ed.). New York: Guilford Press.

Luxenberg, T., Spinazzola, J., & van der Kolk, B. (2001). Complex trauma and the Disorders of Extreme Stress (DESNOS) diagnosis, part one: Assessment. *Directions in Psychiatry*, 21(25), 373–393.

Lynch, S. J., Sunderland, M., Newton, N. C., & Chapman, C. (2021). A systematic review of transdiagnostic risk and protective factors for general and specific psychopathology in young people. *Clinical Psychology Review*, 87, 102036. https://doi.org/10.1016/j.cpr.2021.102036.

Magwai, T., & Xulu, K. R. (2022). Physiological Genomics plays a crucial role in response to stressful life events, the development of aggressive behaviours, and post-traumatic stress disorder (PTSD). *Genes*, 13(2), 300. https://doi.org/10.3390/genes13020300.

Malvaso, C. G., Cale, J., Whitten, T., Day, A., Singh, S., Hackett, L., Delfabbro, P. H., & Ross, S. (2022). Associations between adverse childhood experiences and trauma among young people who offend: A systematic literature review. *Trauma, Violence & Abuse*, 23(5), 1677–1694. https://doi.org/10.1177/15248380211013132.

McKinnon, A., Scheeringa, M. S., Meiser-Stedman, R., Watson, P., De Young, A., & Dalgleish, T. (2019). The dimensionality of proposed DSM-5 PTSD symptoms in trauma-exposed young children. *Journal of Abnormal Child Psychology*, 47(11), 1799–1809. https://doi.org/10.1007/s10802-019-00561-2.

McRae, E. M., Stoppelbein, L., O'Kelley, S. E., Fite, P., & Smith, S. B. (2021). An examination of post-traumatic stress symptoms and aggression among children with a history of adverse childhood experiences. *Journal of Psychopathology and Behavioral Assessment*, 43(3), 657–670. https://doi.org/10.1007/s10862-021-09884-1.

Meiser-Stedman, R., Smith, P., Yule, W., Glucksman, E., & Dalgleish, T. (2017). Posttraumatic stress disorder in young children 3 years posttrauma: Prevalence and longitudinal predictors. *The Journal of Clinical Psychiatry*, 78(3), 334–339. https://doi.org/10.4088/JCP.15m10002.

Mekawi, Y., Carter, S., Brown, B., Martinez de Andino, A., Fani, N., Michopoulos, V., & Powers, A. (2021). Interpersonal trauma and posttraumatic stress disorder among Black women: Does racial discrimination matter? *Journal of Trauma & Dissociation*, 22(2), 154–169. https://doi.org/10.1080/15299732.2020.1869098.

Mercurio, A. E., Hong, F., Amir, C., Tarullo, A. R., Samkavitz, A., Ashy, M., & Malley-Morrison, K. (2022). Relationships among childhood maltreatment, limbic system dysfunction, and eating disorders in college women. *Journal of Interpersonal Violence*, 37(1–2), 520–537. https://doi.org/10.1177/0886260520912590.

Mętel, D., Arciszewska, A., Daren, A., Pionke, R., Cechnicki, A., Frydecka, D., & Gawęda, Ł. (2020). Mediating role of cognitive biases, resilience and depressive symptoms in the relationship between childhood trauma and psychotic-like experiences in young adults. *Early Intervention in Psychiatry*, 14(1), 87–96. *https://doi.org/10.1111/eip.12829.*

Mikolajewski, A. J., & Scheeringa, M. S. (2022). Links between Oppositional Defiant Disorder Dimensions, Psychophysiology, and Interpersonal versus Non-interpersonal Trauma. *Journal of Psychopathology and Behavioral Assessment*, 44(1), 261–275. https://doi.org/10.1007/s10862-021-09930-y.

Moner, N., Soubelet, A., Barbieri, L., & Askenazy, F. (2022). Assessment of PTSD and posttraumatic symptomatology in very young children: A systematic review. *Journal of*

Child and Adolescent Psychiatric Nursing 35(1), 7–23. https://doi.org/10.1111/jcap.12351.

Motsan, S., Bar-Kalifa, E., Yirmiya, K., & Feldman, R. (2021). Physiological and social synchrony as markers of PTSD and resilience following chronic early trauma. *Depression and Anxiety*, 38(1), 89–99. https://doi.org/10.1002/da.23106.

Mysliwiec, V., Brock, M. S., Creamer, J. L., O'Reilly, B. M., Germain, A., & Roth, B. J. (2018). Trauma associated sleep disorder: A parasomnia induced by trauma. *Sleep Medicine Reviews*, 37, 94–104. https://doi.org/10.1016/j.smrv.2017.01.004.

Popovic, D., Schmitt, A., Kaurani, L., Senner, F., Papiol, S., Malchow, B., Fischer, A., Schulze, T. G., Koutsouleris, N., & Falkai, P. (2019). Childhood trauma in schizophrenia: Current findings and research perspectives. *Frontiers in Neuroscience*, 13, 274. https://doi.org/10.3389/fnins.2019.00274.

Rüfenacht, E., Pham, E., Nicastro, R., Dieben, K., Hasler, R., Weibel, S., & Perroud, N. (2021). Link between history of childhood maltreatment and emotion dysregulation in adults suffering from attention deficit/hyperactivity disorder or borderline personality disorder. *Biomedicines*, 9(10), 1469. https://doi.org/10.3390/biomedicines9101469.

Sachser, C., Berliner, L., Holt, T., Jensen, T., Jungbluth, N., Risch, E., Rosner, R., & Goldbeck, L. (2018). Comparing the dimensional structure and diagnostic algorithms between DSM-5 and ICD-11 PTSD in children and adolescents. *European Child & Adolescent Psychiatry*, 27(2), 181–190. https://doi.org/10.1007/s00787-017-1032-9.

Scheeringa, M. S. (2019). Development of a brief screen for symptoms of posttraumatic stress disorder in young children: The young child PTSD screen. *Journal of Developmental and Behavioral Pediatrics*, 40(2), 105–111. https://doi.org/10.1097/DBP.0000000000000639.

Scheeringa, M. S. (2021). Reexamination of diathesis stress and neurotoxic stress theories: A qualitative review of pre-trauma neurobiology in relation to posttraumatic stress symptoms. *International Journal of Methods in Psychiatric Research*, 30(2), e1864. https://doi.org/10.1002/mpr.1864.

Scheeringa, M. S., Zeanah, C. H., & Cohen, J. A. (2011). PTSD in children and adolescents: Toward an empirically based algorithm. *Depression and Anxiety*, 28(9), 770–782. https://doi.org/10.1002/da.20736.

Scheeringa, M. S., Zeanah, C. H., Myers, L., & Putnam, F. W. (2003). New findings on alternative criteria for PTSD in preschool children. *Journal of the American Academy of Child & Adolescent Psychiatry*, 42(5), 561–570. https://doi.org/10.1097/01.CHI.0000046822.95464.14.

Scheeringa, M. S., Zeanah, C. H., Myers, L., & Putnam, F. W. (2005). Predictive validity in a prospective follow-up of PTSD in preschool children. *Journal of the American Academy of Child and Adolescent Psychiatry*, 44(9), 899–906. https://doi.org/10.1097/01.chi.0000169013.81536.71.

Secrist, M. E., Dalenberg, C. J., & Gevirtz, R. (2019). Contributing factors predicting nightmares in children: Trauma, anxiety, dissociation, and emotion regulation. *Psychological Trauma: Theory, Research, Practice, and Policy*, 11(1), 114–121. https://doi.org/10.1037/tra0000387.

Siegel, D. (1956). *Invasion of the body snatchers*. Walter Wanger Productions.

Sousa, C., Mason, W. A., Herrenkohl, T. I., Prince, D., Herrenkohl, R. C., & Russo, M. J. (2018). Direct and indirect effects of child abuse and environmental stress: A lifecourse perspective on adversity and depressive symptoms. *American Journal of Orthopsychiatry*, 88(2), 180–188. https://doi.org/10.1037/ort0000283.

Spinazzola, J., van der Kolk, B., & Ford, J. D. (2018). When nowhere is safe: Interpersonal trauma and attachment adversity as antecedents of posttraumatic stress disorder and developmental trauma disorder. *Journal of Traumatic Stress*, 31(5), 631–642. https://doi.org/10.1002/jts.22320.

Spinazzola, J., van der Kolk, B., & Ford, J. D. (2021). Developmental trauma disorder: A legacy of attachment trauma in victimized children. *Journal of Traumatic Stress*, 34(4), 711–720. https://doi.org/10.1002/jts.22697.

Stanton, K., McDonnell, C. G., Hayden, E. P., & Watson, D. (2020). Transdiagnostic approaches to psychopathology measurement: Recommendations for measure selection, data analysis, and participant recruitment. *Journal of Abnormal Psychology*, 129(1), 21–28. https://doi.org/10.1037/abn0000464.

Stoltz, S., Beijers, R., Smeekens, S., & Deković, M. (2017). Diathesis stress or differential susceptibility?: Testing longitudinal associations between parenting, temperament, and children's problem behavior. *Social Development*, 26(4), 783–796. https://doi.org/10.1111/sode.12237.

Toof, J., Wong, J., & Devlin, J. M. (2020). Childhood trauma and attachment. *The Family Journal*, 28(2), 194–198. https://doi.org/10.1177/1066480720902106.

Tschoeke, S., Bichescu-Burian, D., Steinert, T., & Flammer, E. (2021). History of childhood trauma and association with borderline and dissociative features. *The Journal of Nervous and Mental Disease*, 209(2), 137–143. https://doi.org/10.1097/NMD.0000000000001270.

Tsur, N., Katz, C., & Talmon, A. (2021). The shielding effect of not responding: Peritraumatic responses to child abuse and their links to posttraumatic symptomatology. *Child Abuse & Neglect*, 121, 105224. https://doi.org/10.1016/j.chiabu.2021.105224.

Ulmer-Yaniv, A., Djalovski, A., Yirmiya, K., Halevi, G., Zagoory-Sharon, O., & Feldman, R. (2018). Maternal immune and affiliative biomarkers and sensitive parenting mediate the effects of chronic early trauma on child anxiety. *Psychological Medicine*, 48(6), 1020–1033. https://doi.org/10.1017/S0033291717002550.

Uppendahl, J. R., Alozkan-Sever, C., Cuijpers, P., de Vries, R., & Sijbrandij, M. (2020). Psychological and psychosocial interventions for PTSD, depression and anxiety among children and adolescents in low- and middle-income countries: A meta-analysis. *Frontiers in Psychiatry*, 10, 933. https://doi.org/10.3389/fpsyt.2019.00933.

van der Kolk, B., Pynoos, R., Cicchetti, D., Cloitre, M., D'Andrea, W., Ford, J., & Teicher, M. (2009). Proposal to include a developmental trauma disorder diagnosis for children and adolescents in DSM-V. http://www.traumacenter.org/announcements/dtd_papers_oct_09.pdf.

Van Nieuwenhove, K., & Meganck, R. (2019). Interpersonal features in complex trauma etiology, consequences, and treatment: A literature review. *Journal of Aggression, Maltreatment & Trauma*, 28(8), 903–928. https://doi.org/10.1080/10926771.2017.1405316.

Wamser-Nanney, R., & Chesher, R. E. (2018). Trauma characteristics and sleep impairment among trauma-exposed children. *Child Abuse & Neglect*, 76, 469–479. https://doi.org/10.1016/j.chiabu.2017.11.020.

Williams, B. M., & Levinson, C. A. (2022). A model of self-criticism as a transdiagnostic mechanism of eating disorder comorbidity: A review. *New Ideas in Psychology*, 66, 100949. https://doi.org/10.1016/j.newideapsych.2022.100949.

Wolf, M. R., & Nochajski, T. H. (2022). 'Black Holes' in memory: Childhood autobiographical memory loss in adult survivors of child sexual abuse. *European Journal of Trauma & Dissociation*, 6(1), 100234. https://doi.org/10.1016/j.ejtd.2021.100234.

Woolgar, F., Garfield, H., Dalgleish, T., & Meiser-Stedman, R. (2021). Systematic review and meta-analysis: Prevalence of posttraumatic stress disorder in trauma-exposed preschool-aged children. *Child & Adolescent Psychiatry*, 61(3), 366–377. https://doi.org/10.1016/j.jaac.2021.05.026.

Wozniak, M. (2018). "I" and "Me": The self in the context of consciousness. *Frontiers in Psychology*, 9, 1656. https://doi.org/10.3389/fpsyg.2018.01656.

Zdankiewicz-Ścigała E., & Ścigała, D. K. (2018). Trauma, temperament, alexithymia, and dissociation among persons addicted to alcohol: Mediation model of dependencies. *Frontiers in Psychology*, 9, 1570. https://doi.org/10.3389/fpsyg.2018.01570.

Zdankiewicz-Ścigała, E., & Ścigała, D. K. (2020). Attachment style, early childhood trauma, alexithymia, and dissociation among persons addicted to alcohol: Structural equation model of dependencies. *Frontiers in Psychology*, 10, 2957. https://doi.org/10.3389/fpsyg.2019.02957.

Zhu, W., Chen, Y., & Xia, L. X. (2020). Childhood maltreatment and aggression: The mediating roles of hostile attribution bias and anger rumination. *Personality and Individual Differences*, 162, 110007. https://doi.org/10.1016/j.paid.2020.110007.

3

ATTACHMENT, EXISTENTIAL PSYCHOLOGY, AND DEVELOPMENTAL TRAUMA

How do you define fairness and justice? How do you cope with social injustices that adversely affect you or your loved ones? Did you have an adverse childhood experience? For example, did you experience bullying? Do you forgive those who have hurt you, or do you hold on to anger and resentment? Have these types of experiences impacted how you view yourself, others, and the world?

For children, traumatic events can be confusing, stressful, and distracting, in part because children have limited life experiences and cognitive capacities. They may not be able to communicate to others that they are experiencing anxiety in response to traumatic events. In particular, children may have difficulty identifying and communicating about annihilation anxiety, which refers to an individual's concerns about physical and psychological safety (Kira et al., 2022). Children who experience high levels of annihilation anxiety are likely to be unable to focus on anything other than immediate survival – at the very time when they should be living the best years of their lives.

Introduction to Attachment

Developmental theorists have postulated that early experiences with other people in the world are critical to mastering the fundamental skills needed for adaptive behavior. Scholars such as Erik Erikson surmised that the first five years of life are a model for trust building, independence, and goal-directed behavior (Knight, 2017; Lawford et al., 2020; Mavranezouli et al., 2020; Stern et al., 2018). Likewise, Abraham Maslow theorized that the antecedents of self-actualization (an individual's ability to recognize and value his or her strengths and potential for success) include early positive and supportive experiences with

DOI: 10.4324/9781003304715-3

caregivers, predictably safe environments, and fulfilment of basic needs, such as food, shelter, and love (Bucchio et al., 2021).

John Bowlby's classic theory of attachment is perhaps the most influential model for our understanding of the devastation caused by trauma, including severe neglect that exposes children to unsafe (and possibly life-threatening) circumstances. Attachment theory (Ainsworth et al., 1978; Bowlby, 1958, 1969) refers to the evolutionary bond between an infant and his or her care-giver(s) that, under normal circumstances, is characterized as a warm, recipro-cally reinforcing, predictable, and responsive relationship. According to attachment theorists, in stressful circumstances, such as when infants are sepa-rated from caregivers, children should be able to pursue their caregiver's proximity to cope with psychological distress and return to a state of physiolo-gical equanimity (regulation of the fight-flight-freeze stress-response system). Indeed, in studies of the strange situation paradigm (SSP) (Kondo-Ikemura et al., 2018; Prince et al., 2021; Shakiba & Raby, 2021), securely attached infants often display mild psychological distress upon separation and seek proximity to their caregiver(s) to minimize fear and anxiety. Upon reunifica-tion, they often demonstrate positive emotions and approach their caregiver(s) with open arms. Attachment theorists speculate that securely attached infants have internalized their caregiver(s) as a secure base (i.e., a secure internal working model of self-other; Eller et al., 2022; Grossmann & Grossmann, 2020; Opie et al., 2021; Waters et al., 2017; Zhang et al., 2022) from which they feel safe to separate, explore their environment periodically, and cope effectively. These caregivers often demonstrate reliably sensitive responses to their children, such as responding to their cries and providing them with warmth and physical touch to reconcile their felt distress.

In general, children who are securely attached to caregivers demonstrate positive outcomes with regard to their psychological and physical health. Early attachment security correlates negatively with depression and anxiety and posi-tively with spiritual and religious coping, mindfulness, resilience, and self-reg-ulation (Darling Rasmussen et al., 2019; Dudley et al., 2018; Kerstis et al., 2018; Leman et al., 2018; Tabachnick et al., 2022; Toumbelekis et al., 2021).

Insecure Attachment

Not all infants are securely attached, however. About 39% are what is classified as insecurely attached – insecure-anxious, insecure-avoidant, or insecure-dis-organized (Carr et al., 2018; Puhlmann et al., 2021; Spruit et al., 2020). Inse-cure-anxious infants fearfully hold on to their primary caregiver(s) and protest separation. They often use hyperactivating strategies (e.g., hypervigilance, anxious preoccupation, panic, and aggression), particularly when caregivers are not consistently responsive (Duschinsky & Solomon, 2017; Sood et al., 2022). Insecure-anxious infants tend to intensify their proximity-seeking behaviors (i.

e., clinging) in times of stress so that caregivers are more likely to meet their needs.

In contrast, insecure-avoidant children repress their emotional responses when separated from or reunited with their caregivers and appear not to have emotional responses (i.e., alexithymia). They use deactivating strategies (i.e., cognitive and affective suppression/repression; Murray et al., 2021; Tammilehto et al., 2022) in response to inconsistent and often emotionally unavailable caregivers, including ignoring and disregarding their caregivers upon separation and reunification, regardless of the circumstances. These children strongly prefer autonomy and self-reliance in relationships and experience distress with emotional closeness, vulnerability, and intimacy. These children often have unmet needs and believe their attempts to convey them to caregivers (or others) have little to no impact.

Insecurely attached infants, specifically the disorganized typology, display extreme approach and behavioral avoidance reactions to parental separation and reunification (Dagan et al., 2021; Forslund et al., 2020; Fuentes-Balderrama et al., 2022). These children experience significant psychological distress before, during, and after separation from their caregiver(s). They have difficulty regulating their emotions regardless of the circumstances (e.g., during reunification or separation), and they experience hyperactivation (i.e., anxious) and deactivation (i.e., avoidant) attachment behavioral strategies to cope (Beijers et al., 2021; Gambin et al., 2021; Iwanski et al., 2021; Stenson et al., 2021).

Trauma and Attachment

Trauma, PTSD, and Insecure Attachment

Early traumas – including repeated abuse and neglect – often give rise to insecure attachments (Erkoreka et al., 2022; Paetzold & Rholes, 2021; Peng et al., 2021). Traumatic experiences may disrupt a caregiver's responses to the infant, interfering with reciprocal communication within the dyadic (parent-child) relationship and disrupting the development of a secure attachment. An illustration of this can be seen in parents addicted to alcohol and drugs. Empirical studies suggest that the physiological processes involved in parenting and attachment (e.g., those involving dopamine and the amygdala) are the same neural networks adversely affected by addiction (Liahaugen Flensburg et al., 2022; Liese et al., 2020; Stein et al., 2017; Strathearn et al., 2019). Indeed, individuals who engage in increasing alcohol and drug use typically experience a decreasing interest in maintaining and sustaining a consistent, predictable relationship with their child(ren). Addicted caregivers tend to their children's attachment behaviors negatively and may become less responsive and more frustrated as infants increasingly express their needs. They tend to demonstrate fewer and less consistent responses to infant needs and, instead, increasingly concentrate on the rewarding (and highly addicting) effects of alcohol and drugs. In turn, they often neglect their children and themselves (Giacolini et al., 2021; Hyysalo et al., 2022; Lowell et al., 2021).

Over the last decade, a considerable body of research has examined empirical models of trauma and attachment that also consider the adverse effects of early abuse, neglect, and polyvictimization (i.e., multiple, repeated ACEs; Assini-Meytin et al., 2022; Ford, 2021; Ford & Delker, 2018; Lee et al., 2022; Miedema et al., 2022; Sterzing et al., 2017). The combination of interpersonal trauma and disruption of primary attachment has been shown to interfere with children's mastery of developmental competencies, including emotion regulation, age-appropriate autonomy, self-discovery, language, and communication – all of which are vital for psychosocial development. This notion is compatible with social-cognitive models (i.e., mirror neurons help children imitate behavior and learn from the actions of others; Jahangard et al., 2019; Jeon & Lee, 2018) and the dual representation framework (Bisby et al., 2020; Bryant, 2021), which indicate that traumatic experiences affect multiple cognitive and affective systems. More specifically, these models hold that trauma impacts theory of mind (i.e., perspective taking), empathy, and verbal and perceptual (non-verbal) memory processes via fight-flight-freeze responses to stress and fragmented, incoherent memories.

Attachment and Developmental Trauma

Scholars suggest that insecure attachment itself has adverse impacts on the effects of developmental trauma, originating from multiple factors associated with polyvictimization (e.g., biased – often negative – cognitive appraisals, low self-esteem, social and economic adversity, rejection sensitivity, emotion dysregulation, intrusive thoughts, anxious rumination, sudden shifts in mood, bizarre behaviors; Brumariu et al., 2021; De Paoli et al., 2017; Forslund et al., 2020; Zhou et al., 2021). Scholars have asserted that the diverse outcomes seen in DTD children, including high psychiatric comorbidities, are linked to attachment disturbances arising from early interpersonal trauma and polyvictimization (Ford, 2021; Gawęda et al., 2018). Attachment and trauma-mediated adaptations often occur in the context of other risk factors (e.g., low socioeconomic status [SES], academic problems, and financial caregivers' stress/work-related problems; Donadio et al., 2022; Herstell et al., 2021; Shen et al., 2021; Vowels et al., 2022).

Children who experience ACEs and demonstrate PTSD adaptations are likely to benefit from secure attachments to caregivers. Insecure attachment to primary caregivers is associated with complex developmental trauma in many cross-cultural, longitudinal, and physiological studies (Bosmans et al., 2018; Chatziioannidis et al., 2019; Cimino et al., 2020; Ford et al., 2018; Gray et al., 2018; Sandberg & Refrea, 2022; Spinazzola et al., 2018, 2021). Abusive caregivers – one form of complex developmental trauma – often demonstrate low sensitivity and reflective capacities. Infants with an abusive caregiver are not able to mirror their caregivers.

Children with developmental trauma lack self-esteem and self-efficacy because they were abused and neglected by caregivers, blame themselves for the abuse (or were convinced by others that they were culpable in some way), and developed an insecure attachment and negative internal working model of self and others (Chung et al., 2017; Spinazzola et al., 2018). They have come to view themselves negatively and, in turn, assume that others are unlikely to love and support them regardless of the circumstances. Indeed, these cognitive distortions, referring to maladaptive thoughts about oneself or others, are precipitated by insecure attachment, negative (false) beliefs, and betrayal (Fang et al., 2020; Miller et al., 2017). Scholars have also linked these experiences to higher rates of polyvictimization and intergenerational trauma (Babcock Fenerci & Allen, 2018; Racine et al., 2022; Delker et al., 2018; St. Vil et al., 2021).

Developmental trauma is damaging to children because it is inextricably linked to disruptions in a secure attachment to caregivers during sensitive periods of physiological development. Indeed, research suggests that early traumas cause symptoms of DTD because children essentially lose their capacity to find meaning and purpose in life, which according to existential scholars (e.g., Yalom and Frankl) is just as vital as our need to survive. In other words, children are born with an inherent need to survive and thrive, which underscores their need to find a meaningful place in the world and a sense of belongingness, both of which are mediated by the attachment infants develop to their caregivers. However, children with developmental trauma often lack secure attachment, which limits their attempts to fight for their survival, thereby undermining their strengths and gifts and, in turn, precipitating the high rates of self-injury (e.g., drug abuse, self-mutilation, criminal behavior) and suicide we see in these same children (Khosravani et al., 2017; Spinazzola et al., 2018, 2021). These symptoms may worsen when children re-experience traumatic circumstances, such as those that mirror the original traumas, and when they are overwhelmed, dissociative, and flooded by those reminders.

Indeed, the adverse effects of early repeated abuse and neglect that characterize DTD and attachment disturbances are mediated by physiological disturbances in the nervous system (i.e., corticolimbic structures), including the amygdala, hippocampus, and white matter integrity needed for optimal cognitive capacities (Chen & Ghazali, 2022; Corr et al., 2022; Cruciani et al., 2021; Petrowski et al., 2019; Riem et al., 2019; van Hoof et al., 2019).

Recent studies comparing individuals who experienced trauma and developed measurable symptoms of DTD and PTSD (Spinazzola et al., 2018; van Der Kolk et al., 2019) found that PTSD correlated with higher rates of physical abuse and generalized anxiety; DTD positively correlated with interpersonal violence, insecure attachment, and separation anxiety; and the combination of interpersonal trauma and attachment adversity had cumulative adverse effects on children's physiological and self-regulation capacities. In addition, these effects were independent of PTSD diagnosis.

Developmental Trauma and Worldview Assumptions

A thorough discussion of developmental trauma and attachment would be incomplete without discussing what it means for children to experience a life-threatening event – an event that threatens their safety, security, and emerging ideas about life, love, and relationships. Several prominent scholars, such as Viktor Frankl, Albert Bandura, Irvin Yalom, and Janoff-Bulman, have asserted that individuals are born with foundational schemas or mental representations of the world most prominently influenced by their earliest experiences.

The assumptive world concept refers to the assumptions or beliefs that ground, secure, stabilize, and orient us. In the face of death and trauma, these beliefs are shattered. This is in line with the shattered assumptions theory (Janoff-Bulman, 1992), which posits that individuals inherently view the world as safe, predictable, and meaningful. This theory suggests that trauma gives rise to negative foundational worldviews that are characterized by low optimism and high cynicism (Bai et al., 2021; Khaleque, 2017; Thompson-Hollands et al., 2017), challenging core assumptions about oneself and the world, thereby leading to negative reflections about life (Mazor et al., 2020; Rizeq & McCann, 2021). In other words, traumatic experiences essentially override positive worldview assumptions (about the world's benevolence, meaningfulness, social justice, and one's self-worth) and compromise the self-efficacy and spiritual/existential beliefs that may have helped these individuals cope with ACEs and trauma, positively reappraise their experiences of adversity, and develop transformative resilient adaptations.

Exposure to trauma, especially early, or repeated interpersonal traumas, such as those that cause attachment disturbances in DTD children, also cause children to struggle to manage their concerns about death and dying. Trauma precipitated by multiple, repeated ACEs is often difficult to reconcile. This is in line with the terror management theory (TMT) (Greenberg et al., 1986), which proposes that individuals cope with existential anxiety, including the inevitability of death, by preserving faith in their cultural worldviews, self-esteem, and close interpersonal relationships (Kosloff et al., 2019; Pyszczynski et al., 2021). These adaptive resources have been characterized as an anxiety-buffering system designed to help children, adolescents, and adults cope with fear and stress by providing an organizing framework of the world, including that life is logical, predictable, and fair/just; people are generally kind and trustworthy; and one can exert control over their life circumstances. Experiences of trauma override the anxiety buffering system, contribute to psychological and physiological distress, and worsen responses to trauma and recovery (Vail et al., 2020; Yetzer & Pyszczynski, 2019).

Experiences of developmental trauma may also compromise an individual's belief in God (e.g., that adversity has meaning, value, and spiritual or religious significance).

Such trauma may cause individuals to question whether life is meaningful, whether the world is safe, and whether God can protect them (and their loved ones) from additional traumas (Goodwin et al., 2017; Helm et al., 2019; Vail et al., 2020).

Shattered world assumptions correlate with insecure attachment (Captari et al., 2021), disturbances in self-regulation capacities (Rizeq & McCann, 2021; Smith et al., 2019), high rates of trauma and PTSD (Chung et al., 2017; Chung & Freh, 2019), and psychiatric comorbidities (Mikulincer et al., 2020; Schleider et al., 2021). A negative view of the world and an insecure attachment causes social and psychological disturbances, including mood and behavior problems and difficulty forming close, trusting, dependable relationships. Threats to meaning, self-esteem, and relatedness also can increase susceptibility to anxiety, distress, and emotional difficulties (Bergman et al., 2018; Harvell-Bowman et al., 2022; Lifshin et al., 2021). As such, developmental trauma adaptations reflect maladaptive responses to the inevitability of death precipitated by existential fear and terror, interpersonal (caregiver) betrayal, and insecure attachment (Arredondo & Caparrós, 2019; Yalch & Levendosky, 2018; Zyromski et al., 2018). These individuals tend to use less adaptive psychological defenses against stress (i.e., maladaptive and reality distorting assimilation defenses, such as paranoia, dissociation, codependency, and splitting behaviors; Baryshnikov et al., 2017; Fang et al., 2020; Marshall et al., 2022; Popkirov et al., 2019).

Experiences of trauma increase the recognition that death is inevitable, leading individuals who have experienced such trauma to become preoccupied with questions about the meaning of life and death. This is likely to be overwhelming for children to manage alone. There is evidence indicating that developmental trauma dramatically increases the risk for suicidal behavior, including repeated suicide attempts (Bach et al., 2018; Bai et al., 2021; Khosravani et al., 2017; Thompson et al., 2019; Zatti et al., 2017). Studies have demonstrated how attachment insecurity is specifically associated with developmental trauma and precipitates chronic (often treatment-resistant or refractory) depression leading to self-injury. Early trauma often leads to extreme displays of self-hatred and suicide or resentment and rage towards others, including those who failed to protect them and their caregivers from repeated threats. Some children who experience trauma will develop positive adaptations. However, many will create cynical and distrustful views of others. Children may view the world as unfair and unjust, thereby shifting their view of relationships, possibly limiting their opportunities for positive relationships that have the potential to change their worldviews.

Betrayal Trauma

Contemporary research on developmental trauma suggests that in addition to attachment insecurity, disorganization, and existential despair, DTD negatively correlates with empathy and positively correlates with interpersonal betrayal, which occurs when children and adolescents are betrayed by the adults they depend on for survival (e.g., betrayal trauma theory suggests that trusted adults include caregivers as well as institutions and social systems designed to protect children and families, such as child welfare agencies, schools, religious institutions, and law enforcement; Carroll, 2022; Hocking et al., 2016; Lawson & Akay-Sullivan, 2020; Platt & Freyd, 2015).

Scholars have emphasized the concept of betrayal trauma (Freyd, 1994, 1996) to refer to the lasting adverse effects of a broken bond, such as the relationship between a parent and child or between families and the institutions that protect them. Individuals often respond to interpersonal betrayal by avoiding the person who betrayed them, accepting betrayal (and distrust) as normative in all relationships, and/or developing unhealthy interpersonal interactions, such as aggression and violence against others. Experiences of trauma with high levels of interpersonal betrayal (e.g., caregiver abuse, incest) have been linked to insecure attachment and significant levels of psychological distress (Choi & Kangas, 2020; Wills et al., 2022; Yalch & Levendosky, 2019), and these types of trauma experiences have been found to cause severe, often longstanding psychological disturbances (e.g., shame, psychosis, fear of abandonment, and dissociation; Gómez, 2019; Gómez & Freyd, 2017; Keng et al., 2019; Lawson & Akay-Sullivan, 2020; Zerubavel et al., 2018).

Children who experience betrayal trauma will likely see little value in regulating their behavior, particularly when positive behaviors have been undermined by chaos in the home. Children and adolescents may lose faith in God and choose to live more for the moment than wait for a future that is not guaranteed or that is guaranteed to bring more pain and suffering. Children cannot plan for the future in the way we adults can, such that they cannot readily understand that they will be able to exert more control over their life circumstances. Children are likely questioning if they will make it to adulthood, mainly because they may have developed in the context of pain, suffering, loss, and a lack of positive experiences.

DTD underscores experiences of pervasive interpersonal traumas that occurred early in life for children and adults whose physical, interpersonal/relational, and psychological disturbances originated from insecure attachment, including the disorganized typology. Conceptualizing developmental trauma as an attachment disorder may also help explain the broad, diverse outcomes and comorbidities reported in the literature, including large-scale studies and meta-analyses documenting deleterious effects from early trauma and toxic stress in individuals who experience early abuse, neglect, and disrupted attachment.

Clinical Assessment and Treatment from an Attachment Framework

Attachment theory has been proposed as an integrative framework for assessing and treating individuals who experience early repeated abuse and neglect and who develop measurable symptoms of DTD. Evaluation and treatment procedures have been developed that accommodate classical models of trauma (i.e., PTSD) as well as the diverse responses often seen in individuals who experience early traumatic polyvictimization.

One such model is trauma-focused cognitive behavioral therapy (TF-CBT), which is regarded as one of the most effective treatments for individuals who have experienced early and complex trauma. TF-CBT is a skills-based treatment model that includes strategies based on attachment theory, family therapy, and graded exposure through sequenced (increasingly complex) interventions. TF-CBT is implemented in modules that involve psychoeducation and training on physiological stress and trauma, attachment, and bonding (often with non-offending caregivers); developing a cohesive trauma narrative; improving self-regulation capacities; and responding to perceived threats or danger effectively (and recognizing that such responses originate from trauma). The treatment also includes processing traumas verbally so they can be processed effectively and not repressed, which causes individuals to experience dissociation, psychosis, aggression, and traumatic amnesia.

Rigorous investigations of TF-CBT, including large-scale, multi-site, randomized control trials, have shown that TF-CBT is a valid and reliable treatment (e.g., Jensen et al., 2017; Kameoka et al., 2020; McGuire et al., 2021; Ross et al., 2021). TF-CBT has also been applied effectively to diverse populations (i.e., Culturally Adapted TF-CBT), which underscores intersectional identities, minority stress and trauma, collectivist views of interpersonal relationships, and cultural idioms of stress coping and resilience (Bryant-Davis, 2019; Canale et al., 2022; Latif et al., 2021; Márquez et al., 2020; Peters et al., 2021; Sanchez et al., 2022; Stewart et al., 2021). The positive, long-term gains made by individuals treated with TF-CBT, such as positive reappraisals and enhanced interpersonal communication and coping, are mediated by a broad range of factors, including therapeutic alliance and positive physiological changes (e.g., improved functional connectivity across multiple neural networks; Bryant et al., 2021; Korgaonkar et al., 2020; Santarnecchi et al., 2019) that underlie attention, self-awareness, attachment, memory, and executive functioning.

Conclusions

Developmental trauma has lasting effects because such experiences interrupt attachment security and foundational beliefs about oneself, including one's self-esteem, value and self-worth, acceptance and lovability, and ability to control life circumstances. As such, individuals who have experienced early trauma often develop severe psychological disturbances that compromise their motivation and will to live, their ability to disclose their traumas and seek help from others, and their faith in a higher power. Multiple studies have illustrated the lifelong devastation caused to victims of early trauma, particularly those who experienced polyvictimization. Developmental traumas also adversely affect broad physiological processes and neural networks, such as those responsible for developing healthy relationships. Nevertheless, children, adolescents, and adults who experience trauma can change and develop into healthy, fully functioning adults, particularly when early identification and trauma-informed interventions are used to support them. In the next chapter, I expand on how relationships affect children and families, specifically the systems and institutions that influence victims of trauma and that have the potential to help these individuals recover and live satisfying, meaningful lives.

References

Ainsworth, M. D. S., Blehar, M. C., Waters, E., & Wall, S. (1978). *Patterns of attachment*. Hillsdale, NJ: Erlbaum.

Arredondo, A. Y., & Caparrós, B. (2019). Associations between existential concerns and adverse experiences: A systematic review. *Journal of Humanistic Psychology*, 0022167819846284. https://doi.org/10.1177/0022167819846284.

Assini-Meytin, L. C., Fix, R. L., Green, K. M., Nair, R., & Letourneau, E. J. (2022). Adverse childhood experiences, mental health, and risk behaviors in adulthood: Exploring sex, racial, and ethnic group differences in a nationally representative sample. *Journal of Child & Adolescent Trauma*, 15(3), 833–845. https://doi.org/10. 1007/s40653-021-00424-3.

Babcock Fenerci, R. L., & Allen, B. (2018). From mother to child: Maternal betrayal trauma and risk for maltreatment and psychopathology in the next generation. *Child abuse & neglect*, 82, 1–11. https://doi.org/10.1016/j.chiabu.2018.05.014.

Bach, S. L., Molina, M. A. L., Jansen, K., da Silva, R. A., & Souza, L. D. M. (2018). Suicide risk and childhood trauma in individuals diagnosed with posttraumatic stress disorder. *Trends in Psychiatry and Psychotherapy*, 40(3), 253–257. https://doi.org/10. 1590/2237-6089-2017-0101.

Bai, Q., Huang, S., Hsueh, F. H., & Zhang, T. (2021). Cyberbullying victimization and suicide ideation: A crumbled belief in a just world. *Computers in human behavior*, 120, 106679. https://doi.org/10.1016/j.chb.2021.106679.

Baryshnikov, I., Joffe, G., Koivisto, M., Melartin, T., Aaltonen, K., Suominen, K., Rosenström, T., Näätänen, P., Karpov, B., Heikkinen, M., & Isometsä, E. (2017). Relationships between self-reported childhood traumatic experiences, attachment style, neuroticism and features of borderline personality disorders in patients with mood disorders. *Journal of Affective Disorders*, 210, 82–89. https://doi.org/10.1016/j.jad.2016.12.004.

Beijers, R., Miragall, M., van den Berg, Y., Konttinen, H., & van Strien, T. (2021). Parent-infant attachment insecurity and emotional eating in adolescence: Mediation through emotion suppression and alexithymia. *Nutrients*, 13(5), 1662. https://doi.org/10.3390/nu13051662.

Bergman, Y. S., Bodner, E., & Haber, Y. (2018). The connection between subjective nearness-to-death and depressive symptoms: The mediating role of meaning in life. *Psychiatry Research*, 261, 269–273. https://doi.org/10.1016/j.psychres.2017.12.078.

Bisby, J. A., Burgess, N., & Brewin, C. R. (2020). Reduced memory coherence for negative events and its relationship to posttraumatic stress disorder. *Current Directions in Psychological Science*, 29(3), 267–272. https://doi.org/10.1177/0963721420917691.

Bosmans, G., Young, J. F., & Hankin, B. L. (2018). NR3C1 methylation as a moderator of the effects of maternal support and stress on insecure attachment development. *Developmental Psychology*, 54(1), 29–38. https://doi.org/10.1037/dev0000422.

Bowlby, J. (1958). The nature of the child's tie to his mother. *International Journal of Psychoanalysis*, 39, 350–371.

Bowlby, J. (1969). *Attachment. Attachment and loss: Vol. 1. Loss.* New York: Basic Books.

Brumariu, L. E., Kerns, K. A., Giuseppone, K. R., & Lyons-Ruth, K. (2021). Disorganized/controlling attachments, emotion regulation, and emotion communication in later middle childhood. *Journal of Applied Developmental Psychology*, 76, 101324. https://doi.org/10.1016/j.appdev.2021.101324.

Bryant, R. A. (2021). A critical review of mechanisms of adaptation to trauma: Implications for early interventions for posttraumatic stress disorder. *Clinical Psychology Review*, 85, 101981. https://doi.org/10.1016/j.cpr.2021.101981.

Bryant, R. A., Erlinger, M., Felmingham, K., Klimova, A., Williams, L. M., Malhi, G., ..., & Korgaonkar, M. S. (2021). Reappraisal-related neural predictors of treatment response to cognitive behavior therapy for post-traumatic stress disorder. *Psychological Medicine*, 51(14), 2454–2464. https://doi.org/10.1017/S0033291720001129.

Bryant-Davis, T. (2019). The cultural context of trauma recovery: Considering the posttraumatic stress disorder practice guideline and intersectionality. *Psychotherapy*, 56 (3), 400–408. https://doi.org/10.1037/pst0000241.

Bucchio, J., Jones, V. N., & Dopwell, D. M. (2021). Applying Maslow's Hierarchy of Needs to LGBT foster youth: Practice implications for child welfare professionals and those working in rural settings. *Journal of Social Work Practice*, 35(3), 287–299. https://doi.org/10.1080/02650533.2020.1834372.

Canale, C. A., Hayes, A. M., Yasinski, C., Grasso, D. J., Webb, C., & Deblinger, E. (2022). Caregiver behaviors and child distress in trauma narration and processing sessions of trauma-focused cognitive behavioral therapy (TF-CBT). *Behavior Therapy*, 53 (1), 64–79. https://doi.org/10.1016/j.beth.2021.06.001.

Captari, L. E., Riggs, S. A., & Stephen, K. (2021). Attachment processes following traumatic loss: A mediation model examining identity distress, shattered assumptions, prolonged grief, and posttraumatic growth. *Psychological Trauma: Theory, Research, Practice and Policy*, 13(1), 94–103. https://doi.org/10.1037/tra0000555.

Carr, S. C., Hardy, A., & Fornells-Ambrojo, M. (2018). Relationship between attachment style and symptom severity across the psychosis spectrum: A meta-analysis. *Clinical Psychology Review*, 59, 145–158. https://doi.org/10.1016/j.cpr.2017.12.001.

Carroll, A. R. (2022). Betrayal trauma and resilience in former foster youth. *Emerging adulthood*, 10(2), 459–472. https://doi.org/10.1177/2167696820933126.

Chatziioannidis, S., Andreou, C., Agorastos, A., Kaprinis, S., Malliaris, Y., Garyfallos, G., & Bozikas, V. P. (2019). The role of attachment anxiety in the relationship between childhood trauma and schizophrenia-spectrum psychosis. *Psychiatry Research*, 276, 223–231. https://doi.org/10.1016/j.psychres.2019.05.021.

Chen, Y. Y., & Ghazali, S. R. (2022). Lifetime trauma exposure and PTSD symptoms in relation to health-related behaviors and physiological measures among Malaysian adolescents. *Traumatology*, 28(1), 160–166. https://doi.org/10.1037/trm0000274.

Choi, K. J., & Kangas, M. (2020). Impact of maternal betrayal trauma on parent and child well-being: Attachment style and emotion regulation as moderators. *Psychological Trauma: Theory, Research, Practice, and Policy*, 12(2), 121–130. https://doi.org/10.1037/tra0000492.

Chung, M. C., AlQarni, N., Al Muhairi, S., & Mitchell, B. (2017). The relationship between trauma centrality, self-efficacy, posttraumatic stress and psychiatric co-morbidity among Syrian refugees: Is gender a moderator? *Journal of Psychiatric Research*, 94, 107–115. https://doi.org/10.1016/j.jpsychires.2017.07.001.

Chung, M. C., & Freh, F. M. (2019). The trajectory of bombing-related posttraumatic stress disorder among Iraqi civilians: Shattered world assumptions and altered self-capacities as mediators; attachment and crisis support as moderators. *Psychiatry Research*, 273, 1–8. https://doi.org/10.1016/j.psychres.2019.01.001.

Cimino, S., Carola, V., Cerniglia, L., Bussone, S., Bevilacqua, A., & Tambelli, R. (2020). The μ-opioid receptor gene A118G polymorphism is associated with insecure attachment in children with disruptive mood regulation disorder and their mothers. *Brain and Behavior*, 10(7), e01659. https://doi.org/10.1002/brb3.1659.

Corr, R., Glier, S., Bizzell, J., Pelletier-Baldelli, A., Campbell, A., Killian-Farrell, C., & Belger, A. (2022). Stress-related hippocampus activation mediates the association between polyvictimization and trait anxiety in adolescents. *Social Cognitive and Affective Neuroscience*, 17(8), 767–776. https://doi.org/10.1093/scan/nsab129.

Cruciani, G., Boccia, M., Lingiardi, V., Giovanardi, G., Zingaretti, P., & Spitoni, G. F. (2021). An exploratory study on resting-state functional connectivity in individuals with disorganized attachment: Evidence for key regions in amygdala and hippocampus. *Brain Sciences*, 11(11), 1539. https://doi.org/10.3390/brainsci11111539.

Dagan, O., Groh, A. M., Madigan, S., & Bernard, K. (2021). A lifespan development theory of insecure attachment and internalizing symptoms: Integrating meta-analytic evidence via a testable evolutionary mis/match hypothesis. *Brain Sciences*, 11(9), 1226. https://doi.org/10.3390/brainsci11091226.

Darling Rasmussen, P., Storebø, O. J., Løkkeholt, T., Voss, L. G., Shmueli-Goetz, Y., Bojesen, A. B., Simonsen, E., & Bilenberg, N. (2019). Attachment as a core feature of resilience: A systematic review and meta-analysis. *Psychological Reports*, 122(4), 1259–1296. https://doi.org/10.1177/0033294118785577.

Delker, B. C., Smith, C. P., Rosenthal, M. N., Bernstein, R. E., & Freyd, J. J. (2018). When home is where the harm is: Family betrayal and posttraumatic outcomes in young adulthood. *Journal of Aggression, Maltreatment & Trauma*, 27(7), 720–743. https://doi.org/10.1080/10926771.2017.1382639.

De Paoli, T., Fuller-Tyszkiewicz, M., & Krug, I. (2017). Insecure attachment and maladaptive schema in disordered eating: The mediating role of rejection sensitivity. *Clinical Psychology & Psychotherapy*, 24(6), 1273–1284. https://doi.org/10.1002/cpp.2092.

Donadio, M., Valera, P., & Sinangil, N. (2022). Understanding attachment styles, adverse childhood events, alcohol use, and trauma in Black and Latino Men with criminal justice histories. *Journal of Community Psychology*, 50(5), 2260–2272. https://doi.org/10.1002/jcop.22773.

Dudley, J., Eames, C., Mulligan, J., & Fisher, N. (2018). Mindfulness of voices, self-compassion, and secure attachment in relation to the experience of hearing voices. *The British Journal of Clinical Psychology*, 57(1), 1–17. https://doi.org/10.1111/bjc.12153.

Duschinsky, R., & Solomon, J. (2017). Infant disorganized attachment: Clarifying levels of analysis. *Clinical Child Psychology and Psychiatry*, 22(4), 524–538. https://doi.org/10.1177/1359104516685602.

Eller, J., Magro, S. W., Roisman, G. I., & Simpson, J. A. (2022). The predictive significance of fluctuations in early maternal sensitivity for secure base script knowledge and relationship effectiveness in adulthood. *Journal of Social and Personal Relationships*, 39(10), 3044–3058. https://doi.org/10.1177/02654075221077640.

Erkoreka, L., Zamalloa, I., Rodriguez, S., Muñoz, P., Mendizabal, I., Zamalloa, M. I., Arrue, A., Zumarraga, M., & Gonzalez-Torres, M. A. (2022). Attachment anxiety as mediator of the relationship between childhood trauma and personality dysfunction in borderline personality disorder. *Clinical Psychology & Psychotherapy*, 29(2), 501–511. https://doi.org/10.1002/cpp.2640.

Fang, S., Chung, M. C., & Wang, Y. (2020). The impact of past trauma on psychological distress: The roles of defense mechanisms and alexithymia. *Frontiers in Psychology*, 11, 992. https://doi.org/10.3389/fpsyg.2020.00992.

Ford, J. D. (2021). Polyvictimization and developmental trauma in childhood. *European Journal of Psychotraumatology*, 12(Suppl), 1866394. https://doi.org/10.1080/20008198.2020.1866394.

Ford, J. D., & Delker, B. C. (2018). Polyvictimization in childhood and its adverse impacts across the lifespan: Introduction to the special issue. *Journal of Trauma & Dissociation*, 19(3), 275–288. https://doi.org/10.1080/15299732.2018.1440479.

Ford, J. D., Spinazzola, J., van der Kolk, B., & Grasso, D. J. (2018). Toward an empirically based developmental trauma disorder diagnosis for children: Factor structure, item characteristics, reliability, and validity of the developmental trauma disorder semi-structured interview. *The Journal of Clinical Psychiatry*, 79(5), 17m11675. https://doi.org/10.4088/JCP.17m11675.

Forslund, T., Peltola, M. J., & Brocki, K. C. (2020). Disorganized attachment representations, externalizing behavior problems, and socioemotional competences in early school-age. *Attachment & Human Development*, 22(4), 448–473. https://doi.org/10.1080/14616734.2019.1664603.

Freyd, J. J. (1994). Betrayal trauma: Traumatic amnesia as an adaptive response to childhood abuse. *Ethics & Behavior*, 4(4), 307–329. https://doi.org/10.1207/s15327019eb0404_1.

Freyd, J. J. (1996). *Betrayal trauma: The logic of forgetting childhood abuse*. Cambridge, MA: Harvard University Press.

Fuentes-Balderrama, J., Turnbull-Plaza, B., Ojeda-García, A., Parra-Cardona, J. R., Cruz del Castillo, C., Díaz-Loving, R., & Von Mohr, M. (2022). Insecure attachment to parents as a contributor to internalizing and externalizing problem behaviors in Mexican preadolescents. *Trends in Psychology*, 1–18. https://doi.org/10.1007/s43076-021-00125-8.

Gambin, M., Woźniak-Prus, M., Konecka, A., & Sharp, C. (2021). Relations between attachment to mother and father, mentalizing abilities and emotion regulation in adolescents. *European Journal of Developmental Psychology*, 18(1), 18–37. https://doi.org/10.1080/17405629.2020.1736030.

Gawęda, Ł., Pionke, R., Krężołek, M., Prochwicz, K., Kłosowska, J., Frydecka, D., Misiak, B., Kotowicz, K., Samochowiec, A., Mak, M., Błądziński, P., Cechnicki, A., & Nelson, B. (2018). Self-disturbances, cognitive biases and insecure attachment as mechanisms of the relationship between traumatic life events and psychotic-like experiences in non-clinical adults – A path analysis. *Psychiatry Research*, 259, 571–578. https://doi.org/10.1016/j.psychres.2017.11.009.

Giacolini, T., Conversi, D., & Alcaro, A. (2021). The brain emotional systems in addictions: From attachment to dominance/submission systems. *Frontiers in Human Neuroscience*, 14, 609467. https://doi.org/10.3389/fnhum.2020.609467.

Gómez, J. M. (2019). What's in a betrayal?: Trauma, dissociation, and hallucinations among high-functioning ethnic minority emerging adults. *Journal of Aggression, Maltreatment & Trauma*, 28(10), 1181–1198. https://doi.org/10.1080/10926771.2018. 1494653.

Gómez, J. M., & Freyd, J. J. (2017). High betrayal child sexual abuse and hallucinations: A test of an indirect effect of dissociation. *Journal of Child Sexual Abuse*, 26(5), 507–518. https://doi.org/10.1080/10538712.2017.1310776.

Goodwin, R., Kaniasty, K., Sun, S., & Ben-Ezra, M. (2017). Psychological distress and prejudice following terror attacks in France. *Journal of Psychiatric Research*, 91, 111–115. https://doi.org/10.1016/j.jpsychires.2017.03.001.

Gray, S. A. O., Lipschutz, R. S., & Scheeringa, M. S. (2018). Young children's physiological reactivity during memory recall: Associations with posttraumatic stress and parent physiological synchrony. *Journal of Abnormal Child Psychology*, 46(4), 871–880. https://doi.org/10.1007/s10802-017-0326-1.

Greenberg, J., Pyszczynski, T., & Solomon, S. (1986). The causes and consequences of a need for self-esteem: A terror management theory. In R. F. Baumeister (Ed.), *Public self and private self* (pp. 189–212). New York: Springer.

Grossmann, K., & Grossmann, K. E. (2020). Essentials when studying child-father attachment: A fundamental view on safe haven and secure base phenomena. *Attachment & Human Development*, 22(1), 9–14. https://doi.org/10.1080/14616734.2019. 1589056.

Harvell-Bowman, L. A., Critchfield, K. L., Ndzana, F., Stucker, E., Yocca, C., Wilgus, K., Hurst, A., & Sullivan, K. (2022). Of love and death: Death anxiety, attachment, and suicide as experienced by college students. *OMEGA – Journal of Death and Dying*, 302228221100636. Advance online publication. https://doi.org/ 10.1177/00302228221100636.

Helm, P. J., Lifshin, U., Chau, R., & Greenberg, J. (2019). Existential isolation and death thought accessibility. *Journal of Research in Personality*, 82, 103845. https://doi. org/10.1016/j.jrp.2019.103845.

Herstell, S., Betz, L. T., Penzel, N., Chechelnizki, R., Filihagh, L., Antonucci, L., & Kambeitz, J. (2021). Insecure attachment as a transdiagnostic risk factor for major psychiatric conditions: A meta-analysis in bipolar disorder, depression and schizophrenia spectrum disorder. *Journal of Psychiatric Research*, 144, 190–201. https://doi. org/10.1016/j.jpsychires.2021.10.002.

Hocking, E. C., Simons, R. M., & Surette, R. J. (2016). Attachment style as a mediator between childhood maltreatment and the experience of betrayal trauma as an adult. *Child Abuse & Neglect*, 52, 94–101. https://doi.org/10.1016/j.chiabu.2016.01.001.

Hyysalo, N., Gastelle, M., & Flykt, M. (2022). Maternal pre- and postnatal substance use and attachment in young children: A systematic review and meta-analysis. *Development and Psychopathology*, 34(4), 1231–1248. https://doi.org/10.1017/S0954579421000134.

Iwanski, A., Lichtenstein, L., Mühling, L. E., & Zimmermann, P. (2021). Effects of father and mother attachment on depressive symptoms in middle childhood and adolescence: The mediating role of emotion regulation. *Brain Sciences*, 11(9), 1153. https://doi.org/10.3390/brainsci11091153.

Jahangard, L., Tayebi, M., Haghighi, M., Ahmadpanah, M., Holsboer-Trachsler, E., Sadeghi Bahmani, D., & Brand, S. (2019). Does rTMS on brain areas of mirror neurons lead to higher improvements on symptom severity and empathy compared to the rTMS standard procedure?: Results from a double-blind interventional study in individuals with major depressive disorders. *Journal of Affective Disorders*, 257, 527–535. https://doi.org/10.1016/j.jad.2019.07.019.

Janoff-Bulman, R. (1992). *Shattered assumptions: Towards a new psychology of trauma*. New York: Free Press.

Jensen, T. K., Holt, T., & Ormhaug, S. M. (2017). A follow-up study from a multisite, randomized controlled trial for traumatized children receiving TF-CBT. *Journal of Abnormal Child Psychology*, 45(8), 1587–1597. https://doi.org/10.1007/s10802-017-0270-0.

Jeon, H., & Lee, S.-H. (2018). From neurons to social beings: Short review of the mirror neuron system research and its socio-psychological and psychiatric implications. *Clinical Psychopharmacology and Neuroscience*, 16(1), 18–31. https://doi.org/10.9758/cpn.2018.16.1.18.

Kameoka, S., Tanaka, E., Yamamoto, S., Saito, A., Narisawa, T., Arai, Y., Nosaka, S., Ichikawa, K., & Asukai, N. (2020). Effectiveness of trauma-focused cognitive behavioral therapy for Japanese children and adolescents in community settings: A multisite randomized controlled trial. *European Journal of Psychotraumatology*, 11(1), 1767987. https://doi.org/10.1080/20008198.2020.1767987.

Keng, S. L., Noorahman, N. B., Drabu, S., & Chu, C. M. (2019). Association between betrayal trauma and non-suicidal self-injury among adolescent offenders: Shame and emotion dysregulation as mediating factors. *International Journal of Forensic Mental Health*, 18(4), 293–304. https://doi.org/10.1080/14999013.2018.1552633.

Kerstis, B., Åslund, C., & Sonnby, K. (2018). More secure attachment to the father and the mother is associated with fewer depressive symptoms in adolescents. *Upsala Journal of Medical Sciences*, 123(1), 62–67. https://doi.org/10.1080/03009734.2018.1439552.

Khaleque, A. (2017). Perceived parental hostility and aggression, and children's psychological maladjustment, and negative personality dispositions: A meta-analysis. *Journal of Child and Family Studies*, 26(4), 977–988. https://doi.org/10.1007/s10826-016-0637-9.

Khosravani, V., Kamali, Z., Jamaati Ardakani, R., & Samimi Ardestani, M. (2017). The relation of childhood trauma to suicide ideation in patients suffering from obsessive-compulsive disorder with lifetime suicide attempts. *Psychiatry Research*, 255, 139–145. https://doi.org/10.1016/j.psychres.2017.05.032.

Kira, I. A., Shuweikh, H., Al-Huwailiah, A., El-Wakeel, S. A., Waheep, N. N., Ebada, E. E., & Ibrahim, E. R. (2022). The direct and indirect impact of trauma types and cumulative stressors and traumas on executive functions. *Applied neuropsychology: Adult*, 29(5), 1078–1094. https://doi.org/10.1080/23279095.2020.1848835.

Knight, Z. G. (2017). A proposed model of psychodynamic psychotherapy linked to Erick Erikson's eight stages of psychosocial development. *Clinical Psychology & Psychotherapy*, 24(5), 1047–1058. https://doi.org/10.1002/cpp.2066.

Kondo-Ikemura, K., Behrens, K. Y., Umemura, T., & Nakano, S. (2018). Japanese mothers' prebirth Adult Attachment Interview predicts their infants' response to the Strange Situation Procedure: The strange situation in Japan revisited three decades later. *Developmental Psychology*, 54(11), 2007–2015. https://doi.org/10.1037/dev0000577.

Korgaonkar, M. S., Chakouch, C., Breukelaar, I. A., Erlinger, M., Felmingham, K. L., Forbes, D., Williams, L.M., & Bryant, R. A. (2020). Intrinsic connectomes underlying response to trauma-focused psychotherapy in post-traumatic stress disorder. *Translational Psychiatry*, 10(1), 1–11. https://doi.org/10.1038/s41398-020-00938-8.

Kosloff, S., Anderson, G., Nottbohm, A., & Hoshiko, B. (2019). Proximal and distal terror management defenses: A systematic review and analysis. In C. Routledge & M.

Vess (Eds.), *Handbook of terror management theory* (pp. 31–63). London: Elsevier Academic Press. https://doi.org/10.1016/B978-0-12-811844-3.00002-0.

Latif, M., Husain, M. I., Gul, M., Naz, S., Irfan, M., Aslam, M., Awan, F., Sharif, A., Rathod, S., Farooq, S., Ayub, M., & Naeem, F. (2021). Culturally adapted trauma-focused CBT-based guided self-help (CatCBT GSH) for female victims of domestic violence in Pakistan: Feasibility randomized controlled trial. *Behavioural and Cognitive Psychotherapy*, 49(1), 50–61. https://doi.org/10.1017/S1352465820000685.

Lawford, H. L., Astrologo, L., Ramey, H. L., & Linden-Andersen, S. (2020). Identity, intimacy, and generativity in adolescence and young adulthood: A test of the psychosocial model. *Identity*, 20(1), 9–21. https://doi.org/10.1080/15283488.2019.1697271.

Lawson, D. M., & Akay-Sullivan, S. (2020). Considerations of Dissociation, Betrayal Trauma, and Complex Trauma in the Treatment of Incest. *Journal of Child Sexual Abuse*, 29(6), 677–696. https://doi.org/10.1080/10538712.2020.1751369.

Lee, N., Pigott, T. D., Watson, A., Reuben, K., O'Hara, K., Massetti, G., Fang, X., & Self-Brown, S. (2022). Childhood polyvictimization and associated health outcomes: A systematic scoping review. *Trauma, Violence & Abuse*, 15248380211073847. Advance online publication. https://doi.org/10.1177/15248380211073847.

Leman, J., Hunter, W. III, Fergus, T., & Rowatt, W. (2018). Secure attachment to God uniquely linked to psychological health in a national, random sample of American adults. *International Journal for the Psychology of Religion*, 28(3), 162–173. https://doi.org/10.1080/10508619.2018.1477401.

Liahaugen Flensburg, O., Richert, T., & Väfors Fritz, M. (2022). Parents of adult children with drug addiction dealing with shame and courtesy stigma. *Drugs: Education, Prevention and Policy*, 1–10. https://doi.org/10.1080/09687637.2022.2099249.

Liese, B. S., Kim, H. S., & Hodgins, D. C. (2020). Insecure attachment and addiction: Testing the mediating role of emotion dysregulation in four potentially addictive behaviours. *Addictive Behaviors*, 107, 106432. https://doi.org/10.1016/j.addbeh.2020.106432.

Lifshin, U., Horner, D. E., Helm, P. J., Solomon, S., & Greenberg, J. (2021). Self-esteem and immortality: Evidence regarding the terror management hypothesis that high self-esteem is associated with a stronger sense of symbolic immortality. *Personality and Individual Differences*, 175, 110712. https://doi.org/10.1016/j.paid.2021.110712.

Lowell, A. F., Peacock-Chambers, E., Zayde, A., DeCoste, C. L., McMahon, T. J., & Suchman, N. E. (2021). Mothering from the inside out: Addressing the intersection of addiction, adversity, and attachment with evidence-based parenting intervention. *Current Addiction Reports*, 8(4), 605–615. https://doi.org/10.1007/s40429-021-00389-1.

Márquez, Y. I., Deblinger, E., & Dovi, A. T. (2020). The value of trauma-focused cognitive behavioral therapy (TF-CBT) in addressing the therapeutic needs of trafficked youth: A case study. *Cognitive and Behavioral Practice*, 27(3), 253–269. https://doi.org/10.1016/j.cbpra.2019.10.001.

Marshall, C., Langevin, R., & Cabecinha-Alati, S. (2022). Victim-to-victim intergenerational cycles of child maltreatment: A systematic scoping review of theoretical frameworks. *International Journal of Child And Adolescent Resilience*, 9(1). https://doi.org/10.54488/ijcar.2022.283.

Mavranezouli, I., Megnin-Viggars, O., Daly, C., Dias, S., Welton, N. J., Stockton, S., Bhutan, G., Grey, N., Leach, J., Greenberg, N., Katona, C., El-Leithy, S., & Pilling, S. (2020). Psychological treatments for post-traumatic stress disorder in adults: A network meta-analysis. *Psychological Medicine*, 50(4), 542–555. https://doi.org/10.1017/S0033291720000070.

Mazor, Y., Gelkopf, M., & Roe, D. (2020). Posttraumatic growth in psychosis: Challenges to the assumptive world. *Psychological Trauma: Theory, Research, Practice, and Policy*, 12(1), 3–10. https://doi.org/10.1037/tra0000443.

McGuire, A., Steele, R. G., & Singh, M. N. (2021). Systematic review on the application of trauma-focused cognitive behavioral therapy (TF-CBT) for preschool-aged children. *Clinical Child and Family Psychology Review*, 24(1), 20–37. https://doi.org/10.1007/s10567-020-00334-0.

Miedema, S. S., Le, V. D., Chiang, L., Ngann, T., & Wu Shortt, J. (2022). Adverse childhood experiences and intimate partner violence among youth in Cambodia: A latent class analysis. *Journal of Interpersonal Violence*, 38(1–2), 1446–1472. https://doi.org/10.1177/08862605221090573.

Mikulincer, M., Lifshin, U., & Shaver, P. R. (2020). Towards an anxiety-buffer disruption approach to depression: Attachment anxiety and worldview threat heighten death-thought accessibility and depression-related feelings. *Journal of Social and Clinical Psychology*, 39(4), 238–273. https://doi.org/10.1521/jscp.2020.39.4.238.

Miller, A. B., Williams, C., Day, C., & Esposito-Smythers, C. (2017). Effects of cognitive distortions on the link between dating violence exposure and substance problems in clinically hospitalized youth. *Journal of Clinical Psychology*, 73(6), 733–744. https://doi.org/10.1002/jclp.22373.

Murray, C. V., Jacobs, J. I., Rock, A. J., & Clark, G. I. (2021). Attachment style, thought suppression, self-compassion and depression: Testing a serial mediation model. *PloS one*, 16(1), e0245056. https://doi.org/10.1371/journal.pone.0245056.

Opie, J. E., McIntosh, J. E., Esler, T. B., Duschinsky, R., George, C., Schore, A., Kothe, E. J., Tan, E. S., Greenwood, C. J., & Olsson, C. A. (2021). Early childhood attachment stability and change: A meta-analysis. *Attachment & Human Development*, 23(6), 897–930. https://doi.org/10.1080/14616734.2020.1800769.

Paetzold, R. L., & Rholes, W. S. (2021). The link from child abuse to dissociation: The roles of adult disorganized attachment, self-concept clarity, and reflective functioning. *Journal of Trauma & Dissociation*, 22(5), 615–635. https://doi.org/10.1080/15299732.2020.1869654.

Peng, W., Liu, Z., Liu, Q., Chu, J., Zheng, K., Wang, J., Wei, H., Zhong, M., Ling, Y., & Yi, J. (2021). Insecure attachment and maladaptive emotion regulation mediating the relationship between childhood trauma and borderline personality features. *Depression and Anxiety*, 38(1), 28–39. https://doi.org/10.1002/da.23082.

Peters, W., Rice, S., Cohen, J., Murray, L., Schley, C., Alvarez-Jimenez, M., & Bendall, S. (2021). Trauma-focused cognitive-behavioral therapy (TF-CBT) for interpersonal trauma in transitional-aged youth. *Psychological Trauma: Theory, Research, Practice and Policy*, 13(3), 313–321. https://doi.org/10.1037/tra0001016.

Petrowski, K., Wintermann, G. B., Hübner, T., Smolka, M. N., & Donix, M. (2019). Neural responses to faces of attachment figures and unfamiliar faces: Associations with organized and disorganized attachment representations. *The Journal of Nervous and Mental Disease*, 207(2), 112–120. https://doi.org/10.1097/NMD.0000000000000931.

Platt, M. G., & Freyd, J. J. (2015). Betray my trust, shame on me: Shame, dissociation, fear, and betrayal trauma. *Psychological Trauma: Theory, Research, Practice and Policy*, 7(4), 398–404. https://doi.org/10.1037/tra0000022.

Popkirov, S., Flasbeck, V., Schlegel, U., Juckel, G., & Brüne, M. (2019). Childhood trauma and dissociative symptoms predict frontal EEG asymmetry in borderline personality disorder. *Journal of Trauma & Dissociation*, 20(1), 32–47. https://doi.org/10.1080/15299732.2018.1451808.

Prince, E. B., Ciptadi, A., Tao, Y., Rozga, A., Martin, K. B., Rehg, J., & Messinger, D. S. (2021). Continuous measurement of attachment behavior: A multimodal view of the strange situation procedure. *Infant Behavior & Development*, 63, 101565. https://doi.org/10.1016/j.infbeh.2021.101565.

Puhlmann, L. M., Derome, M., Morosan, L., Kilicel, D., Vrtička, P., & Debbané, M. (2021). Longitudinal associations between self-reported attachment dimensions and neurostructural development from adolescence to early adulthood. *Attachment & Human Development*, 25(1), 162–180. https://doi.org/10.1080/14616734.2021.1993628.

Pyszczynski, T., Lockett, M., Greenberg, J., & Solomon, S. (2021). Terror management theory and the COVID-19 pandemic. *Journal of Humanistic Psychology*, 61(2), 173–189. https://doi.org/10.1177/0022167820959488.

Racine, N., Zhu, J., Hartwick, C., & Madigan, S. (2022). Differences in demographic, risk, and protective factors in a clinical sample of children who experienced sexual abuse only vs. poly-victimization. *Frontiers in Psychiatry*, 12, 2425. https://doi.org/10.3389/fpsyt.2021.789329.

Riem, M. M. E., van Hoof, M. J., Garrett, A. S., Rombouts, S. A. R. B., van der Wee, N. J. A., van IJzendoorn, M. H., & Vermeiren, R. R. J. M. (2019). General psychopathology factor and unresolved-disorganized attachment uniquely correlated to white matter integrity using diffusion tensor imaging. *Behavioural Brain Research*, 359, 1–8. https://doi.org/10.1016/j.bbr.2018.10.014.

Rizeq, J., & McCann, D. (2021). The cognitive, emotional, and behavioral sequelae of trauma exposure: An integrative approach to examining trauma's effect. *Psychological trauma: theory, research, practice and policy*, 15(2), 313–321. https://doi.org/10.1037/tra0001152.

Ross, S. L., Sharma-Patel, K., Brown, E. J., Huntt, J. S., & Chaplin, W. F. (2021). Complex trauma and Trauma-Focused Cognitive-Behavioral Therapy: How do trauma chronicity and PTSD presentation affect treatment outcome? *Child Abuse & Neglect*, 111, 104734. https://doi.org/10.1016/j.chiabu.2020.104734.

Sanchez, A. L., Comer, J. S., & LaRoche, M. (2022). Enhancing the responsiveness of family-based CBT through culturally informed case conceptualization and treatment planning. *Cognitive and Behavioral Practice*, 29(4), 750–770. https://doi.org/10.1016/j.cbpra.2021.04.003.

Sandberg, D. A., & Refrea, V. (2022). Adult attachment as a mediator of the link between interpersonal trauma and international classification of diseases (ICD)-11 complex posttraumatic stress disorder symptoms among college men and women. *Journal of Interpersonal Violence*, 37(23–24), NP22528–NP22548. https://doi.org/10.1177/08862605211072168.

Santarnecchi, E., Bossini, L., Vatti, G., Fagiolini, A., La Porta, P., Di Lorenzo, G., Siracusano, A., Rossi, S., & Rossi, A. (2019). Psychological and brain connectivity changes following trauma-focused CBT and EMDR treatment in single-episode PTSD patients. *Frontiers in psychology*, 10, 129. https://doi.org/10.3389/fpsyg.2019.00129.

Schleider, J. L., Woerner, J., Overstreet, C., Amstadter, A. B., & Sartor, C. E. (2021). Interpersonal trauma exposure and depression in young adults: Considering the role of world assumptions. *Journal of Interpersonal Violence*, 36(13–14), 6596–6620. https://doi.org/10.1177/0886260518819879.

Shakiba, N., & Raby, K. L. (2021). Attachment dimensions and cortisol responses during the strange situation among young children adopted internationally. *Attachment & Human Development*, 25(1), 89–103. https://doi.org/10.1080/14616734.2021.1896445.

Shen, F., Soloski, K., & Liu, Y. (2021). Adolescent parental attachment and intimate relationship in adulthood: An investigation of contextual factors and long-term outcomes of child sexual abuse. *Children and Youth Services Review*, 122, 105869. https://doi.org/10.1016/j.childyouth.2020.105869.

Smith, A. J., Holohan, D. R., & Jones, R. T. (2019). Emotion regulation difficulties and social cognitions predicting PTSD severity and quality of life among treatment seeking combat veterans. *Military Behavioral Health*, 7(1), 73–82. https://doi.org/10.1080/21635781.2018.1540314.

Sood, M., Carnelley, K. B., & Newman-Taylor, K. (2022). How does insecure attachment lead to paranoia?: A systematic critical review of cognitive, affective, and behavioural mechanisms. *The British Journal of Clinical Psychology*, 61(3), 781–815. https://doi.org/10.1111/bjc.12361.

Spinazzola, J., van der Kolk, B., & Ford, J. D. (2018). When nowhere is safe: Interpersonal trauma and attachment adversity as antecedents of posttraumatic stress disorder and developmental trauma disorder. *Journal of Traumatic Stress*, 31(5), 631–642. https://doi.org/10.1002/jts.22320.

Spinazzola, J., van der Kolk, B., & Ford, J. D. (2021). Developmental trauma disorder: A legacy of attachment trauma in victimized children. *Journal of Traumatic Stress*, 34(4), 711–720. https://doi.org/10.1002/jts.22697.

Spruit, A., Goos, L., Weenink, N., Rodenburg, R., Niemeyer, H., Stams, G. J., & Colonnesi, C. (2020). The relation between attachment and depression in children and adolescents: A multilevel meta-analysis. *Clinical Child and Family Psychology Review*, 23(1), 54–69. https://doi.org/10.1007/s10567-019-00299-9.

St. Vil, N. M., Carter, T., & Johnson, S. (2021). Betrayal trauma and barriers to forming new intimate relationships among survivors of intimate partner violence. *Journal of interpersonal violence*, 36(7–8), NP3495–NP3509. https://doi.org/10.1177/0886260518779596.

Stein, M. D., Conti, M. T., Kenney, S., Anderson, B. J., Flori, J. N., Risi, M. M., & Bailey, G. L. (2017). Adverse childhood experience effects on opioid use initiation, injection drug use, and overdose among persons with opioid use disorder. *Drug and Alcohol Dependence*, 179, 325–329. https://doi.org/10.1016/j.drugalcdep.2017.07.007.

Stenson, A. F., van Rooij, S. J. H., Carter, S. E., Powers, A., & Jovanovic, T. (2021). A legacy of fear: Physiological evidence for intergenerational effects of trauma exposure on fear and safety signal learning among African Americans. *Behavioural Brain Research*, 402, 113017. https://doi.org/10.1016/j.bbr.2020.113017.

Stern, J. A., Fraley, R. C., Jones, J. D., Gross, J. T., Shaver, P. R., & Cassidy, J. (2018). Developmental processes across the first two years of parenthood: Stability and change in adult attachment style. *Developmental Psychology*, 54(5), 975–988. https://doi.org/10.1037/dev0000481.

Sterzing, P. R., Ratliff, G. A., Gartner, R. E., McGeough, B. L., & Johnson, K. C. (2017). Social ecological correlates of polyvictimization among a national sample of transgender, genderqueer, and cisgender sexual minority adolescents. *Child Abuse & Neglect*, 67, 1–12. https://doi.org/10.1016/j.chiabu.2017.02.017.

Stewart, R. W., Orengo-Aguayo, R., Wallace, M., Metzger, I. W., & Rheingold, A. A. (2021). Leveraging technology and cultural adaptations to increase access and engagement among trauma-exposed African American youth: Exploratory study of school-based telehealth delivery of trauma-focused cognitive behavioral therapy. *Journal of Interpersonal Violence*, 36(15–16), 7090–7109. https://doi.org/10.1177/0886260519831380.

Strathearn, L., Mertens, C. E., Mayes, L., Rutherford, H., Rajhans, P., Xu, G., Potenza, M. N., & Kim, S. (2019). Pathways relating the neurobiology of attachment to drug addiction. *Frontiers in Psychiatry*, 10, 737. https://doi.org/10.3389/fpsyt.2019.00737.

Tabachnick, A. R., He, Y., Zajac, L., Carlson, E. A., & Dozier, M. (2022). Secure attachment in infancy predicts context-dependent emotion expression in middle childhood. *Emotion*, 22(2), 258–269. https://doi.org/10.1037/emo0000985.

Tammilehto, J., Bosmans, G., Kuppens, P., Flykt, M., Peltonen, K., Kerns, K. A., & Lindblom, J. (2022). Dynamics of attachment and emotion regulation in daily life: uni- and bidirectional associations. *Cognition & Emotion*, 36(6), 1109–1131. https://doi.org/10.1080/02699931.2022.2081534.

Thompson, M. P., Kingree, J. B., & Lamis, D. (2019). Associations of adverse childhood experiences and suicidal behaviors in adulthood in a U.S. nationally representative sample. *Child: Care, Health and Development*, 45(1), 121–128. https://doi.org/10.1111/cch.12617.

Thompson-Hollands, J., Jun, J. J., & Sloan, D. M. (2017). The association between peritraumatic dissociation and PTSD symptoms: The mediating role of negative beliefs about the self. *Journal of Traumatic Stress*, 30(2), 190–194. https://doi.org/10.1002/jts.22179.

Toumbelekis, M., Liddell, B. J., & Bryant, R. A. (2021). Secure attachment priming protects against relapse of fear in young adults. *Translational psychiatry*, 11, 584. https://doi.org/10.1038/s41398-021-01715-x.

Vail, K. E. III, Reed, D. E. II, Goncy, E. A., Cornelius, T., & Edmondson, D. (2020). Anxiety buffer disruption: Self-evaluation, death anxiety, and stressor appraisals among low and high posttraumatic stress symptom samples. *Journal of Social and Clinical Psychology*, 39(5), 353–382. https://doi.org/10.1521/jscp.2020.39.5.353.

van Der Kolk, B., Ford, J. D., & Spinazzola, J. (2019). Comorbidity of developmental trauma disorder (DTD) and post-traumatic stress disorder: Findings from the DTD field trial. *European Journal of Psychotraumatology*, 10(1), 1562841. https://doi.org/10.1080/20008198.2018.1562841.

van Hoof, M. J., Riem, M., Garrett, A., Pannekoek, N., van der Wee, N., van IJzendoorn, M., & Vermeiren, R. (2019). Unresolved-disorganized attachment is associated with smaller hippocampus and increased functional connectivity beyond psychopathology. *Journal of Traumatic Stress*, 32(5), 742–752. https://doi.org/10.1002/jts.22432.

Vowels, L. M., Carnelley, K. B., & Stanton, S. C. E. (2022). Attachment anxiety predicts worse mental health outcomes during COVID-19: Evidence from two studies. *Personality and Individual Differences*, 185, 111256. https://doi.org/10.1016/j.paid.2021.111256.

Waters, T. E., Ruiz, S. K., & Roisman, G. I. (2017). Origins of secure base script knowledge and the developmental construction of attachment representations. *Child Development*, 88(1), 198–209. https://doi.org/10.1111/cdev.12571.

Wills, C., Cuevas, C. A., & Sabina, C. (2022). The role of the victim-offender relationship on psychological distress among Latinx women: A betrayal trauma perspective. *Psychological Trauma: Theory, Research, Practice, and Policy*, 14(1), 20–28. https://doi.org/10.1037/tra0000923.

Yalch, M. M., & Levendosky, A. A. (2018). Influence of betrayal trauma on death anxiety. *The Humanistic Psychologist*, 46(4), 390–398. https://doi.org/10.1037/hum 0000115.

Yalch, M. M., & Levendosky, A. A. (2019). Influence of betrayal trauma on borderline personality disorder traits. *Journal of Trauma & Dissociation*, 20(4), 392–401. https://doi. org/10.1080/15299732.2019.1572042.

Yetzer, A. M., & Pyszczynski, T. (2019). Terror management theory and psychological disorder: Ineffective anxiety-buffer functioning as a transdiagnostic vulnerability factor for psychopathology. In C. Routledge & M. Vess (Eds.), *Handbook of terror management theory* (pp. 417–447). London: Elsevier Academic Press. https://doi.org/10.1016/B978-0-12-811844-3.00018-4.

Zatti, C., Rosa, V., Barros, A., Valdivia, L., Calegaro, V. C., Freitas, L. H., Cereser, K. M. M., Rocha, N. S. D., Bastos, A. G., & Schuch, F. B. (2017). Childhood trauma and suicide attempt: A meta-analysis of longitudinal studies from the last decade. *Psychiatry Research*, 256, 353–358. https://doi.org/10.1016/j.psychres.2017.06.082.

Zerubavel, N., Messman-Moore, T. L., DiLillo, D., & Gratz, K. L. (2018). Childhood sexual abuse and fear of abandonment moderate the relation of intimate partner violence to severity of dissociation. *Journal of Trauma & Dissociation*, 19(1), 9–24. https://doi.org/10.1080/15299732.2017.1289491.

Zhang, X., Li, J., Xie, F., Chen, X., Xu, W., & Hudson, N. W. (2022). The relationship between adult attachment and mental health: A meta-analysis. *Journal of Personality and Social Psychology*, 123(5), 1089–1137. https://doi.org/10.1037/pspp0000437.

Zhou, X., Zhen, R., & Wu, X. (2021). Insecure attachment to parents and PTSD among adolescents: The roles of parent-child communication, perceived parental depression, and intrusive rumination. *Development and Psychopathology*, 33(4), 1290–1299. https://doi.org/10.1017/S0954579420000498.

Zyromski, B., Dollarhide, C. T., Aras, Y., Geiger, S., Oehrtman, J. P., & Clarke, H. (2018). Beyond complex trauma: An existential view of adverse childhood experiences. *The Journal of Humanistic Counseling*, 57, 156–172. https://doi.org/10.1002/johc.12080.

4
DEVELOPMENTAL TRAUMA AND BRONFENBRENNER'S SOCIOECOLOGICAL MODEL

Trauma as a Response to Systemic Problems

Most of the research on DTD has come from the individual level (i.e., client/ patient) and, as such, has not adequately addressed the broad range of theoretical (systemic) perspectives needed to fully understand the issues at play in this disorder. More recently, scholars have asserted that with DTD patients the emphasis on an individual illness perspective may have contributed to victim shaming and blaming (Hansford & Jobson, 2022; Heberle et al., 2020; Selwyn et al., 2021). Instead, research should be highlighting the institutions and social systems, including policies and procedures (or lack thereof), that worsen DTD symptoms or have the potential to mitigate adverse outcomes with a high impact on individuals, families, and communities.

Scholars have increasingly advanced a social and systemic view of medical and psychological disorders that underscores large-scale mitigation of early stress and trauma (e.g., by supporting children and families, addressing food and housing insecurity, etc.), particularly within high-risk populations. Scholars in the social sciences have also advanced conceptual frameworks of trauma and developmental trauma to include diverse theoretical and empirical approaches that underscore the intersection of health, culture, and diversity. As part of this work, scholars have discussed culture-specific constructs, such as collective trauma, intergenerational violence, and cultural betrayal (Bower et al., 2021; Gómez, 2021; Moleiro, 2018; Ranjbar et al., 2020).

The increased focus on social and cultural influences on trauma and recovery from trauma has given rise to cultural constructs such as collective (cultural) trauma (Hirschberger, 2018). Collective trauma refers to events that pervasively affect individuals from disenfranchised communities and often cause

DOI: 10.4324/9781003304715-4

psychological disturbances, such as substance abuse, mood disturbances, low self-esteem, reactive aggression, and violence (Gómez, 2019; Metzger et al., 2021; Stephens et al., 2021). Experiences of racism and discrimination, violence against women, political torture and captivity, and genocide are examples of collective traumas (scholars use terms like historical, political, and intergenerational trauma, race-based PTSD, and acculturation and migration trauma to describe experiences of trauma in diverse populations; Jore et al., 2020; Matthies-Boon, 2017; Pumariega et al., 2022). Scholars have also highlighted the experiences of racial and ethnic minorities living in impoverished inner-city communities (e.g., alcohol abuse, drug addiction, homelessness, underperforming school systems, community violence, etc.; Garcia et al., 2019; Kirkinis et al., 2021; Liang et al., 2020; Matheson et al., 2019; Skewes & Blume, 2019).

Introduction to Bronfenbrenner's Model

Urie Bronfenbrenner developed a systemic, ecological framework of human development that expanded mainstream ideas about early development (Eriksson et al., 2018; Halsall et al., 2018; Hapunda et al., 2017; Probst et al., 2018; Xia et al., 2020). The ecological systems approach considers multiple levels of analysis reflecting factors that have immediate and direct effects on children (i. e., microsystems) and broader social and political, historical, and economic contexts. Bronfenbrenner used terms such as *mesosystems, exosystems*, and *chronosystems* to underscore the degree to which early development is influenced by broad social contexts that extend beyond an individual's biological constitution, attachment, psychological symptoms, and interpersonal relationships.

According to the social-ecological framework, mental health (and illness) is influenced by individual risks and resources as well as broader social, economic, and political circumstances, including, but not limited to, the economy, mainstream policies and laws, and family/social and community stressors and supports (Cramer & Kapusta, 2017; Reupert, 2017). Research suggests, for example, that adverse (or unstable) economic conditions contribute to financial stress/insecurity, unemployment and low quality of life, and high rates of alcohol abuse, depression/anxiety, and interpersonal violence (Cunradi et al., 2021; Doran & Kinchin, 2017; Nesoff et al., 2021).

Informed by Bronfenbrenner's model, scholars now recognize that psychological disturbances arise from multi-level influences and that their mitigation will require systemic change, advocacy, and social justice efforts (Finan & Yap, 2021; Lewis et al., 2021; Ungar & Theron, 2020). Evaluation and treatment of children and families affected by developmental trauma require addressing diverse external factors that may perpetuate or exacerbate maladaptive coping and impairments in functioning (Diab et al., 2018; Obasaju & LiVecchi, 2018; Salter & Hall, 2022; Zhu et al., 2020). A critical aspect of the socio-ecological framework that distinguishes it from other mainstream views of mental illness is that psychological disturbances arise not from the individual per se (e.g., traumatic events, psychiatric symptoms, and disorders) but rather from disturbances in the social systems that influence them (for example, normalizing sexual violence against girls, toxic masculinity, heteronormativity; Brown et al., 2020; Bryant-Davis, 2019; El-Khodary et al., 2020; El-Khodary & Samara, 2020; Ingram et al., 2019; Moleiro, 2018).

Comic Book Realism

For many years now, scholars have used the graphic novel medium to analyze social, psychological, and political issues affecting individuals and families. Indeed, comic book realism theory suggests that graphic novels provide meaningful representations of many factors that affect individuals and families in real life, including culture and identity, gender norms, intergroup relationships, race, and sexual orientations (Bosqui et al., 2020; Brodie & Ingram, 2021; Lev-Wiesel & First, 2018; McGunnigle, 2018; O'Roark & Grant, 2018; Schulte & Frederick, 2020). I invite you to explore comic book realism in more detail through consideration of a common type of character within comic books – mutants – and how their experiences tend to parallel many of the experiences of individuals who have gone through developmental traumas.

Comic Book Realism: The X-Men

The X-Men (a superhero film series based on the Marvel Comics superhero team of the same name) are a group of mutant superheroes and protagonists with unique abilities. Professor Charles Xavier and Magneto are two of the most powerful (Omega level) mutants, and their powers include telepathy and the ability to control the earth's magnetic field. Professor Charles Xavier advocates for peace and social justice and believes that humans and mutants can live and work together peacefully. In fact, he created a school for gifted youth (i.e., mutants) dedicated to supporting humanity and working with government leaders to establish policies that would allow mutants and humans to live in harmony (for example, working to abolish anti-mutant sentiments requiring mutants to register with the government for surveillance).

Magneto was a child victim of the Holocaust, forcibly separated from his parents, who died by execution. Magneto escaped the Holocaust; however, the traumatic loss of his family caused him to view all people as culpable for his (and his family's) pain and suffering. He vowed to protect mutants from being revictimized by humans. Magneto used his magnetic powers to manipulate ferrous metals and objects with magnetic properties into weapons of mass destruction and would use deadly force to defend mutant kind.

One of Professor Xavier's most notable students is Jean Grey, a powerful and highly empathic being with telepathic and telekinetic abilities. Jean's abilities first became evident when she experienced trauma after losing her best friend, who died in a car accident. Her powers were amplified, however, when she was possessed by a cosmic force known as the Phoenix Force. This force amplified her powers but also caused her to re-experience trauma, dissociate from reality, and develop multiple personalities, including the dark phoenix, an evil entity consumed by a desire to destroy the world.

Ororo Munroe, also known as Storm, possesses the ability to control the weather. Like Magneto and Jean, Ororo also had a history of ACEs and early repeated trauma, including poverty, residing in orphanages, and homelessness. At age five, a plane crash destroyed her home, and her parents were killed, but she survived and was later discovered buried under rubble near her parents' lifeless bodies. Ororo's experiences of trauma gave rise to behavioral problems, such as stealing and joining street gangs, and she later developed severe claustrophobia that affected her as an adolescent and adult.

These characteristics highlight conditions known to affect individuals with trauma and DTD, such as social alienation and rejection sensitivity, intergroup conflict, discrimination, internalized prejudice, unethical medical experimentation, unplanned or unwanted pregnancies, social hierarchies, ideas of normal and abnormal, and genocide and violence (Deman, 2020; Doran, 2020; Fradkin et al., 2016; Smith, 2017).

Conceptualization of Trauma from an Ecological Systems Framework

Scholars have expanded the traumatic stress framework to incorporate a socioecological perspective that underscores family, community, and cultural systems perspectives (Chavez- Dueñas et al., 2019; Collings et al., 2022; Kartal et al., 2018; Monteith et al., 2019; Newton, 2019). Responses to trauma can vary (sometimes dramatically) because of social and political circumstances (Cummings et al., 2017; O'Neill et al., 2016; Sangalang & Vang, 2017; Yatham et al., 2018) and cultural influences, such as cultural conceptualizations of trauma (for example, whether it may be more acceptable to disclose trauma by reporting physical health symptoms instead of acknowledging psychological problems). Responses to trauma also depend on an individual's or group's unique physical characteristics, including skin color, racial background, gender, and sexual orientation as well as family, ethnocultural, and community membership, including majority or minority group status, religious beliefs and practices, socioeconomic resources, and political affiliations (Carter et al., 2017; Cave et al., 2020; Guerra et al., 2021; Livingston et al., 2019; Loyd et al., 2019; Quinn, 2022; Strompolis et al., 2019; Wamser-Nanney & Cherry, 2018).

The ecological systems framework, conceptualized by Bronfenbrenner and contemporary scholars, suggests that the social and systemic impacts affecting children and families are best understood when considered by four differentiated and highly influential systems (Adu & Oudshoorn, 2020; Atilola, 2017; Diab et al., 2018; Minh et al., 2017; Vélez-Agosto et al., 2017; Walker et al., 2019).

The first analysis level is *microsystems*, which underscores children's closest interpersonal relationships. Relationships at this level are limited to those where the child is directly interacting with the other individual(s) (e.g., caregivers, peers, siblings, teachers). *Mesosystems* refer to interactions between individuals from the microsystems level and include interpersonal exchanges between siblings, parents, teachers, and healthcare providers, for example. According to the ecological framework, when children's teachers and caregivers have established positive and supportive relationships, for example, this will presumably also positively influence children's relationships with caregivers and teachers (Johns et al., 2018; Moore et al., 2018; Moses & Villodas, 2017; Quin et al., 2018; Timshel et al., 2017). Negative relationships or adversarial exchanges between individuals within microsystems, however, are likely to result in negative parenting and/or teaching practices that increase the risk of negative experiences and outcomes for the child.

Exosystems refer to relationships between social systems that influence children and their families. These systems include a caregiver's workplace, neighborhood, or community as well as laws and statutes, mass media, and the economy. For example, caregivers who spend considerable time at work because of high work demands or who experience workplace bullying will have less time to spend with one another and their children, or they will displace their frustration from work at home with their loved ones (Greene et al., 2020; Griffith, 2022; Hong et al., 2018; Lee et al., 2022; Mikolajczak et al., 2018). When they do so, they may displace their frustrations on their children or other loved ones.

Media messages on gender, race, physical attractiveness, lifestyle, and popular culture are examples of exosystems that influence individuals who have experienced developmental trauma. Negative media messages, including frequent coverage of violence, rape, and trauma, can cause individuals to experience (and re-experience) depression, isolation, and trauma (Holman et al., 2020; Hopwood & Schutte, 2017; Pfefferbaum et al., 2021; Thompson et al., 2019). In addition, mass media can cause individuals from minority communities to develop psychological problems from viewing their communities being attacked. Hate crimes against racial, sexual, and religious minorities, for example, are on the rise and continue to affect the communities that experience them (Cramer et al., 2018; Tessler et al., 2020; Xu et al., 2021; Zhang et al., 2022).

Macrosystems refer to social and cultural norms, values, beliefs, and attitudes, including cultural identity and heritage, and social and economic resources. For example, within collectivist (non-Western) cultures, problems are often resolved within the family (Katzenstein & Fontes, 2017; Reyes et al., 2020; Sawrikar & Katz, 2017). Individuals from these groups may tend to distrust healthcare providers, and prayer and religious coping (e.g., attending church services, confessing sins, special baths, and cleaning rituals) may be more appropriate approaches to recovery (Calloway & Creed, 2022; Fripp & Carlson, 2017; Klest et al., 2019; Mosher et al., 2017; Range et al., 2018; Smith et al., 2019). The macrosystem highlights the diverse range of within-group differences, such as those linked to racial, ethnic, sexual, and religious identities, as well as the broader impacts of historical stressors, protective factors, and coping resources.

Chronosystems, the final level of analysis in Bronfenbrenner's ecological systems framework, include social and historical events, such as life transitions, natural disasters, caregiver separation/divorce, unemployment, and incarceration. These events adversely affect children and families and may contribute to placement in foster care, homelessness, and social instability, which may also give rise to violence, including violence against oneself (e.g., cutting, suicide attempts, drug use) and/or others. An example of a chronosystem circumstance is homelessness (Brothers et al., 2020; Crosby et al., 2018; Monteith et al., 2019; Sample & Ferguson, 2020; Santa Maria et al., 2018). As many as 2.5 million youths per year experience homelessness. Along with losing their homes, community, friends, routines, and sense of stability and safety, many homeless youths are also victims of violence or other traumatic events. While coming from various backgrounds, research suggests that most of these youth have experienced early and multiple traumas (Dawson-Rose et al., 2020; DiGuiseppi et al., 2020; Petering et al., 2017; Tyler & Schmitz, 2018). Their responses to these events have been shaped – at least in part – by age, gender, ethnicity, and/or sexual orientation. Their history of trauma, in turn, often causes significant mental health problems, including depression, anxiety disorders, PTSD, suicidal ideation, attachment issues, and substance abuse disorders. Once they arrive on the street, many youths are re-traumatized.

Trauma, Culture, and Diversity

In some cultures, it is considered inappropriate for a person to talk about their feelings openly, acknowledge weakness to others, or pay attention to their traumatic experiences, which would imply a psychiatric disorder that possibly goes against cultural norms (Chang et al., 2017; Herron et al., 2020; Schunk et al., 2022). Doing so may result in experiencing additional traumas, cultural shame, and stigma (Wojcik et al., 2019). Responses to trauma are mediated by social, political, and cultural influences, such as cultural conceptualizations of masculinity and femininity, acceptable norms of behavior and trauma, or whether it may be more appropriate to appear invulnerable and, thus, inflict suffering on others. Researchers have increasingly acknowledged the universality of trauma, including its broad impact on individuals and across diverse communities and populations, as well as the diverse range of adaptations and behavioral expressions resulting from differing cultural beliefs, attitudes, and acceptable norms of behavior (including possible departures from what may be considered abnormal or indicative of illness).

Trauma and Gender

From a social and cultural perspective, men are socialized to embody masculinity (Affleck et al., 2018; Neilson et al., 2020; Brown et al., 2020; Elder et al., 2017), which may include normalizing interpersonal aggression and violence and minimizing the expression of emotional vulnerability or any other signs of perceived weakness. Scholars have asserted that toxic masculinity, for example, maintains men's perceived dominance over women by subordinating and discouraging characteristics associated with weakness. Consequently, boys and men who experience sexual abuse, physical assaults, and neglect (e.g., food insecurity, masked depression, and fear) may avoid disclosing these experiences to authority figures because of shame and embarrassment (Easton & Kong, 2017; Hlavka, 2017; MacGinley et al., 2019; Parent et al., 2019; Sivagurunathan et al., 2019). They may also be concerned that others will view them negatively, including being weak and incapable of defending themselves and others. This may lead to re-victimization by other men who adhere to more traditional (and biased) views of gender. For some men of color, this may explain their high rates of substance abuse, anger and aggression, and legal troubles. As a result, racial and ethnic minorities, particularly those living in urban communities, often do not recognize or effectively treat DTD symptoms, which likely intersect with high poverty rates, substance abuse, and crime.

Trauma and Social Discrimination

Research suggests that minority groups, especially children living in impoverished communities as well as racial and sexual minorities, are disproportionately exposed to abuse, neglect, trauma, and violence. They are also at increased risk for repeated trauma and re-victimization. Developmental trauma and the marginalization of disenfranchised communities continue to be oppressive societal issues that negatively affect individuals' and groups' health and well-being. For decades, social discrimination – defined as perceived discriminatory behaviors and practices against subjugated groups (e.g., racial and sexual minorities, individuals with disabilities, religious groups) – has attracted substantial interest among researchers, healthcare providers, and policymakers because it is a significant cause of cumulative stress and illness and a prominent social determinant of health and well-being. Research has shown that racial and sexual minorities, who are subject to higher rates of social discrimination, are at greater risk than other groups for stress-related illness, substance abuse, depression, and suicide (Cyrus, 2017; Ghabrial, 2017; Goodwill et al., 2021; Madubata et al., 2022; Oh et al., 2019; Ramirez & Paz Galupo, 2019).

Experiences of discrimination and microaggressions, such as ignoring or undermining bias and hostility against minority groups and undermining their strengths and resilience by focusing exclusively on negative stereotypes, have measurable adverse effects on communities of color. For example, negative biases, racial microaggressions, and hate crimes against Asian Americans, including assaults and vandalism in response to the COVID-19 pandemic, have led many Asian communities to experience anxiety, anger, and psychological distress (Tessler et al., 2020; Xu et al., 2021; Zhang et al., 2022).

Numerous studies demonstrate that lesbian, gay, bisexual, transgender, queer, intersex, asexual, and others (LGBTQIA+) children and adolescents are likely to experience abuse by peers, caregivers, and individuals within their communities (Berger et al., 2019; Pollitt et al., 2018; Taliaferro & Muehlenkamp, 2017). Research on the experiences of LGBTQIA+ children and youth living in various countries around the globe suggests that, in addition to lacking adequate social and legal protections for sexual and gender minorities, abuse by caregivers, peers, and school personnel is common (Lamontagne et al., 2018; Müller et al., 2021; Smith, 2018). However, such abuse may be dismissed because of fear of cultural shame and stigma. Oppression and cultural norms that perpetuate stigma and discrimination limit the availability of social support among sexual minorities and, in turn, contribute to adverse mental and sexual health outcomes (Alessi et al., 2017; Ching et al., 2018; Ciocca et al., 2017; Jauregui et al., 2021; Sugarman et al., 2018). These children often report feeling that they have nowhere to turn to cope with psychological distress, which places them at cumulative risk for poor mental health outcomes including depression, suicide, substance use (and misuse), and failure in school and at work (Alessi et al., 2016; Garcia et al., 2020; Ogunbajo et al., 2019; Pereira et al., 2022; Su et al., 2018).

Researchers have found that the health consequences associated with trauma are cumulative and pose a higher risk for individuals who belong to multiple minority groups. This is consistent with intersectional theories of trauma, which underscore that cumulative stressors tend to be higher for those belonging to multiple minority groups (Ching et al., 2018).

Concluding Thoughts

From an ecological framework, development is conceptualized as a dynamic process whereby children actively influence and are highly influenced by environmental contexts, which intersect with multiple systems, including family, peers, and, more broadly, academic and cultural norms and values. All levels of analysis have relevance to developmental trauma. Developmental trauma adaptations depend on a broad range of factors, as discussed in this chapter, including an individual's cultural contexts, socioeconomic status, ethnicity or race, geographic location, and other circumstances unique to each individual. The ecological systems framework carefully considers the overarching contexts that influence children and families and that are embedded in the systems proposed by Bronfenbrenner's multilevel framework. Individuals from cultural groups often share a common (collective) identity as well as values, beliefs, and responses to stress and trauma. An ecological framework also encourages us to advocate for trauma victims by addressing health disparities, inequities in criminal justice, government policies, and mental health systems that have adverse effects on the individual or potentially change their developmental trajectory for the better. From a public health perspective, laws and social and institutional policies are needed to effectively monitor and enforce trauma-informed practices, such as those that aim to prevent the escalation of trauma. We must continue to recognize that ACEs and interpersonal traumas are systemic problems that will require systemic efforts for meaningful change to occur – namely, a paradigm shift in how healthcare providers and individuals in positions of power understand the impact of and take actionable steps against trauma in all its forms. Thus, individual reactions to experiences of trauma should be validated and respected, and the opportunity to examine (or re-examine) such reactions should be done carefully, considering the individual and their relational, cultural, and sociopolitical history.

References

Adu, J., & Oudshoorn, A. (2020). The deinstitutionalization of psychiatric hospitals in Ghana: An application of Bronfenbrenner's social-ecological model. *Issues in Mental Health Nursing*, 41(4), 306–314. https://doi.org/10.1080/01612840.2019.1666327.

Affleck, W., Thamotharampillai, U., Jeyakumar, J., & Whitley, R. (2018). "If One Does Not Fulfil His Duties, He Must Not Be a Man": Masculinity, Mental Health and Resilience Amongst Sri Lankan Tamil Refugee Men in Canada. *Culture, Medicine and Psychiatry*, 42(4), 840–861. https://doi.org/10.1007/s11013-018-9592-9.

Alessi, E. J., Kahn, S., & Chatterji, S. (2016). 'The darkest times of my life': Recollections of child abuse among forced migrants persecuted because of their sexual orientation and gender identity. *Child Abuse & Neglect*, 51, 93–105. https://doi.org/10.1016/j.chiabu.2015.10.030.

Alessi, E. J., Kahn, S., & Van Der Horn, R. (2017). A qualitative exploration of the premigration victimization experiences of sexual and gender minority refugees and asylees in the United States and Canada. *Journal of Sex Research*, 54(7), 936–948. https://doi.org/10.1080/00224499.2016.1229738.

Atilola, O. (2017). Child mental-health policy development in sub-Saharan Africa: Broadening the perspectives using Bronfenbrenner's ecological model. *Health Promotion International*, 32(2), 380–391. https://doi.org/10.1093/heapro/dau065.

Berger, C., Poteat, V. P., & Dantas, J. (2019). Should I report?: The role of general and sexual orientation-specific bullying policies and teacher behavior on adolescents' reporting of victimization experiences. *Journal of School Violence*, 18(1), 107–120. https://doi.org/10.1080/15388220.2017.1387134.

Bosqui, T., Mayya, A., Younes, L., Baker, M. C., & Annan, I. M. (2020). Disseminating evidence-based research on mental health and coping to adolescents facing adversity in Lebanon: A pilot of a psychoeducational comic book 'Somoud'. *Conflict and Health*, 14, 1–10. https://doi.org/10.1186/s13031-020-00324-7.

Bower, K. L., Lewis, D. C., Bermúdez, J. M., & Singh, A. A. (2021). Narratives of generativity and resilience among LGBT older adults: Leaving positive legacies despite social stigma and collective trauma. *Journal of Homosexuality*, 68(2), 230–251. https://doi.org/10.1080/00918369.2019.1648082.

Brodie, Z. P., & Ingram, J. (2021). The dark triad of personality and hero/villain status as predictors of parasocial relationships with comic book characters. *Psychology of Popular Media*, 10(2), 230–242. https://doi.org/10.1037/ppm0000323.

Brothers, S., Lin, J., Schonberg, J., Drew, C., & Auerswald, C. (2020). Food insecurity among formerly homeless youth in supportive housing: A social-ecological analysis of a structural intervention. *Social Science & Medicine*, 245, 112724. https://doi.org/10.1016/j.socscimed.2019.112724.

Brown, C. S., Biefeld, S. D., & Elpers, N. (2020). A bioecological theory of sexual harassment of girls: Research synthesis and proposed model. *Review of General Psychology*, 24(4), 299–320. https://doi.org/10.1177/1089268020954363.

Bryant-Davis, T. (2019). The cultural context of trauma recovery: Considering the posttraumatic stress disorder practice guideline and intersectionality. *Psychotherapy*, 56(3), 400–408. https://doi.org/10.1037/pst0000241.

Calloway, A., & Creed, T. A. (2022). Enhancing CBT consultation with multicultural counseling principles. *Cognitive and Behavioral Practice*, 29(4), 787–795. https://doi.org/10.1016/j.cbpra.2021.05.007.

Carter, R. T., Johnson, V. E., Roberson, K., Mazzula, S. L., Kirkinis, K., & Sant-Barket, S. (2017). Race-based traumatic stress, racial identity statuses, and psychological functioning: An exploratory investigation. *Professional Psychology: Research and Practice*, 48(1), 30–37. https://doi.org/10.1037/pro0000116.

Cave, L., Cooper, M. N., Zubrick, S. R., & Shepherd, C. C. J. (2020). Racial discrimination and child and adolescent health in longitudinal studies: A systematic review. *Social Science & Medicine*, 250, 112864. https://doi.org/10.1016/j.socscimed.2020.112864.

Chang, M. X.-L., Jetten, J., Cruwys, T., & Haslam, C. (2017). Cultural identity and the expression of depression: A social identity perspective. *Journal of Community & Applied Social Psychology*, 27(1), 16–34. https://doi.org/10.1002/casp.2291.

Chavez-Dueñas, N. Y., Adames, H. Y., Perez-Chavez, J. G., & Salas, S. P. (2019). Healing ethno-racial trauma in Latinx immigrant communities: Cultivating hope, resistance, and action. *American Psychologist*, 74(1), 49–62. https://doi.org/10.1037/amp0000289.

Ching, T. H. W., Lee, S. Y., Chen, J., So, R. P., & Williams, M. T. (2018). A model of intersectional stress and trauma in Asian American sexual and gender minorities. *Psychology of Violence*, 8(6), 657–668. https://doi.org/10.1037/vio0000204.

Ciocca, G., Niolu, C., Déttore, D., Antonelli, P., Conte, S., Tuziak, B., Limoncin, E., Mollaioli, D., Carosa, E., Gravina, G. L., Di Sante, S., Di Lorenzo, G., Fisher, A. D., Maggi, M., Lenzi, A., Siracusano, A., & Jannini, E. A. (2017). Cross-cultural and sociodemographic correlates of homophobic attitude among university students in three European countries. *Journal of Endocrinological Investigation*, 40(2), 227–233. https://doi.org/10.1007/s40618-016-0554-1.

Collings, S., Wright, A. C., McLean, L., & Buratti, S. (2022). Trauma-informed family contact practice for children in out-of-home care. *The British Journal of Social Work*, 52(4), 1837–1858. https://doi.org/10.1093/bjsw/bcab147.

Cramer, R. J., & Kapusta, N. D. (2017). A social-ecological framework of theory, assessment, and prevention of suicide. *Frontiers in Psychology*, 8, 1756. https://doi.org/10.3389/fpsyg.2017.01756.

Cramer, R. J., Wright, S., Long, M. M., Kapusta, N. D., Nobles, M. R., Gemberling, T. M., & Wechsler, H. J. (2018). On hate crime victimization: Rates, types, and links with suicide risk among sexual orientation minority special interest group members. *Journal of Trauma & Dissociation*, 19(4), 476–489. https://doi.org/10.1080/15299732.2018.1451972.

Crosby, S. D., Hsu, H.-T., Jones, K., & Rice, E. (2018). Factors that contribute to help-seeking among homeless, trauma-exposed youth: A social-ecological perspective. *Children and Youth Services Review*, 93, 126–134. https://doi.org/10.1016/j.childyouth.2018.07.015.

Cummings, E. M., Merrilees, C. E., Taylor, L. K., & Mondi, C. F. (2017). Developmental and social-ecological perspectives on children, political violence, and armed conflict. *Development and Psychopathology*, 29(1), 1–10. https://doi.org/10.1017/S0954579416001061.

Cunradi, C. B., Caetano, R., Ponicki, W. R., & Alter, H. J. (2021). Interrelationships of economic stressors, mental health problems, substance use, and intimate partner violence among Hispanic emergency department patients: The role of language-based acculturation. *International Journal of Environmental Research and Public Health*, 18(22), 12230. https://doi.org/10.3390/ijerph182212230.

Cyrus, K. (2017). Multiple minorities as multiply marginalized: Applying the minority stress theory to LGBTQ people of color. *Journal of Gay & Lesbian Mental Health*, 21(3), 194–202. https://doi.org/10.1080/19359705.2017.1320739.

Dawson-Rose, C., Shehadeh, D., Hao, J., Barnard, J., Khoddam-Khorasani, L. L., Leonard, A., Clark, K., Kersey, E., Mousseau, H., Frank, J., Miller, A., Carrico, A., Schustack, A., & Cuca, Y. P. (2020). Trauma, substance use, and mental health symptoms in transitional age youth experiencing homelessness. *Public Health Nursing*, 37(3), 363–370. https://doi.org/10.1111/phn.12727.

Deman, J. A. (2020). Busting Loose: Ms. Marvel and post-rape trauma in X-Men comics. *Journal of Graphic Novels and Comics*, 11(4), 412–424. https://doi.org/10.1080/21504857.2020.1757477.

Diab, S. Y., Palosaari, E., & Punamäki, R. L. (2018). Society, individual, family, and school factors contributing to child mental health in war: The ecological-theory perspective. *Child Abuse & Neglect*, 84, 205–216. https://doi.org/10.1016/j.chiabu.2018.07.033.

DiGuiseppi, G. T., Davis, J. P., Christie, N. C., & Rice, E. (2020). Polysubstance use among youth experiencing homelessness: The role of trauma, mental health, and social network composition. *Drug and Alcohol Dependence*, 216, 108228. https://doi.org/10.1016/j.drugalcdep.2020.108228.

Doran, C. M., & Kinchin, I. (2017). A review of the economic impact of mental illness. *Australian Health Review*, 43(1), 43–48. https://doi.org/10.1071/AH16115.

Doran, F. (2020). Alone amidst X-men: Rogue, sexuality, and mental illness. *Journal of Graphic Novels and Comics*, 11(4), 425–437. https://doi.org/10.1080/21504857.2020.1758183.

Easton, S. D., & Kong, J. (2017). Mental health indicators fifty years later: A population-based study of men with histories of child sexual abuse. *Child Abuse & Neglect*, 63, 273–283. https://doi.org/10.1016/j.chiabu.2016.09.011.

Edgcomb, J. B., Sorter, M., Lorberg, B., & Zima, B. T. (2020). Psychiatric readmission of children and adolescents: A systematic review and meta-analysis. *Psychiatric Services*, 71(3), 269–279. https://doi.org/10.1176/appi.ps.201900234.

Elder, W. B., Domino, J. L., Mata-Galán, E. L., & Kilmartin, C. (2017). Masculinity as an avoidance symptom of posttraumatic stress. *Psychology of Men & Masculinity*, 18(3), 198–207. https://doi.org/10.1037/men0000123.

El-Khodary, B., & Samara, M. (2020). The relationship between multiple exposures to violence and war trauma, and mental health and behavioural problems among Palestinian children and adolescents. *European Child & Adolescent Psychiatry*, 29(5), 719–731. https://doi.org/10.1007/s00787-019-01376-8.

El-Khodary, B., Samara, M., & Askew, C. (2020). Traumatic events and PTSD among Palestinian children and adolescents: The effect of demographic and socioeconomic factors. *Frontiers in Psychiatry*, 11, Article 4. https://doi.org/10.3389/fpsyt.2020. 00004.

Eriksson, M., Ghazinour, M., & Hammarström, A. (2018). Different uses of Bronfenbrenner's ecological theory in public mental health research: What is their value for guiding public mental health policy and practice? *Social Theory & Health*, 16(4), 414–433. https://doi.org/10.1057/s41285-018-0065-6.

Finan, S. J., & Yap, M. B. (2021). Engaging parents in preventive programs for adolescent mental health: A socio-ecological framework. *Journal of Family Theory & Review*, 13(4), 515–527. https://doi.org/10.1111/jftr.12440.

Fradkin, C., Weschenfelder, G. V., & Yunes, M. A. (2016). Shared adversities of children and comic superheroes as resources for promoting resilience: Comic superheroes are an untapped resource for empowering vulnerable children. *Child Abuse & Neglect*, 51, 407–415. https://doi.org/10.1016/j.chiabu.2015.10.010.

Fripp, J. A., & Carlson, R. G. (2017). Exploring the influence of attitude and stigma on participation of African American and Latino populations in mental health services. *Journal of Multicultural Counseling and Development*, 45(2), 80–94. https://doi.org/10. 1002/jmcd.12066.

Garcia, G. M., David, E. J. R., & Mapaye, J. C. (2019). Internalized racial oppression as a moderator of the relationship between experiences of racial discrimination and mental distress among Asians and Pacific Islanders. *Asian American Journal of Psychology*, 10(2), 103–112. https://doi.org/10.1037/aap0000124.

Garcia, J., Vargas, N., Clark, J. L., Magaña Álvarez, M., Nelons, D. A., & Parker, R. G. (2020). Social isolation and connectedness as determinants of well-being: Global evidence mapping focused on LGBTQ youth. *Global Public Health*, 15(4), 497–519. https:// doi.org/10.1080/17441692.2019.1682028.

Ghabrial, M. A. (2017). "Trying to figure out where we belong": Narratives of racialized sexual minorities on community, identity, discrimination, and health. *Sexuality Research & Social Policy: A Journal of the NSRC*, 14(1), 42–55. https://doi.org/10. 1007/s13178-016-0229-x.

Gómez, J. M. (2019). What's the harm?: Internalized prejudice and cultural betrayal trauma in ethnic minorities. *American Journal of Orthopsychiatry*, 89(2), 237–247. https:// doi.org/10.1037/ort0000367.

Gómez, J. M. (2021). Cultural betrayal as a dimension of traumatic harm: Violence and PTSS among ethnic minority emerging adults. *Journal of Child & Adolescent Trauma*, 14(3), 347–356. https://doi.org/10.1007/s40653-020-00314-0.

Goodwill, J. R., Taylor, R. J., & Watkins, D. C. (2021). Everyday discrimination, depressive symptoms, and suicide ideation among African American men. *Archives of Suicide Research*, 25(1), 74–93. https://doi.org/10.1080/13811118.2019.1660287.

Greene, C. A., Haisley, L., Wallace, C., & Ford, J. D. (2020). Intergenerational effects of childhood maltreatment: A systematic review of the parenting practices of adult survivors of childhood abuse, neglect, and violence. *Clinical Psychology Review*, 80, 101891. https://doi.org/10.1016/j.cpr.2020.101891.

Griffith, A. K. (2022). Parental burnout and child maltreatment during the COVID-19 pandemic. *Journal of Family Violence*, 37(5), 725–731. https://doi.org/10.1007/s10896-020-00172-2.

Guerra, C., Arredondo, V., Saavedra, C., Pinto-Cortez, C., Benguria, A., & Orrego, A. (2021). Gender differences in the disclosure of sexual abuse in Chilean adolescents. *Child Abuse Review*, 30(3), 210–225. https://doi.org/10.1002/car.2672.

Halsall, T., Manion, I., & Henderson, J. (2018). Examining integrated youth services using the bioecological model: Alignments and opportunities. *International Journal of Integrated Care*, 18(4), 10. https://doi.org/10.5334/ijic.4165.

Hansford, M., & Jobson, L. (2022). Sociocultural context and the posttraumatic psychological response: Considering culture, social support, and posttraumatic stress disorder. *Psychological Trauma: Theory, Research, Practice and Policy*, 14(4), 669–679. https://doi.org/10.1037/tra0001009.

Hapunda, G., Abubakar, A., & van de Vijver, F. (2017). Applying the bioecological model to understand factors contributing to psychosocial well-being and healthcare of children and adolescents with diabetes mellitus. *South African Journal of Diabetes and Vascular Disease*, 14(1), 11–17. https://hdl.handle.net/10520/EJC-94d31a9cf.

Heberle, A. E., Obus, E. A., & Gray, S. A. (2020). An intersectional perspective on the intergenerational transmission of trauma and state-perpetrated violence. *Journal of Social Issues*, 76(4), 814–834. https://doi.org/10.1111/josi.12404.

Herron, R. V., Ahmadu, M., Allan, J. A., Waddell, C. M., & Roger, K. (2020). "Talk about it": Changing masculinities and mental health in rural places? *Social Science & Medicine*, 258, 113099. https://doi.org/10.1016/j.socscimed.2020.113099.

Hirschberger, G. (2018). Collective trauma and the social construction of meaning. *Frontiers in Psychology*, 9, 1441. https://doi.org/10.3389/fpsyg.2018.01441.

Hlavka, H. R. (2017). Speaking of stigma and the silence of shame: Young men and sexual victimization. *Men and Masculinities*, 20(4), 482–505. https://doi.org/10.1177/1097184X16652656.

Holman, E. A., Garfin, D. R., Lubens, P., & Silver, R. C. (2020). Media exposure to collective trauma, mental health, and functioning: Does it matter what you see? *Clinical Psychological Science*, 8(1), 111–124. https://doi.org/10.1177/2167702619858300.

Hong, J. S., Kim, D. H., Thornberg, R., Kang, J. H., & Morgan, J. T. (2018). Correlates of direct and indirect forms of cyberbullying victimization involving South Korean adolescents: An ecological perspective. *Computers in Human Behavior*, 87, 327–336. https://doi.org/10.1016/j.chb.2018.06.010.

Hopwood, T. L., & Schutte, N. S. (2017). Psychological outcomes in reaction to media exposure to disasters and large-scale violence: A meta-analysis. *Psychology of Violence*, 7(2), 316–327. https://doi.org/10.1037/vio0000056.

Ingram, K. M., Davis, J. P., Espelage, D. L., Hatchel, T., Merrin, G. J., Valido, A., & Torgal, C. (2019). Longitudinal associations between features of toxic masculinity and bystander willingness to intervene in bullying among middle school boys. *Journal of School Psychology*, 77, 139–151. https://doi.org/10.1016/j.jsp.2019.10.007.

Jauregui, J. C., Mwochi, C. R., Crawford, J., Jadwin-Cakmak, L., Okoth, C., Onyango, D. P., & Harper, G. W. (2021). Experiences of violence and mental health concerns among sexual and gender minority adults in western Kenya. *LGBT Health*, 8(7), 494–501. https://doi.org/10.1089/lgbt.2020.0495.

Johns, M. M., Beltran, O., Armstrong, H. L., Jayne, P. E., & Barrios, L. C. (2018). Protective factors among transgender and gender variant youth: A systematic review by socioecological level. *The Journal of Primary Prevention*, 39(3), 263–301. https://doi.org/10.1007/s10935-018-0508-9.

Jore, T., Oppedal, B., & Biele, G. (2020). Social anxiety among unaccompanied minor refugees in Norway: The association with pre-migration trauma and post-migration acculturation related factors. *Journal of Psychosomatic Research*, 136, 110175. https://doi.org/10.1016/j.jpsychores.2020.110175.

Kartal, D., Alkemade, N., Eisenbruch, M., & Kissane, D. (2018). Traumatic exposure, acculturative stress and cultural orientation: the influence on PTSD, depressive and anxiety symptoms among refugees. *Social Psychiatry and Psychiatric Epidemiology*, 53(9), 931–941.

Katzenstein, D., & Fontes, L. A. (2017). Twice Silenced: The underreporting of child sexual abuse in Orthodox Jewish communities. *Journal of Child Sexual Abuse*, 26(6), 752–767. https://doi.org/10.1080/10538712.2017.1336505.

Kirkinis, K., Pieterse, A. L., Martin, C., Agiliga, A., & Brownell, A. (2021). Racism, racial discrimination, and trauma: A systematic review of the social science literature. *Ethnicity & Health*, 26(3), 392–412. https://doi.org/10.1080/13557858.2018.1514453.

Klest, B., Tamaian, A., & Boughner, E. (2019). A model exploring the relationship between betrayal trauma and health: The roles of mental health, attachment, trust in healthcare systems, and nonadherence to treatment. *Psychological Trauma: Theory, Research, Practice and Policy*, 11(6), 656–662. https://doi.org/10.1037/tra0000453.

Lamontagne, E., d'Elbée, M., Ross, M. W., Carroll, A., Plessis, A. D., & Loures, L. (2018). A socioecological measurement of homophobia for all countries and its public health impact. *European Journal of Public Health*, 28(5), 967–972. https://doi.org/10.1093/eurpub/cky023.

Lee, S. J., Ward, K. P., Lee, J. Y., & Rodriguez, C. M. (2022). Parental social isolation and child maltreatment risk during the COVID-19 pandemic. *Journal of Family Violence*, 37(5), 813–824. https://doi.org/10.1007/s10896-020-00244-3.

Lev-Wiesel, R., & First, M. (2018). Willingness to disclose child maltreatment: CSA vs other forms of child abuse in relation to gender. *Child Abuse & Neglect*, 79, 183–191. https://doi.org/10.1016/j.chiabu.2018.02.010.

Lewis, F. J., Tor, S., Rappleyea, D., Didericksen, K. W., & Sira, N. (2021). Behavioral health and refugee youth in primary care: An ecological systems perspective of the complexities of care. *Children and Youth Services Review*, 120, 105599. https://doi.org/10.1016/j.childyouth.2020.105599.

Liang, Y., Zhou, Y., Ruzek, J. I., & Liu, Z. (2020). Patterns of childhood trauma and psychopathology among Chinese rural-to-urban migrant children. *Child Abuse & Neglect*, 108, 104691. https://doi.org/10.1016/j.chiabu.2020.104691.

Livingston, N. A., Berke, D. S., Ruben, M. A., Matza, A. R., & Shipherd, J. C. (2019). Experiences of trauma, discrimination, microaggressions, and minority stress among trauma-exposed LGBT veterans: Unexpected findings and unresolved service gaps.

Psychological Trauma: Theory, Research, Practice, and Policy, 11(7), 695–703. https://doi.org/10.1037/tra0000464.

Loyd, A. B., Hotton, A. L., Walden, A. L., Kendall, A. D., Emerson, E., & Donenberg, G. R. (2019). Associations of ethnic/racial discrimination with internalizing symptoms and externalizing behaviors among juvenile justice-involved youth of color. *Journal of Adolescence*, 75, 138–150. https://doi.org/10.1016/j.adolescence.2019.07.012.

MacGinley, M., Breckenridge, J., & Mowll, J. (2019). A scoping review of adult survivors' experiences of shame following sexual abuse in childhood. *Health & Social Care in the Community*, 27(5), 1135–1146. https://doi.org/10.1111/hsc.12771.

Madubata, I., Spivey, L. A., Alvarez, G. M., Neblett, E. W., & Prinstein, M. J. (2022). Forms of racial/ethnic discrimination and suicidal ideation: A prospective examination of African-American and Latinx youth. *Journal of Clinical Child and Adolescent Psychology*, 51(1), 23–31. https://doi.org/10.1080/15374416.2019.1655756.

Matheson, K., Foster, M. D., Bombay, A., McQuaid, R. J., & Anisman, H. (2019). Traumatic experiences, perceived discrimination, and psychological distress among members of various socially marginalized groups. *Frontiers in Psychology*, 10, 416. https://doi.org/10.3389/fpsyg.2019.00416.

Matthies-Boon, V. (2017). Shattered worlds: Political trauma amongst young activists in post-revolutionary Egypt. *The Journal of North African Studies*, 22(4), 620–644. https://doi.org/10.1080/13629387.2017.1295855.

McGunnigle, C. (2018). The difference between heroes and monsters: Marvel monsters and their transition into the superhero genre. *University of Toronto Quarterly*, 87(1), 110–135. https://doi.org/10.3138/utq.87.1.110.

Metzger, I. W., Anderson, R. E., Are, F., & Ritchwood, T. (2021). Healing interpersonal and racial trauma: Integrating racial socialization into trauma-focused cognitive behavioral therapy for African American youth. *Child Maltreatment*, 26(1), 17–27. https://doi.org/10.1177/1077559520921457.

Mikolajczak, M., Brianda, M. E., Avalosse, H., & Roskam, I. (2018). Consequences of parental burnout: Its specific effect on child neglect and violence. *Child Abuse & Neglect*, 80, 134–145. https://doi.org/10.1016/j.chiabu.2018.03.025.

Minh, A., Muhajarine, N., Janus, M., Brownell, M., & Guhn, M. (2017). A review of neighborhood effects and early child development: How, where, and for whom, do neighborhoods matter? *Health & Place*, 46, 155–174. https://doi.org/10.1016/j.healthplace.2017.04.012.

Moleiro, C. (2018). Culture and psychopathology: New perspectives on research, practice, and clinical training in a globalized world. *Frontiers in Psychiatry*, 9, 366. https://doi.org/10.3389/fpsyt.2018.00366.

Monteith, L. L., Brownstone, L. M., Gerber, H. R., Soberay, K. A., & Bahraini, N. H. (2019). Understanding suicidal self-directed violence among men exposed to military sexual trauma: An ecological framework. *Psychology of Men & Masculinities*, 20(1), 23–35. https://doi.org/10.1037/men0000141.

Moore, G. F., Cox, R., Evans, R. E., Hallingberg, B., Hawkins, J., Littlecott, H. J., Long, S. J., & Murphy, S. (2018). School, peer and family relationships and adolescent substance use, subjective wellbeing and mental health symptoms in Wales: A cross sectional study. *Child Indicators Research*, 11(6), 1951–1965. https://doi.org/10.1007/s12187-017-9524-1.

Moses, J. O., & Villodas, M. T. (2017). The potential protective role of peer relationships on school engagement in at-risk adolescents. *Journal Of Youth and Adolescence*, 46 (11), 2255–2272. https://doi.org/10.1007/s10964-017-0644-1.

Mosher, D. K., Hook, J. N., Captari, L. E., Davis, D. E., DeBlaere, C., & Owen, J. (2017). Cultural humility: A therapeutic framework for engaging diverse clients. *Practice Innovations*, 2(4), 221–233. https://doi.org/10.1037/pri0000055.

Müller, A., Daskilewicz, K., Kabwe, M. L., Mmolai-Chalmers, A., Morroni, C., Muparamoto, N., Muula, A.S., Odira, V., & Zimba, M. (2021). Experience of and factors associated with violence against sexual and gender minorities in nine African countries: a cross-sectional study. *BMC Public Health*, 21(1), 1–11. https://doi.org/10. 1186/s12889-021-10314-w.

Neilson, E. C., Singh, R. S., Harper, K. L., & Teng, E. J. (2020). Traditional masculinity ideology, posttraumatic stress disorder (PTSD) symptom severity, and treatment in service members and veterans: A systematic review. *Psychology of Men & Masculinities*, 21(4), 578–592. https://doi.org/10.1037/men0000257.

Nesoff, E. D., Gutkind, S., Sirota, S., McKowen, A. L., & Veldhuis, C. B. (2021). Mental health and economic stressors associated with high-risk drinking and increased alcohol consumption early in the COVID-19 pandemic in the United States. *Preventive Medicine*, 153, 106854. https://doi.org/10.1016/j.ypmed.2021.106854.

Newton, B. J. (2019). Understanding child neglect in Aboriginal families and communities in the context of trauma. *Child & Family Social Work*, 24(2), 218–226. https://doi.org/10.1111/cfs.12606.

Obasaju, M., & LiVecchi, P. (2018). Exploring the use of an integrative and ecological framework when treating children with trauma. *Journal of Infant, Child & Adolescent Psychotherapy*, 17(4), 252–264. https://doi.org/10.1080/15289168.2018.1526023.

Ogunbajo, A., Anyamele, C., Restar, A. J., Dolezal, C., & Sandfort, T. G. M. (2019). Substance use and depression among recently migrated African gay and bisexual men living in the United States. *Journal of Immigrant and Minority Health*, 21(6), 1224–1232. https://doi.org/10.1007/s10903-018-0849-8.

Oh, H., Stickley, A., Koyanagi, A., Yau, R., & DeVylder, J. E. (2019). Discrimination and suicidality among racial and ethnic minorities in the United States. *Journal of Affective Disorders*, 245, 517–523. https://doi.org/10.1016/j.jad.2018.11.059.

O'Neill, L., Fraser, T., Kitchenham, A., & McDonald, V. (2016). Hidden burdens: A review of intergenerational, historical and complex trauma, implications for indigenous families. *Journal of Child & Adolescent Trauma*, 11(2), 173–186. https://doi.org/10. 1007/s40653-016-0117-9.

O'Roark, B., & Grant, W. (2018). Games superheroes play: Teaching game theory with comic book favorites. *The Journal of Economic Education*, 49(2), 180–193. https://doi.org/10.1080/00220485.2018.1438861.

Parent, M. C., Gobble, T. D., & Rochlen, A. (2019). Social media behavior, toxic masculinity, and depression. *Psychology of Men & Masculinities*, 20(3), 277–287. https://doi.org/10.1037/men0000156.

Pereira, H., De Vries, B., Esgalhado, G., & Serrano, J. P. (2022). Loneliness perceptions in older Portuguese gay and bisexual men. *Journal of Homosexuality*, 69(6), 985–1003. https://doi.org/10.1080/00918369.2021.1901504.

Petering, R., Rhoades, H., Winetrobe, H., Dent, D., & Rice, E. (2017). Violence, trauma, mental health, and substance use among homeless youth Juggalos. *Child Psychiatry & Human Development*, 48(4), 642–650. https://doi.org/10.1007/s10578-016-0689-5.

Pfefferbaum, B., Nitiéma, P., & Newman, E. (2021). The association of mass trauma media contact with depression and anxiety: A meta-analytic review. *Journal of Affective Disorders Reports*, 3, 100063. https://doi.org/10.1016/j.jadr.2020.100063.

Pollitt, A. M., Mallory, A. B., & Fish, J. N. (2018). Homophobic bullying and sexual minority youth alcohol use: Do sex and race/ethnicity matter? *LGBT Health*, 5(7), 412–420. https://doi.org/10.1089/lgbt.2018.0031.

Probst, T. M., Sinclair, R. R., Sears, L. E., Gailey, N. J., Black, K. J., & Cheung, J. H. (2018). Economic stress and well-being: Does population health context matter? *Journal of Applied Psychology*, 103(9), 959–979. https://doi.org/10.1037/apl0000309.

Pumariega, A. J., Jo, Y., Beck, B., & Rahmani, M. (2022). Trauma and US minority children and youth. *Current Psychiatry Reports*, 24(4), 285–295. https://doi.org/10.1007/s11920-022-01336-1.

Quin, D., Heerde, J. A., & Toumbourou, J. W. (2018). Teacher support within an ecological model of adolescent development: Predictors of school engagement. *Journal of School Psychology*, 69, 1–15. https://doi.org/10.1016/j.jsp.2018.04.003.

Quinn, K. G. (2022). Applying an intersectional framework to understand syndemic conditions among young Black gay, bisexual, and other men who have sex with men. *Social Science & Medicine*, 295, 112779. https://doi.org/10.1016/j.socscimed.2019.112779.

Ramirez, J. L., & Paz Galupo, M. (2019). Multiple minority stress: The role of proximal and distal stress on mental health outcomes among lesbian, gay, and bisexual people of color. *Journal of Gay & Lesbian Mental Health*, 23(2), 145–167. https://doi.org/10.1080/19359705.2019.1568946.

Range, B., Gutierrez, D., Gamboni, C., Hough, N. A., & Wojciak, A. (2018). Mass trauma in the African American community: Using multiculturalism to build resilient systems. *Contemporary Family Therapy: An International Journal*, 40(3), 284–298. https://doi.org/10.1007/s10591-017-9449-3.

Ranjbar, N., Erb, M., Mohammad, O., & Moreno, F. A. (2020). Trauma-informed care and cultural humility in the mental health care of people from minoritized communities. *Focus*, 18(1), 8–15. https://doi.org/10.1176/appi.focus.20190027.

Reupert, A. (2017). A socio-ecological framework for mental health and well-being. *Advances in Mental Health*, 15(2), 105–107. https://doi.org/10.1080/18387357.2017.1342902.

Reyes, A. T., Constantino, R. E., Cross, C. L., Tan, R. A., & Bombard, J. N. (2020). Resilience, trauma, and cultural norms regarding disclosure of mental health problems among foreign-born and US-born Filipino American women. *Behavioral Medicine*, 46 (3–4), 217–230. https://doi.org/10.1080/08964289.2020.1725413.

Salter, M., & Hall, H. (2022). Reducing shame, promoting dignity: A model for the primary prevention of complex post-traumatic stress disorder. *Trauma, Violence & Abuse*, 23(3), 906–919. https://doi.org/10.1177/1524838020979667.

Sample, K., & Ferguson, K. M. (2020). It shouldn't be this hard: Systemic, situational, and intrapersonal barriers to exiting homelessness among homeless young adults. *Qualitative Social Work: Research and Practice*, 19(4), 580–598. https://doi.org/10.1177/1473325019836280.

Sangalang, C. C., & Vang, C. (2017). Intergenerational trauma in refugee families: A systematic review. *Journal of Immigrant and Minority Health*, 19(3), 745–754. https://doi.org/10.1007/s10903-016-0499-7.

Santa Maria, D., Padhye, N., Yang, Y., Gallardo, K., Santos, G. M., Jung, J., & Businelle, M. (2018). Drug use patterns and predictors among homeless youth: Results of an ecological momentary assessment. *The American Journal of Drug and Alcohol Abuse*, 44(5), 551–560. https://doi.org/10.1080/00952990.2017.1407328.

Sawrikar, P., & Katz, I. (2017). Barriers to disclosing child sexual abuse (CSA) in ethnic minority communities: A review of the literature and implications for practice in Australia. *Children and Youth Services Review*, 83, 302–315. https://doi.org/10.1016/j.childyouth.2017.11.011.

Schulte, W., & Frederick, N. (2020). Black Panther and black agency: Constructing cultural nationalism in comic books featuring Black Panther, 1973–1979. *Journal of Graphic Novels and Comics*, 11(3), 296–314. https://doi.org/10.1080/21504857.2019.1569081.

Schunk, F., Trommsdorff, G., & König-Teshnizi, D. (2022). Regulation of positive and negative emotions across cultures: Does culture moderate associations between emotion regulation and mental health? *Cognition & Emotion*, 36(2), 352–363. https://doi.org/10.1080/02699931.2021.1997924.

Selwyn, C. N., Lathan, E. C., Richie, F., Gigler, M. E., & Langhinrichsen-Rohling, J. (2021). Bitten by the system that cared for them: Towards a trauma-informed understanding of patients' healthcare engagement. *Journal of Trauma & Dissociation*, 22(5), 636–652. https://doi.org/10.1080/15299732.2020.1869657.

Skewes, M. C., & Blume, A. W. (2019). Understanding the link between racial trauma and substance use among American Indians. *American Psychologist*, 74(1), 88–100. https://doi.org/10.1037/amp0000331.

Sivagurunathan, M., Orchard, T., MacDermid, J. C., & Evans, M. (2019). Barriers and facilitators affecting self-disclosure among male survivors of child sexual abuse: The service providers' perspective. *Child Abuse & Neglect*, 88, 455–465. https://doi.org/10.1016/j.chiabu.2018.08.015.

Smith, D. E. (2018). Homophobic and transphobic violence against youth: The Jamaican context. *International Journal of Adolescence and Youth*, 23(2), 250–258. https://doi.org/10.1080/02673843.2017.1336106.

Smith, S. T. (2017). A likely Jew: Magneto, the holocaust, and comic-book history. *Studies in American Jewish Literature*, 36(1), 1–39. https://doi.org/10.5325/studamerjewilite.36.1.0001.

Smith, T. B., Lyon, R. C., & O'Grady, K. (2019). Integration or separation?: Addressing religious and spiritual issues in multicultural counseling: A national survey of college counselors. *Journal of College Counseling*, 22(3), 194–210. https://doi.org/10.1002/jocc.12137.

Stephens, M., Curry, G., & Stephens, S. (2021). Empathizing with black women's experiences at the intersections of collective trauma, isolation, anxiety, depression, and HIV/AIDS amid a global pandemic: Narratives of two community based organization (CBO) service providers. *Journal of Underrepresented & Minority Progress*, 5(SI), 67–82. https://doi.org/10.32674/jump.v5iSI.3114.

Strompolis, M., Tucker, W., Crouch, E., & Radcliff, E. (2019). The intersectionality of adverse childhood experiences, race/ethnicity, and income: Implications for policy. *Journal of Prevention & Intervention in the Community*, 47(4), 310–324. https://doi.org/10.1080/10852352.2019.1617387.

Su, X., Zhou, A. N., Li, J., Shi, L. E., Huan, X., Yan, H., & Wei, C. (2018). Depression, loneliness, and sexual risk-taking among HIV-negative/unknown men who have sex with men in China. *Archives of Sexual Behavior*, 47(7), 1959–1968. https://doi.org/10.1007/s10508-017-1061-y.

Sugarman, D. B., Nation, M., Yuan, N. P., Kuperminc, G. P., Hassoun Ayoub, L., & Hamby, S. (2018). Hate and violence: Addressing discrimination based on race, ethnicity, religion, sexual orientation, and gender identity. *Psychology of Violence*, 8(6), 649–656. https://doi.org/10.1037/vio0000222.

Taliaferro, L. A., & Muehlenkamp, J. J. (2017). Nonsuicidal self-injury and suicidality among sexual minority youth: Risk factors and protective connectedness factors. *Academic Pediatrics*, 17(7), 715–722. https://doi.org/10.1016/j.acap.2016.11.002.

Tessler, H., Choi, M., & Kao, G. (2020). The anxiety of being Asian American: Hate crimes and negative biases during the COVID-19 pandemic. *American Journal of Criminal Justice*, 45(4), 636–646. https://doi.org/10.1007/s12103-020-09541-5.

Thompson, E. J., Anderson, V. A., Hearps, S. J. C., McCarthy, M. C., Mihalopoulos, C., Nicholson, J. M., Rayner, M., & Muscara, F. (2017). Posttraumatic stress symptom severity and health service utilization in trauma-exposed parents. *Health Psychology*, 36(8), 779–786. https://doi.org/10.1037/hea0000476.

Thompson, R. R., Jones, N. M., Holman, E. A., & Silver, R. C. (2019). Media exposure to mass violence events can fuel a cycle of distress. *Science Advances*, 5(4), eaav3502. https://doi.org/10.1126/sciadv.aav3502.

Timshel, I., Montgomery, E., & Dalgaard, N. T. (2017). A systematic review of risk and protective factors associated with family related violence in refugee families. *Child Abuse & Neglect*, 70, 315–330. https://doi.org/10.1016/j.chiabu.2017.06.023.

Tyler, K. A., & Schmitz, R. M. (2018). A comparison of risk factors for various forms of trauma in the lives of lesbian, gay, bisexual and heterosexual homeless youth. *Journal of Trauma & Dissociation, 19*(4), 431–443. https://doi.org/10.1080/15299732.2018.1451971.

Ungar, M., & Theron, L. (2020). Resilience and mental health: How multisystemic processes contribute to positive outcomes. *The Lancet Psychiatry*, 7(5), 441–448. https://doi.org/10.1016/S2215-0366(19)30434-30431.

Vélez-Agosto, N. M., Soto-Crespo, J. G., Vizcarrondo-Oppenheimer, M., Vega-Molina, S., & García Coll, C. (2017). Bronfenbrenner's bioecological theory revision: Moving culture from the macro into the micro. *Perspectives on Psychological Science*, 12 (5), 900–910. https://doi.org/10.1177/1745691617704397.

Walker, M., Nixon, S., Haines, J., & McPherson, A. C. (2019). Examining risk factors for overweight and obesity in children with disabilities: A commentary on Bronfenbrenner's ecological systems framework. *Developmental Neurorehabilitation*, 22(5), 359–364. https://doi.org/10.1080/17518423.2018.1523241.

Wamser-Nanney, R., & Cherry, K. E. (2018). Children's trauma-related symptoms following complex trauma exposure: Evidence of gender differences. *Child Abuse & Neglect*, 77, 188–197. https://doi.org/10.1016/j.chiabu.2018.01.009.

Wojcik, K. D., Cox, D. W., & Kealy, D. (2019). Adverse childhood experiences and shame- and guilt-proneness: Examining the mediating roles of interpersonal problems in a community sample. *Child Abuse & Neglect*, 98, 104233. https://doi.org/10.1016/j.chiabu.2019.104233.

Xia, M., Li, X., & Tudge, J. R. (2020). Operationalizing Urie Bronfenbrenner's process-person-context-time model. *Human Development*, 64(1), 10–20. https://doi.org/10.1159/000507958.

Xu, J., Sun, G., Cao, W., Fan, W., Pan, Z., Yao, Z., & Li, H. (2021). Stigma, discrimination, and hate crimes in Chinese-speaking world amid COVID-19 pandemic. *Asian Journal of Criminology*, 16(1), 51–74. https://doi.org/10.1007/s11417-020-09339-8.

Yatham, S., Sivathasan, S., Yoon, R., da Silva, T. L., & Ravindran, A. V. (2018). Depression, anxiety, and post-traumatic stress disorder among youth in low and middle income countries: a review of prevalence and treatment interventions. *Asian Journal of Psychiatry*, 38, 78–91. https://doi.org/10.1016/j.ajp.2017.10.029.

Zhang, Y., Zhang, L., & Benton, F. (2022). Hate Crimes against Asian Americans. *American Journal of Criminal Justice*, 47(3), 441–461. https://doi.org/10.1007/s12103-020-09602-9.

Zhu, P., Lau, J., & Navalta, C. P. (2020). An ecological approach to understanding pervasive and hidden shame in complex trauma. *Journal of Mental Health Counseling*, 42(2), 155–169. http://dx.doi.org/10.17744/mehc.42.2.05.

5

APPLICATION OF BRONFENBRENNER'S SOCIOECOLOGICAL MODEL TO VIOLENCE

Domestic violence is likely to be familiar to most readers because of its widespread prevalence and impact. According to the National Coalition Against Domestic Violence (NCADV), 1 in 4 women and 1 in 9 men experience domestic violence, and 1 in 15 children are exposed to intimate partner violence (IPV) each year, with 90% of these children directly witnessing the abuse and violence. Scholars have described domestic violence as a public health problem, a social justice matter, and as a human rights violation that disproportionately affects women and children worldwide. Research suggests, for example, that domestic violence rates increased dramatically during the COVID-19 pandemic across the globe, including in Germany, India, Spain, France, Brazil, Africa, Canada, and the USA (Ertan et al., 2020; Kourti et al., 2021; Ortega Pacheco & Martínez Rudas, 2021; Piquero et al., 2021). Actual rates were likely higher than reported given the tendency for victims to underreport violence.

Domestic violence is a pervasive social problem with broad, multifaceted effects on individuals, families, and communities. More specifically, violence intersects with the individual, family, social, and economic circumstances that both adversely impact children who experience developmental traumas and have the potential to help these children recover from ACEs, repeated abuse and neglect, and violence. As an illustration, consider the following story of Isaiah, a 13-year-old child who experienced early repeated abuse, neglect, and IPV exposure and whose family was adversely affected by broad social and economic stressors (Grasso, 2022).

Isaiah is a 13-year-old child who experienced early severe abuse, neglect, and violence exposure. In fact, the abuse began when his mother, Sandra, was pregnant with him. During her pregnancy, Sandra was abused on numerous

DOI: 10.4324/9781003304715-5

occasions by his soon-to-be father, George. As an infant, Isaiah was also abused and threatened by his father. Isaiah also witnessed his parents struggle with addiction. When Isaiah was 6, he got in the middle of an altercation between his caregivers in an attempt to defend his mother and suffered an injury as a result (a concussion). Eventually, Isaiah's father left home, and Isaiah's mother began a new relationship with a man named Joseph. Joseph and Sandra had two children together, Juliana and Dimitri. Unfortunately, the abuse did not end for Isaiah and his family. Isaiah and his siblings experienced emotional neglect and severe IPV, which were worsened by a broad range of socioecological factors, including the COVID-19 pandemic, employment instability (Joseph was laid off, and Sandra lost work hours), and the family's growing frustration with Isaiah, who had trouble adjusting to virtual learning. To cope with stress, Isaiah's caregivers abused alcohol, which worsened matters. Eventually, the police and CPS intervened, and Isaiah was placed into foster care, where he experienced additional traumas including separation from his siblings.

Isaiah's story highlights the complexities of working with children and families who experience polyvictimization and depend on support from others, such as law enforcement, school personnel, social workers, and caregiver advocates, to assist them in preventing further abuse and neglect and in recovering from their traumas. Isaiah was eventually evaluated and treated from a trauma-informed care framework, which helped to reconceptualize his symptoms (i.e., aggression, ADHD, and oppositional defiant disorder) as characteristic of children who have experienced DTD.

Trauma and Violence

Domestic violence can manifest itself in explicit physical and sexual acts (e.g., kicking, hair pulling, punching or slapping, spitting) as well as through psychological means, such as behaviors characterized by intimidation and coercive control (for example, threatening a child and his or her mother with additional abuse if they contact law enforcement; Dworkin et al., 2019; Haselschwerdt et al., 2019). More specifically, domestic violence, or interpersonal violence, defined as the deliberate abuse of power to intimidate or harm another person or persons emotionally or physically, is linked to several mental health problems, including psychological distress, substance abuse, and relational (interpersonal) trauma (Ford et al., 2020; Hauw et al., 2021; Russell et al., 2020; Talevi et al., 2019). Some scholars use the terms domestic and intimate partner violence interchangeably, although others differentiate them to describe whether individuals live together (domestic violence) or not (IPV).

Domestic violence is key to understanding the developmental trauma framework (Ford, 2017; Spinazzola et al., 2021). Being an early childhood victim of IPV, such as physical or sexual abuse, bullying, or assault, often results in both acute and chronic forms of stress that, especially for young children and adolescents, disrupt attachment, self-awareness, behavioral regulation, and coping capacities (Bonache et al., 2019; Lee et al., 2021; Speranza et al., 2022; Spinazzola et al., 2018; Theall et al., 2017; Tussey et al., 2021) and, in turn, increases the likelihood of interpersonal trauma, DTD, and complex PTSD in adulthood. More specifically, domestic violence or IPV against women (IPVAW) plays a significant role in the development of DTD because it negatively impacts children's relationship models, compromises their safety and self-regulation capacities, and normalizes violence as a way to cope with fear, insecurity, anger, and frustration (Jung et al., 2019; Kim et al., 2019). Indeed, studies suggest these children develop insecure attachment patterns without effective interventions or surrogate attachment figures, and these adverse effects are longstanding and multifactorial (Boeckel et al., 2017). Some children may cope with their fear by joining the abusive parent in inflicting IPV (Burck et al., 2019; Hernández et al., 2020; Ibabe, 2019) because they cannot cope with the victimized parent's inability to protect themselves and the child (and his or her siblings). Studies have demonstrated that children exposed to violence in the home are at greater risk of developing measurable symptoms of anxiety, depression, sleep disturbances, and aggression (Gallegos et al., 2021; Gardner et al., 2019; Lee et al., 2020; LeMoult et al., 2020; Narayan et al., 2017). This is particularly true for children for whom responsive, trauma-informed interventions are unavailable.

Because children with DTD rely on anger and aggression as a primary coping strategy in response to psychological distress, they develop limited social problem-solving skills, including resolving conflicts and communicating their needs effectively. In working with DTD individuals, I have been struck by the degree of stigma and shame these individuals experience, which they often find difficult to convey to others because they fear being negatively judged or viewed as weak and incapable of helping themselves (which would mean, in turn, that they are incapable of helping themselves and their caregivers and siblings when violence occurs in the home or when they are re-victimized by sexual abuse). Although we often consider anger and aggression maladaptive, for children with DTD, it is the primary coping strategy that has kept them alive. In other words, anger is an emotion that allows children to effectively "turn off" their physiological fear and anxiety (i.e., fight response mediated by norepinephrine) and act to defend themselves and others. Anger is associated with heightened attention and focus (including the abuse and exploitation of others at risk for victimization), perceived control, and goal-directed problem solving. It can heighten one's understanding and awareness of one's core values and beliefs, and, if communicated effectively and justified by the circumstances, anger can help reconcile interpersonal conflicts, increase cooperation, and enhance creativity and emotional intelligence (self-awareness by understanding that anger is masking deep emotional pain and suffering). Anger can also help children affected by DTD succeed in school (because anger positively influences persistence and determination with support) and in the workplace (studies of individuals who have experienced anger and aggression and who were able to manage their anger effectively have shown that anger is a motivating force that can lead to positive justice-oriented careers such counseling, psychology, government, social work, and law). The point here is that we should not give up on children who are perceived to be challenging or who are experiencing self-regulation difficulties because of ACEs and early traumas. These individuals have unimaginable potential if we work to understand and support them.

Conceptualizing Violence from a Socioecological Framework

Bronfenbrenner's ecological systems theory is valuable to our analysis of developmental trauma and violence because violence is linked to broad social, economic, psychological, legal, and cultural factors (Gatfield et al., 2022; Jegatheesan et al., 2020; McKay, 2022; Mora et al., 2022; Pokharel et al., 2020). Responses to violence may differ given one's gender, culture, and country, including in contexts of forced labor, child marriage, commercial trafficking, and exploitation of children and adolescents. For example, in some cultures the power between a mother and father is unequal and, as such, women, more often than men, lack voice, authority, and self-determination (Song et al., 2021; Stephens & Eaton, 2020; Yalley & Olutayo, 2020). In such cultures, it may be considered disrespectful for women to express their feelings, particularly concerning private family matters, regardless of the circumstances. Women may be required to submit to men and may be discouraged from expressing their individual needs. Children may also be expected to speak only when spoken to and to respect the family's hierarchy. Violence against women, however, continues to be maintained by structural and cultural factors that implicitly disempower women and children (Serrano-Montilla et al., 2020; Sikweyiya et al., 2020; Tekkas Kerman & Betrus, 2020).

Regrettably, some victims may sustain injuries and health problems from physical and sexual violence, such as traumatic head injuries, bone fractures, chronic pain/migraines, sexually transmitted infections, and unintended pregnancies resulting from rape. These adverse health effects increase the likelihood of high-risk pregnancies, including perinatal exposure to HIV and AIDS as well as premature and low-birth-weight infants, which contribute to developmental trauma. These children may experience developmental disturbances, such as developmental delays, learning disabilities, and longstanding health problems.

An ecological framework of trauma and violence also considers systemic issues, such as the failure of institutions to monitor and enforce policies and procedures effectively (e.g., minimizing or denying that abuse occurred to protect perpetrators; lessening negative consequences, including on institutions; or avoiding reporting obligations, institutional monitoring/auditing, or public disclosure). An ecological framework of trauma and violence also highlights vicarious and secondary traumas experienced as a result of interactions with child protection service workers and administrators, healthcare providers, first responders, and law enforcement (Heward-Belle et al., 2018; Laing, 2017). In responding to reports of child abuse and neglect, psychiatric emergencies, or violent circumstances, for example, these individuals may experience traumas from witnessing severe forms of violence, caring for victims, or coping with anger, helplessness, guilt, and possible losses (of victims) in the process. Traditional approaches, which focus exclusively on the patient and his or her mental health symptoms, may underappreciate this type of trauma.

Early Interpersonal Violence Exposure

Children exposed to early violence develop mental and physical health problems that may be elusive to others (for example, in psychological, medical, and forensic evaluation; Bailey & Brown, 2020; Becker-Haimes et al., 2021; John et al., 2019), mainly when adaptations to extreme violence give rise to complex developmental traumas. Early exposure to violence, ACEs, and DTD have been linked to negative emotionality, somatization, poor school performance, engagement in fire setting, and animal cruelty (Baglivio et al., 2017; Blodgett & Lanigan, 2018; Bright et al., 2018; Jegatheesan et al., 2020; Stempel et al., 2017; Watt et al., 2021), and these traumatic experiences precipitate stress/substance-abuse mediated psychiatric disturbances, such as hallucinations and delusions (Croft et al., 2019; Liu et al., 2021; Medjkane et al., 2020; Setién-Suero et al., 2020), conduct disorder in children and adolescents, and antisocial personality disorder in adults (Bright et al., 2018; DeLisi et al., 2019; Stoffel et al., 2019).

These responses to trauma may be less volitional and more behavioral expressions of cognitive and neurological problems. Children, as well as adolescents and adults who experienced trauma as children, may also experience cognitive impairments associated with interpersonal violence exposure from chronic stress (giving rise to ADHD-like symptoms and behaviors) or from sustaining injuries while trying to defend one of their caregivers or siblings from being (re)victimized (i.e., abusive head trauma [AHT], anoxic-hypoxic head injuries; Nemeth et al., 2019; Sayrs et al., 2022). Individuals who experience head injuries from domestic violence often forego medical treatment. However, these same individuals experience long-term cognitive disturbances, problems at school and work, and antisocial/criminal behavior (e.g., learning disabilities, developmental delays, epilepsy, or visual and auditory processing problems; Anderst et al., 2018; Miller Ferguson et al., 2017; Kelly et al., 2017; Keenen et al., 2019; Nuño et al., 2018; Pendharkar et al., 2022). Poor receptive and expressive language, low physiological arousal (including for rewarding, positively reinforcing events and circumstances) as well as memory disturbances have been linked to early repeated interpersonal violence (Cassiers et al., 2018; Sherin & Nemeroff, 2022).

As a result, individuals with indications of DTD are at heightened risk for school problems and often fail to respond to traditional interventions effectively (e.g., behavior modification, applied behavioral analysis) because of cognitive and physiological changes associated with trauma that cause them to be less influenced by positive and negative reinforcers (reinforcing desirable behaviors in children by giving them attention, verbal praise, and toys/games that they enjoy when they demonstrate positive behaviors or removing things they enjoy less, such as chores). However, these children, adolescents, and adults are also less likely to seek support from others, including healthcare providers, because they feel ashamed and embarrassed; they use denial, alcohol, and drugs to cope; or they engage in violence and eventually come to the attention of law enforcement. This is likely to be worsened by addiction to hard drugs, like crack cocaine, methamphetamines, and opioids (Halpern et al., 2018; Huang et al., 2021), or legal responses by law enforcement that demand compliance and control and that focus far less on rehabilitation and recovery from trauma and addiction.

It is particularly important to identify children who are experiencing developmental trauma within the context of early interpersonal violence exposure. Early interpersonal violence exposure occurs during sensitive periods of development and is highly predictive of – and serves as a pathway to – poverty, prison, disease, and drugs (Jones et al., 2018; Woodhall-Melnik et al., 2018). This progression is in part due to dissociative responses to trauma that increase the risk for repeated perpetration of violence in adulthood (i.e., intergenerational violence that is worsened by physical and emotional problems as well as by neglect and traumatic loss). Systematic reviews and meta-analyses, for example, suggest that witnessing or being a victim of early violence predictably gives rise to violence in adulthood, which is worsened by substance abuse disorders, neurological disturbances, accumulated legal records, and high recidivism rates (Fazel et al., 2018).

Children exposed to early interpersonal violence may demonstrate acute distress reactions and symptoms consistent with PTSD conceptualizations of trauma, such as nightmares, enuresis, or encopresis (bedwetting), problems concentrating, increased mood disturbances, separation anxiety, and preoccupation with safety (associated with flight-flight-freeze adaptations; Dunn et al., 2017). Most individuals with symptoms characteristic of DTD, however, particularly those who have been polyvictimized (physical, verbal, sexual abuse; bullying at school; loss of a caregiver or caregivers; experiences of violence at home and in their communities), have delayed responses to trauma or may appear asymptomatic when classical PTSD symptoms are considered in the absence of DTD or may appear seemingly normal to others. However, they suffer from profound anxiety levels, particularly when returning home from school or work and facing another day of violence, substance abuse, and sleeplessness.

Effects of Community Violence on DTD Children

Children with symptoms characteristic of developmental trauma often experience abuse, neglect, and violence in many settings that is perpetrated by siblings, family, peers, and adults in their communities. Recent studies examining exposure to violence found that while children who experienced PTSD report high levels of physical abuse, DTD children are uniquely affected by high levels of family and community violence and impaired caregivers (i.e., insecure attachment to parents who are less sensitive and responsive to their children's needs; Spinazzola et al., 2018, 2021). Scholars have used the term "toxic triad" to describe the experiences of children who have experienced trauma and have caregivers who exposed them to domestic violence, addiction, and poorly managed parental mental illness (Fuller-Thomson et al., 2021). These circumstances place children at high risk for chronic and debilitating medical problems (mediated by physiological stress and dysregulation of the pituitary-adrenal stress pathway; Ross et al., 2021), psychological disturbances (e.g., DTD, self-mutilation, traumatic psychosis, addiction, antisocial behaviors; Dargis & Koenigs, 2017), and psychosocial adversities (e.g., school failure, housing instability, incarceration; Newman et al., 2022).

Although we have discussed violence that occurs mainly in the home, interpersonal violence also occurs in one's neighborhood and community, including witnessing or being the victim of violent assault, gang-on-gang violence, or neighborhood shootings (Chen & Lee, 2021; Lee et al., 2020; Pickover et al., 2021). Children with DTD are at higher risk for community violence (Pierre et al., 2020; Yearwood et al., 2021). These children ultimately have no safe place to recover from their psychological traumas because they live in dangerous circumstances at home, school, and within their communities. These children may also suffer from food insecurity and substandard living conditions (e.g., unkempt homes, environmental pollution exposure, insect and rodent infestations). However, they may have difficulty asking for help because they may not know where to begin (e.g., whether they should ask for food when living in a home with violence, drugs, and sexual abuse victimization). Research suggests, for example, that children who experience community violence are more likely to develop depression and substance abuse in adulthood than children who experience low early adversity (Cabanis et al., 2021; Dawson-Rose et al., 2020; Lee et al., 2020; Tache et al., 2020).

Children affected by community violence may also ask themselves troubling questions about whether they will (or even should) live a long life and whether they should care enough to put forth the effort to change their ways, including behaviors that mirror their earlier experiences of violence and abuse at the hands of their caregivers. Children may struggle to reconcile these thoughts, which likely cause them to ruminate, dissociate, and experience anger as they hope others will be able to see they are struggling and help them. At the same time, they may be asking whether they should use a weapon (knife or gun) to hurt others before others hurt them.

Trauma and Violence in Multiple Minority Communities

Low-income children and families are disproportionally affected by interpersonal violence, developmental trauma, and polyvictimization, which intersects with race, ethnicity, culture, and sexual orientation (Castro-Ramirez et al., 2021; Maguire-Jack et al., 2021; Pahl et al., 2020; Travers et al., 2022). Families living in low-income communities, including poverty-stricken nations, may also experience mass shootings, terrorism, bombings, and hate crimes against racial, sexual, and religious minorities, which may or may not be adequately addressed by those in positions of power. Indeed, studies continue to demonstrate the cumulative effects of early trauma and violence that are inextricably linked to poor social and economic circumstances worldwide (Gaylord-Harden et al., 2017; Yearwood et al., 2019, 2021).

Research suggests that minority groups, especially children living in low SES conditions as well as racial and sexual minorities, are disproportionately exposed to trauma and violence (Douglas et al., 2021; Ragavan et al., 2020; Richards et al., 2021; Roesch et al., 2021). The results of a recent study with sexual minorities (Brewerton et al., 2022), for example, showed higher rates of early childhood abuse, IPV, and trauma compared to gender-conforming adults. Racial minorities are at greater risk than non-minorities for witnessing domestic violence and experiencing high rates of trauma (Maguire-Jack et al., 2020; Wamser-Nanney et al., 2021). As a result, urban communities often do not recognize or effectively treat DTD symptoms, which likely intersect with high poverty rates, substance abuse, and crime.

LGBTQIA+ individuals are affected by extreme violence, such as exposure to hate crimes, which have been demonstrated to contribute to high suicide rates (Malta et al., 2020; Meyer et al., 2021; Mitchell et al., 2020). They are also over-represented in child welfare systems, as demonstrated by the higher rates of out-of-home placements (i.e., foster care settings) for sexual minority children compared to heterosexual youth (Fish et al., 2019). Research has identified differences between same-sex domestic violence and other-sex domestic violence, including internalized and externalized stressors associated with being a sexual minority that interact with domestic violence to create or exacerbate vulnerabilities, higher risk for complex trauma experiences, and difficulties accessing services (Antebi-Gruszka & Scheer, 2021; Scheer & Poteat, 2021).

A Socioecological Framework of Child Abuse Investigation and Parenting Capacity Evaluation

When child abuse, neglect, or domestic violence is suspected, there are state and federal guidelines that child protection service (CPS) workers follow to ensure the safety and well-being of alleged victims and their siblings. In general, CPS workers conduct an investigation within 24 to 72 hours, interviewing and evaluating all individuals involved, including victims and alleged perpetrators of abuse. Regional diagnostic and treatment centers (RDTCs) and child advocacy centers (CACs) often conduct these investigations, which include multi-disciplinary interviews and evaluations by law enforcement, pediatricians, psychologists, social workers, and child/family advocates in collaboration with family and criminal courts. State and federal policies and practice guidelines provide objective frameworks so that individuals who evaluate families affected by traumas (determining the broad impact of abuse on children's psychological, medical, and interpersonal well-being; evaluating a caregiver's parenting capacity; and determining a child's best interest, such as whether they should remain with their family of origin or be placed with kin or into foster care) can do so with standardized procedures, measurement tools, and evaluation practices (refer to the Child Welfare Information Gateway for these and other resources used; Children's Bureau, 2023).

Children and families affected by trauma may find their experiences with CPS troubling and possibly traumatizing. Caregivers must prove their ability to meet their child's social, economic, emotional, and physical needs, such as adequate housing, food, and healthcare coverage (likely because they have failed to do so in the past). This can give rise to highly contentious interactions between caregivers (e.g., custody disputes), family members (e.g., when family members get involved in supporting a child's mother or father), and professionals (e.g., lawyers defending their clients during court hearings).

Determining a child's best interest, a caregiver's parenting capacity, and the evaluation and treatment procedures designed for complex and developmental traumas must also carefully consider systemic factors, including immigration, racism and discrimination, stigma, and socioeconomic disparities. For example, one parent may have more financial resources than the other, and they may be able to hire multiple attorneys and pursue long-term litigation and appeals while the other caregiver is barely making ends meet. They must also understand and respond to the power differential that exists between individuals affected by trauma and the providers and social systems/institutions that exert influence over them (e.g., when determining whether a child should remain with their family of origin after experiencing abuse or whether they should be put in an out-of-home placement setting). When carrying out their work, healthcare providers, child welfare advocates, and legal system personnel depend on guidance provided by policies and procedures designed to mitigate trauma. In the next section, I discuss some of these policies and procedures in detail, including trauma-responsive policies and legal practices.

Trauma and Violence Victimization-Perpetration

Trauma-informed research, practice, policies, and procedures must also understand the relationships between violence victimization and perpetration. An overriding theme in empirical studies investigating interpersonal trauma and violence is that perpetrators model for children that relationships should be characterized by willful use of power and control because they have been raised to normalize violence as a means to coping and survival. Social and ecological theories of interpersonal violence suggest that children who experience early violence are at higher risk for perpetrating violence and for being revictimized by multiple interpersonal traumas because they dissociate or use alcohol and drugs to cope with emotional pain and numbing, because the systems put in place to protect them failed to do so, and because they were never provided with more healthy and stable relationship models. Research suggests, for example, that male perpetrators of IPV experience severe forms of physical punishment (often at the hands of their father or a male caregiver) compounded by neglect and witnessing family psychological and physical violence (including witnessing their mother be assaulted severely and observing measurable changes in her ability to function either because of traumatic head injury or severe depression; St. Ivany et al., 2018; Teva et al., 2021). Current literature demonstrates a specific pattern in male batterers compared to other criminals, brain alterations in female victims who have suffered post-traumatic stress disorder, and volumetric global changes and alterations in many brain regions in child victims, which may increase their vulnerability to psychopathology.

Research demonstrates that individuals who use violence to cope with psychological distress often experience complex traumas, insecure attachments, personality disturbances, and substance abuse, all of which contribute to normalizing violence (Jung et al., 2019). Interpersonal violence perpetration correlates with low empathy as well as narcissistic and antisocial personality disorders, which are also indicative of developmental trauma, multigenerational violence, and polyvictimization. However, men and women are influenced by violence differently, at least in terms of how they express psychological distress and trauma. For example, experiences of sexual abuse positively predict interpersonal violence and the normalization of coercive control in relationships for women, not men. Furthermore, survivors of sexual abuse are often blamed, violated, and sometimes distrusted by their families, friends, and legal systems, which leave girls and women fending for themselves. Male children are more likely to experience abuse within their communities, and they are also more likely to delay disclosing their abuse or forego disclosure and legal action because of shame, guilt, lack of family support, and stigma (Coburn et al., 2019). Male victims of intimate partner violence experience stereotypes, social expectations, and norms that cause them to deny or underreport abuse, including severe assault (Hine et al., 2022). Croatia is a European country with one of the highest prevalence of domestic violence (DV) against women and without a strategy related to male victims. Men were more likely to suffer psychological abuse. Men were less likely to report abuse to the police and misdemeanor or felony courts (Peraica et al., 2021).

Trauma-Informed Care for Judicial Systems and Policymakers

Scholars have increasingly asserted a growing need for public health responses to trauma, such as those characterized by multicultural trauma-informed care systems, to highlight intersectional approaches, social justice, and organizational and community capacity building (Bassuk et al., 2020; Franklin et al., 2020; Hampton-Anderson et al., 2021; James, 2020; Quintas & Sousa, 2021). This is particularly important for DTD children and families, given the high addiction rates, interpersonal violence, incarceration, and recidivism. Children and families affected by violence often require the support of police officers to assist them in maintaining safety and security, including those living in shelters (Sullivan et al., 2018). Developing violence prevention programs, establishing safe and supportive places for children and families to recover from trauma, and developing and maintaining sound, evidence-based policies, practices, and laws are vital to these efforts.

Domestic violence interventions from law enforcement are subject to change (sometimes dramatically) over time (i.e., chronosystems). They differ by state and country with regard to the level of protection afforded to victims and the support services provided to them (e.g., domestic violence restraining orders [DVROs], mandatory reporting laws, temporary housing, arrests for IPV without a need for a warrant). In 1994, for example, domestic violence protections improved with the passage of the Violence Against Women Act (VAWA) and the Gun Control Act (GCA), which recognized domestic violence as a crime, limited the availability of weapons for perpetrators of IPV, and offered victims of federal violence rights and protections (Sullivan et al., 2021). Nevertheless, national (and international) studies of legal policies, procedures, and practices associated with domestic violence suggest that there are significant problems with current domestic violence investigations, including fidelity to practice models, adherence to procedural laws, a lack of congressional bills designed for trauma-informed care, and failure to comply with human rights standards (e.g., Chin & Cunningham, 2019; Purtle & Lewis, 2017; Zeoli et al., 2019).

In many circumstances, however, victims of domestic violence, often a child's mother, may deny the abuse to law enforcement either because they were threatened with severe consequences, including homicide against her and her children, or because they may be worried about losing children to the foster care system, children they may experience additional traumas (e.g., traumatic separation, institutional abuse). Extended families, who may be able to support caregivers and their children, may have also been subjected to violence and intimidation, leaving victims isolated and dependent on the abuser and children at a higher risk for developmental trauma. Children in these circumstances often have to carry the additional burden of ensuring the safety of their caregivers and siblings as well as their own safety. However, they may be suffering emotionally, experiencing additional problems at school and within their communities, and feeling unable to express their fears to others because doing so might make them a burden. As such, scholars urge widespread use of trauma-informed principles and practices, including by legal systems, such as juvenile justice centers and family and criminal courts.

Trauma-informed policies, such as those published by the Substance Abuse Mental Health Services Administration (SAMHSA), underscore values of safety, trust, transparency, collaboration, empowerment, choice, and intersectional systems-based practices for implementation in medical and behavioral health service settings as well as juvenile justice, youth-serving community centers, schools, and workplaces (Bowen & Irish, 2022; Branson et al., 2017; Champine et al., 2021; Purtle, 2020). This framework reflects an awareness of the universality of trauma and differentiated effects by gender; racial, sexual, and religious minorities spanning skin color; language; acculturation; and health. From a policy perspective, however, research suggests a need for developmentally informed, strength-based policies that highlight positive adaptations to ACEs and trauma (Masten & Barnes, 2018). A trauma-informed perspective and a focus on assets and growth opportunities are relevant to various local, state, federal, and international policies that aim to help individuals to recover and thrive in response to trauma and violence. Creating cost-effective, multilevel, strength-based policies and programs may also help to create environments that prevent psychological traumas or that respond with an appreciation for an individual's felt powerfulness, stigma, and fear of being revictimized in ways that mirror their early traumatic circumstances (Briesch et al., 2020; Champine et al., 2022; Figley & Burnette, 2017; Hamby et al., 2020; Hecht et al., 2018; Matlin et al., 2019; McCrea et al., 2019).

Conclusions

In this chapter, I discussed developmental trauma and violence from a socioecological framework. Early interpersonal violence intersects with a broad range of neurobehavioral disturbances in children that are mediated by social and cultural factors, including institutional responses and interventions. With the widespread implementation of trauma-informed care, individuals who have experienced trauma may get the help that they need, particularly when others (including those in positions of power) understand and respond to trauma effectively. Policymakers should continue to work to develop trauma-informed violence prevention programs and resources that emphasize the measurement of primary and secondary outcomes (individual, social, legal) from a socioecological framework. Trauma-informed care policies must also conceptualize individual responses to trauma as stemming from intergenerational and historical traumas and the failure of social systems and institutions to recognize and respond to traumatic re-enactments effectively. The adverse effects of early trauma, including traumatic experiences by family members who experienced poverty, discrimination, and ineffective evaluation and treatments, may be improved by carefully examining the developmental, systemic, and cultural implications of complex trauma and the kinds of support needed to help these same individuals thrive. Informed support for individuals and families combined with trauma-informed, anti-stigmatizing mental health and social justice advocacy at a systems level is critical to breaking traumatic adaptations to adversity affecting individuals and communities.

References

Anderst, J. D., Carpenter, S. L., Presley, R., Berkoff, M. C., Wheeler, A. P., Sidonio, R. F., Jr, & Soucie, J. M. (2018). Relevance of abusive head trauma to intracranial hemorrhages and bleeding disorders. *Pediatrics*, 141(5), e20173485. https://doi.org/10.1542/peds. 2017-3485.

Antebi-Gruszka, N., & Scheer, J. R. (2021). Associations between trauma-informed care components and multiple health and psychosocial risks among LGBTQ survivors of intimate partner violence. *Journal of Mental Health Counseling*, 43(2), 139–156. https:// doi.org/10.17744/mehc.43.2.04.

Baglivio, M. T., Wolff, K. T., DeLisi, M., Vaughn, M. G., & Piquero, A. R. (2017). Juvenile animal cruelty and firesetting behaviour. *Criminal Behaviour and Mental Health: CBMH*, 27(5), 484–500. https://doi.org/10.1002/cbm.2018.

Bailey, T. D., & Brown, L. S. (2020). Complex trauma: Missed and misdiagnosis in forensic evaluations. *Psychological Injury and Law*, 13(2), 109–123. https://doi.org/10. 1007/s12207-020-09383-w.

Bassuk, E. L., Hart, J. A., & Donovan, E. (2020). Resetting policies to end family homelessness. *Annual Review of Public Health*, 41, 247–263. https://doi.org/10.1146/a nnurev-publhealth-040119-094256.

Becker-Haimes, E. M., Wislocki, K., DiDonato, S., Beidas, R. S., & Jensen-Doss, A. (2021). Youth trauma histories are associated with under-diagnosis and under-treatment of co-occurring youth psychiatric symptoms. *Journal of Clinical Child and Adolescent Psychology*, 53, 1–12. https://doi.org/10.1080/15374416.2021.1923020.

Blodgett, C., & Lanigan, J. D. (2018). The association between adverse childhood experience (ACE) and school success in elementary school children. *School Psychology Quarterly*, 33(1), 137–146. https://doi.org/10.1037/spq0000256.

Boeckel, M. G., Wagner, A., & Grassi-Oliveira, R. (2017). The effects of intimate partner violence exposure on the maternal bond and PTSD symptoms of children. *Journal of Interpersonal Violence*, 32(7), 1127–1142. https://doi.org/10.1177/ 0886260515587667.

Bonache, H., Gonzalez-Mendez, R., & Krahé, B. (2019). Adult attachment styles, destructive conflict resolution, and the experience of intimate partner violence. *Journal of Interpersonal Violence*, 34(2), 287–309. https://doi.org/10.1177/0886260516640776.

Bowen, E. A., & Irish, A. (2022). Trauma and principles of trauma-informed care in the U.S. federal legislative response to the opioid epidemic: A policy mapping analysis. *Psychological Trauma: Theory, Research, Practice and Policy*, 14(7), 1158–1166. https:// doi.org/10.1037/tra0000568.

Branson, C. E., Baetz, C. L., Horwitz, S. M., & Hoagwood, K. E. (2017). Trauma-informed juvenile justice systems: A systematic review of definitions and core components. *Psychological Trauma: Theory, Research, Practice, and Policy*, 9(6), 635–646. https://doi.org/10.1037/tra0000255.

Brewerton, T. D., Suro, G., Gavidia, I., & Perlman, M. M. (2022). Sexual and gender minority individuals report higher rates of lifetime traumas and current PTSD than cisgender heterosexual individuals admitted to residential eating disorder treatment. *Eating and Weight Disorders: EWD*, 27(2), 813–820. https://doi.org/10.1007/s40519-021-01222-4.

Briesch, A. M., Chafouleas, S. M., Nissen, K., & Long, S. (2020). A review of state-level procedural guidance for implementing multitiered systems of support for behavior (MTSS-B). *Journal of Positive Behavior Interventions*, 22(3), 131–144. https://doi.org/10.1177/1098300719884707.

Bright, M. A., Huq, M. S., Spencer, T., Applebaum, J. W., & Hardt, N. (2018). Animal cruelty as an indicator of family trauma: Using adverse childhood experiences to look beyond child abuse and domestic violence. *Child Abuse & Neglect*, 76, 287–296. https://doi.org/10.1016/j.chiabu.2017.11.011.

Burck, D., Walsh, D., & Lynch, D. (2019). Silenced mothers: Exploring definitions of adolescent-to-parent violence and implications for practice. *Advances in Social Work and Welfare Education*, 21(1), 7–18.

Cabanis, M., Outadi, A., & Choi, F. (2021). Early childhood trauma, substance use and complex concurrent disorders among adolescents. *Current Opinion in Psychiatry*, 34(4), 393–399. https://doi.org/10.1097/YCO.0000000000000718.

Cassiers, L. L., Sabbe, B. G., Schmaal, L., Veltman, D. J., Penninx, B. W., & Van Den Eede, F. (2018). Structural and functional brain abnormalities associated with exposure to different childhood trauma subtypes: A systematic review of neuroimaging findings. *Frontiers in Psychiatry*, 9, 329. https://doi.org/10.3389/fpsyt.2018.00329.

Castro-Ramirez, F., Al-Suwaidi, M., Garcia, P., Rankin, O., Ricard, J. R., & Nock, M. K. (2021). Racism and poverty are barriers to the treatment of youth mental health concerns. *Journal of Clinical Child and Adolescent Psychology*, 50(4), 534–546. https://doi.org/10.1080/15374416.2021.1941058.

Champine, R. B., Hoffman, E. E., Matlin, S. L., Strambler, M. J., & Tebes, J. K. (2022). "What does it mean to be trauma-informed?": A mixed-methods study of a trauma-informed community initiative. *Journal of Child and Family Studies*, 31(2), 459–472. https://doi.org/10.1007/s10826-021-02195-9

Chen, W. Y., & Lee, Y. (2021). Mother's exposure to domestic and community violence and its association with child's behavioral outcomes. *Journal of Community Psychology*, 49(7), 2623–2638. https://doi.org/10.1002/jcop.22508.

Children's Bureau. (2023). *Child Welfare Information Gateway*. https://www.childwelfare.gov.

Chin, Y. M., & Cunningham, S. (2019). Revisiting the effect of warrantless domestic violence arrest laws on intimate partner homicides. *Journal of Public Economics*, 179, 104072. https://doi.org/10.1016/j.jpubeco.2019.104072.

Coburn, P. I., Harvey, M. B., Anderson, S. F., Price, H. L., Chong, K., & Connolly, D. A. (2019). Boys abused in a community setting: An analysis of gender, relationship, and delayed prosecutions in cases of child sexual abuse. *Journal of Child Sexual Abuse*, 28(5), 586–607. https://doi.org/10.1080/10538712.2019.1580329.

Croft, J., Heron, J., Teufel, C., Cannon, M., Wolke, D., Thompson, A., Houtepen, L., & Zammit, S. (2019). Association of trauma type, age of exposure, and frequency in childhood and adolescence with psychotic experiences in early adulthood. *JAMA Psychiatry*, 76(1), 79–86. https://doi.org/10.1001/jamapsychiatry.2018.3155.

Dargis, M., & Koenigs, M. (2017). Witnessing domestic violence during childhood is associated with psychopathic traits in adult male criminal offenders. *Law and Human Behavior*, 41(2), 173–179. https://doi.org/10.1037/lhb0000226.

Dawson-Rose, C., Shehadeh, D., Hao, J., Barnard, J., Khoddam-Khorasani, L. L., Leonard, A., Clark, K., Kersey, E., Mousseau, H., Frank, J., Miller, A., Carrico, A., Schustack, A., & Cuca, Y. P. (2020). Trauma, substance use, and mental health symptoms in transitional age youth experiencing homelessness. *Public Health Nursing*, 37(3), 363–370. https://doi.org/10.1111/phn.12727.

DeLisi, M., Drury, A. J., & Elbert, M. J. (2019). The etiology of antisocial personality disorder: The differential roles of adverse childhood experiences and childhood psychopathology. *Comprehensive Psychiatry*, 92, 1–6. https://doi.org/10.1016/j.comppsych.2019.04.001.

Douglas, R. D., Alvis, L. M., Rooney, E. E., Busby, D. R., & Kaplow, J. B. (2021). Racial, ethnic, and neighborhood income disparities in childhood posttraumatic stress and grief: Exploring indirect effects through trauma exposure and bereavement. *Journal of Traumatic Stress*, 34(5), 929–942. https://doi.org/10.1002/jts.22732.

Dunn, E. C., Nishimi, K., Powers, A., & Bradley, B. (2017). Is developmental timing of trauma exposure associated with depressive and post-traumatic stress disorder symptoms in adulthood? *Journal of Psychiatric Research*, 84, 119–127. https://doi.org/10.1016/j.jpsychires.2016.09.004.

Dworkin, E. R., Brill, C. D., & Ullman, S. E. (2019). Social reactions to disclosure of interpersonal violence and psychopathology: A systematic review and meta-analysis. *Clinical Psychology Review*, 72, 101750. https://doi.org/10.1016/j.cpr.2019.101750.

Ertan, D., El-Hage, W., Thierrée, S., Javelot, H., & Hingray, C. (2020). COVID-19: Urgency for distancing from domestic violence. *European Journal of Psychotraumatology*, 11(1), 1800245. https://doi.org/10.1080/20008198.2020.1800245.

Fazel, S., Smith, E. N., Chang, Z., & Geddes, J. R. (2018). Risk factors for interpersonal violence: An umbrella review of meta-analyses. *The British Journal of Psychiatry*, 213(4), 609–614. https://doi.org/10.1192/bjp.2018.145.

Figley, C. R., & Burnette, C. E. (2017). Building bridges: Connecting systemic trauma and family resilience in the study and treatment of diverse traumatized families. *Traumatology*, 23(1), 95–101. https://doi.org/10.1037/trm0000089.

Fish, J. N., Baams, L., Wojciak, A. S., & Russell, S. T. (2019). Are sexual minority youth overrepresented in foster care, child welfare, and out-of-home placement?: Findings from nationally representative data. *Child Abuse & Neglect*, 89, 203–211. https://doi.org/10.1016/j.chiabu.2019.01.005.

Ford, J. D. (2017). Complex trauma and developmental trauma disorder in adolescence. *Adolescent Psychiatry*, 7(4), 220–235. https://doi.org/10.2174/2210676608666180112160419.

Ford, J. D., Grasso, D. J., Jones, S., Works, T., & Andemariam, B. (2020). Interpersonal violence exposure and chronic pain in adult sickle cell patients. *Journal of Interpersonal Violence*, 35(3–4), 924–942. https://doi.org/10.1177/0886260517691521.

Franklin, C. A., Garza, A. D., Goodson, A., & Bouffard, L. A. (2020). Police perceptions of crime victim behaviors: A trend analysis exploring mandatory training and knowledge of sexual and domestic violence survivors' trauma responses. *Crime & Delinquency*, 66(8), 1055–1086. https://doi.org/10.1177/0011128719845148.

Fuller-Thomson, E., Sawyer, J.-L., & Agbeyaka, S. (2021). The toxic triad: Childhood exposure to parental domestic violence, parental addictions, and parental mental illness as factors associated with childhood physical abuse. *Journal of Interpersonal Violence*, 36(17–18), NP9015–NP9034. https://doi.org/10.1177/0886260519853407.

Gallegos, A. M., Trabold, N., Cerulli, C., & Pigeon, W. R. (2021). Sleep and interpersonal violence: A systematic review. *Trauma, Violence, & Abuse*, 22(2), 359–369. https://doi.org/10.1177/1524838019852633.

Gardner, M. J., Thomas, H. J., & Erskine, H. E. (2019). The association between five forms of child maltreatment and depressive and anxiety disorders: A systematic review and meta-analysis. *Child Abuse & Neglect*, 96, 104082. https://doi.org/10.1016/j.chiabu.2019.104082.

Gatfield, E., O'Leary, P., Meyer, S., & Baird, K. (2022). A multitheoretical perspective for addressing domestic and family violence: Supporting fathers to parent without harm. *Journal of Social Work*, 22(4), 876–895. https://doi.org/10.1177/14680173211028562.

Gaylord-Harden, N. K., So, S., Bai, G. J., Henry, D. B., & Tolan, P. H. (2017). Examining the pathologic adaptation model of community violence exposure in male adolescents of color. *Journal of Clinical Child and Adolescent Psychology*, 46(1), 125–135. https://doi.org/10.1080/15374416.2016.1204925.

Grasso, D. J. (2022). A trauma-informed approach to assessment, case conceptualisation, and treatment planning for youth exposed to intimate partner violence. *Journal of Health Service Psychology*, 48(1), 3–11. https://doi.org/10.1007/s42843-021-00053-2.

Halpern, S. C., Schuch, F. B., Scherer, J. N., Sordi, A. O., Pachado, M., Dalbosco, C., Fara, L., Pechansky, L., Kessler, F., & Von Diemen, L. (2018). Child maltreatment and illicit substance abuse: A systematic review and meta-analysis of longitudinal studies. *Child Abuse Review*, 27(5), 344–360. https://doi.org/10.1002/car.2534.

Hamby, S., Taylor, E., Mitchell, K., Jones, L., & Newlin, C. (2020). Poly-victimization, trauma, and resilience: Exploring strengths that promote thriving after adversity. *Journal of Trauma & Dissociation*, 21(3), 376–395. https://doi.org/10.1080/15299732.2020.1719261.

Hampton-Anderson, J. N., Carter, S., Fani, N., Gillespie, C. F., Henry, T. L., Holmes, E., Lamis, D. A., LoParo, D., Maples-Keller, J. L., Powers, A., Sonu, S., & Kaslow, N. J. (2021). Adverse childhood experiences in African Americans: Framework, practice, and policy. *American Psychologist*, 76(2), 314–325. https://doi.org/10.1037/amp0000767.

Haselschwerdt, M. L., Hlavaty, K., Carlson, C., Schneider, M., Maddox, L., & Skipper, M. (2019). Heterogeneity within domestic violence exposure: Young adults' retrospective experiences. *Journal of Interpersonal Violence*, 34(7), 1512–1538. https://doi.org/10.1177/0886260516651625.

Hauw, M. E., Revranche, M., Kovess-Masfety, V., & Husky, M. M. (2021). Sexual and nonsexual interpersonal violence, psychiatric disorders, and mental health service use. *Journal of Traumatic Stress*, 34(2), 416–426. https://doi.org/10.1002/jts.22638.

Hecht, A. A., Biehl, E., Buzogany, S., & Neff, R. A. (2018). Using a trauma-informed policy approach to create a resilient urban food system. *Public Health Nutrition*, 21(10), 1961–1970. https://doi.org/10.1017/S1368980018000198.

Hernández, A., Martín, A. M., Hess-Medler, S., & García-García, J. (2020). What goes on in this house do not stay in this house: Family variables related to adolescent-to-parent offenses. *Frontiers in Psychology*, 11, 581761. https://doi.org/10.3389/fpsyg.2020.581761.

Heward-Belle, S., Laing, L., Humphreys, C., & Toivonen, C. (2018). Intervening with children living with domestic violence: Is the system safe? *Australian Social Work*, 71(2), 135–147. https://doi.org/10.1080/0312407X.2017.1422772.

Hine, B., Bates, E. A., & Wallace, S. (2022). "I have guys call me and say 'I can't be the victim of domestic abuse'": Exploring the experiences of telephone support providers for male victims of domestic violence and abuse. *Journal of Interpersonal Violence*, 37(7–8), NP5594–NP5625. https://doi.org/10.1177/0886260520944551.

Huang, C., Yuan, Q., Zhang, L., Wang, L., Cui, S., Zhang, K., & Zhou, X. (2021). Associations between childhood trauma and the age of first-time drug use in methamphetamine-dependent patients. *Frontiers in Psychiatry*, 12, 658205. https://doi.org/10.3389/fpsyt.2021.658205.

Ibabe, I. (2019). Adolescent-to-parent violence and family environment: The perceptions of same reality? *International Journal of Environmental Research and Public Health*, 16(12), 2215. https://doi.org/10.3390/ijerph16122215.

St. Ivany, A., Kools, S., Sharps, P., & Bullock, L. (2018). Extreme control and instability: Insight into head injury from intimate partner violence. *Journal of Forensic Nursing*, 14 (4), 190–205. https://doi.org/10.1097/JFN.0000000000000220.

James, C. (2020). Towards trauma-informed legal practice: A review. *Psychiatry, Psychology, and Law*, 27(2), 275–299. https://doi.org/10.1080/13218719.2020. 1719377.

Jegatheesan, B., Enders-Slegers, M. J., Ormerod, E., & Boyden, P. (2020). Understanding the link between animal cruelty and family violence: The bioecological systems model. *International Journal of Environmental Research and Public Health*, 17(9), 3116. https://doi.org/10.3390/ijerph17093116.

John, S. G., Brandt, T. W., Secrist, M. E., Mesman, G. R., Sigel, B. A., & Kramer, T. L. (2019). Empirically-guided assessment of complex trauma for children in foster care: A focus on appropriate diagnosis of attachment concerns. *Psychological Services*, 16 (1), 120–133. https://doi.org/10.1037/ser0000263.

Jones, M. S., Worthen, M. G., Sharp, S. F., & McLeod, D. A. (2018). Bruised inside out: The adverse and abusive life histories of incarcerated women as pathways to PTSD and illicit drug use. *Justice Quarterly*, 35(6), 1004–1029. https://doi.org/10. 1080/07418825.2017.1355009.

Jung, H., Herrenkohl, T. I., Skinner, M. L., Lee, J. O., Klika, J. B., & Rousson, A. N. (2019). Gender differences in intimate partner violence: A predictive analysis of IPV by child abuse and domestic violence exposure during early childhood. *Violence Against Women*, 25(8), 903–924. https://doi.org/10.1177/1077801218796329.

Keenan, H. T., Presson, A. P., Clark, A. E., Cox, C. S., & Ewing-Cobbs, L. (2019). Longitudinal developmental outcomes after traumatic brain injury in young children: Are infants more vulnerable than toddlers? *Journal of Neurotrauma*, 36(2), 282–292. https://doi.org/10.1089/neu.2018.5687.

Kelly, P., Thompson, J. M. D., Koh, J., Ameratunga, S., Jelleyman, T., Percival, T. M., Elder, H., & Mitchell, E. A. (2017). Perinatal risk and protective factors for pediatric abusive head trauma: A multicenter case-control study. *The Journal of Pediatrics*, 187, 240–246.e4. https://doi.org/10.1016/j.jpeds.2017.04.058.

Kim, J., Lee, B., & Farber, N. B. (2019). Where do they learn violence?: The roles of three forms of violent socialization in childhood. *Children and Youth Services Review*, 107, 104494. https://doi.org/10.1016/j.childyouth.2019.104494.

Kourti, A., Stavridou, A., Panagouli, E., Psaltopoulou, T., Spiliopoulou, C., Tsolia, M., Sergentanis, T. N., & Tsitsika, A. (2021). Domestic violence during the COVID-19 pandemic: A systematic review. *Trauma, Violence & Abuse*, 15248380211038690. Advance online publication. https://doi.org/10.1177/15248380211038690.

Laing, L. (2017). Secondary victimization: Domestic violence survivors navigating the family law system. *Violence Against Women*, 23(11), 1314–1335. https://doi.org/10.1177/1077801216659942.

Lee, H., Kim, Y., & Terry, J. (2020). Adverse childhood experiences (ACEs) on mental disorders in young adulthood: Latent classes and community violence exposure. *Preventive Medicine*, 134, 106039. https://doi.org/10.1016/j.ypmed.2020.106039.

Lee, J. M., Kim, J., Hong, J. S., & Marsack-Topolewski, C. N. (2021). From bully victimization to aggressive behavior: Applying the problem behavior theory, theory of stress and coping, and general strain theory to explore potential pathways. *Journal of Interpersonal Violence*, 36(21–22),10314–10337. https://doi.org/10.1177/0886260519884679.

LeMoult, J., Humphreys, K. L., Tracy, A., Hoffmeister, J. A., Ip, E., & Gotlib, I. H. (2020). Meta-analysis: Exposure to early life stress and risk for depression in childhood and adolescence. *Journal of the American Academy of Child and Adolescent Psychiatry*, 59 (7), 842–855. https://doi.org/10.1016/j.jaac.2019.10.011.

Liu, J., Mahendran, R., Chong, S. A., & Subramaniam, M. (2021). Elucidating the impact of childhood, adulthood, and cumulative lifetime trauma exposure on psychiatric symptoms in early schizophrenia spectrum disorders. *Journal of Traumatic Stress*, 34(1), 137–148. https://doi.org/10.1002/jts.22607.

Maguire-Jack, K., Font, S., Dillard, R., Dvalishvili, D., & Barnhart, S. (2021). Neighborhood poverty and adverse childhood experiences over the first 15 years of life. *International Journal on Child Maltreatment: Research, Policy and Practice*, 4(1), 93–114. https://doi.org/10.1007/s42448-021-00072-y.

Maguire-Jack, K., Lanier, P., & Lombardi, B. (2020). Investigating racial differences in clusters of adverse childhood experiences. *American Journal of Orthopsychiatry*, 90(1), 106–114. https://doi.org/10.1037/ort0000405.

Malta, M., Gomes de Jesus, J., LeGrand, S., Seixas, M., Benevides, B., Silva, M. D. D., Lana, J. S., Huynh, H. V., Belden, C. M., & Whetten, K. (2020). 'Our life is pointless … ': Exploring discrimination, violence and mental health challenges among sexual and gender minorities from Brazil. *Global Public Health*, 15(10), 1463–1478. https://doi.org/10.1080/17441692.2020.1767676.

Masten, A. S., & Barnes, A. J. (2018). Resilience in children: Developmental perspectives. *Children*, 5(7), 98. https://doi.org/10.3390/children5070098.

Matlin, S. L., Champine, R. B., Strambler, M. J., O'Brien, C., Hoffman, E., Whitson, M., Kolka, L., & Tebes, J. K. (2019). A community's response to adverse childhood experiences: Building a resilient, trauma-informed community. *American Journal of Community Psychology*, 64(3–4), 451–466. https://doi.org/10.1002/ajcp.12386.

McCrea, K. T., Richards, M., Quimby, D., Scott, D., Davis, L., Hart, S., Thomas, A., & Hopson, S. (2019). Understanding violence and developing resilience with African American youth in high-poverty, high-crime communities. *Children and Youth Services Review*, 99, 296–307. https://doi.org/10.1016/j.childyouth.2018.12.018.

McKay, T. (2022). Toward a social ecology of Johnson's types: Exploring pathways to situational couple violence and coercive controlling violence among returning prisoners. *Journal of Family Violence*, 1–14. https://doi.org/10.1007/s10896-022-00444-z.

Medjkane, F., Notredame, C. E., Sharkey, L., D'Hondt, F., Vaiva, G., & Jardri, R. (2020). Association between childhood trauma and multimodal early-onset hallucinations. *The British Journal of Psychiatry: The Journal of Mental Science*, 216(3), 156–158. https://doi.org/10.1192/bjp.2019.266.

Meyer, I. H., Russell, S. T., Hammack, P. L., Frost, D. M., & Wilson, B. D. (2021). Minority stress, distress, and suicide attempts in three cohorts of sexual minority adults: A US probability sample. *PLoS One*, 16(3), e0246827. https://doi.org/10.1371/journal.pone.0246827.

Miller Ferguson, N., Sarnaik, A., Miles, D., Shafi, N., Peters, M. J., Truemper, E., Vavilala, M. S., Bell, M. J., Wisniewski, S. R., Luther, J. F., Hartman, A. L., Kochanek, P. M., & Investigators of the Approaches and Decisions in Acute Pediatric Traumatic Brain Injury (ADAPT) Trial. (2017). Abusive head trauma and mortality: An analysis from an international comparative effectiveness study of children with severe traumatic brain injury. *Critical Care Medicine*, 45(8), 1398–1407. https://doi.org/10.1097/CCM.0000000000002378.

Mitchell, K. J., Jones, L. M., Turner, H. A., Hamby, S., Farrell, A., Cuevas, C., & Daly, B. (2020). Exposure to multiple forms of bias victimization on youth and young adults: Relationships with trauma symptomatology and social support. *Journal of Youth and Adolescence*, 49(10), 1961–1975. https://doi.org/10.1007/s10964-020-01304-z.

Mora, A. S., Ceballo, R., & Cranford, J. A. (2022). Latino/a adolescents facing neighborhood dangers: An examination of community violence and gender-based harassment. *American Journal of Community Psychology*, 69(1–2), 18–32. https://doi.org/10.1002/ajcp.12556.

Narayan, A. J., Labella, M. H., Englund, M. M., Carlson, E. A., & Egeland, B. (2017). The legacy of early childhood violence exposure to adulthood intimate partner violence: Variable- and person-oriented evidence. *Journal of Family Psychology*, 31(7), 833–843. https://doi.org/10.1037/fam0000327.

Nemeth, J. M., Mengo, C., Kulow, E., Brown, A., & Ramirez, R. (2019). Provider perceptions and domestic violence (DV) survivor experiences of traumatic and anoxic-hypoxic brain injury: Implications for DV advocacy service provision. *Journal of Aggression, Maltreatment & Trauma*, 28(6), 744–763. https://doi.org/10.1080/10926771.2019.1591562.

Newman, M., Fedina, L., Nam, B., DeVylder, J., & Alleyne-Green, B. (2022). Associations between interpersonal violence, psychological distress, and suicidal ideation among formerly incarcerated men and women. *Journal of Interpersonal Violence*, 37(3–4), NP2338–NP2359. https://doi.org/10.1177/0886260520933045.

Nuño, M., Ugiliweneza, B., Zepeda, V., Anderson, J. E., Coulter, K., Magana, J. N., Drazin, D., & Boakye, M. (2018). Long-term impact of abusive head trauma in young children. *Child Abuse & Neglect*, 85, 39–46. https://doi.org/10.1016/j.chiabu.2018.08.011.

Ortega Pacheco, Y. J., & Martínez Rudas, M. (2021). Domestic violence and COVID-19 in Colombia. *Psychiatry Research*, 300, 113925. https://doi.org/10.1016/j.psychres.2021.113925.

Pahl, K., Williams, S. Z., Lee, J. Y., Joseph, A., & Blau, C. (2020). Trajectories of violent victimization predicting PTSD and comorbidities among urban ethnic/racial minorities. *Journal of Consulting and Clinical Psychology*, 88(1), 39–47. https://doi.org/10.1037/ccp0000449.

Pendharkar, H., Jabeen, S., Pruthi, N., Narasinga Rao, K. V. L. N., Shukla, D., Kamble, N., Jangam, K. V., Kommu, J. V. S., Kandavel, T., & Amudhan, S. (2022). Abusive head trauma in India: Imaging raises the curtain. *International Journal of Injury Control and Safety Promotion*, 29(1), 103–111. https://doi.org/10.1080/17457300.2021.2007955.

Peraica, T., Kovačić Petrović, Z., Barić, Ž., Galić, R., & Kozarić-Kovačić, D. (2021). Gender differences among domestic violence help-seekers: socio-demographic characteristics, types and duration of violence, perpetrators, and interventions. *Journal of Family Violence*, 36, 429–442. https://doi.org/10.1007/s10896-020-00207-8.

Pickover, A. M., Bhimji, J., Sun, S., Evans, A., Allbaugh, L. J., Dunn, S. E., & Kaslow, N. J. (2021). Neighborhood disorder, social support, and outcomes among violence-exposed African American women. *Journal of Interpersonal Violence*, 36(7–8), NP3716–NP3737. https://doi.org/10.1177/0886260518779599.

Pierre, C. L., Burnside, A., & Gaylord-Harden, N. K. (2020). A longitudinal examination of community violence exposure, school belongingness, and mental health among African-American adolescent males. *School Mental Health: A Multidisciplinary Research and Practice Journal*, 12(2), 388–399. https://doi.org/10.1007/s12310-020-09359-w.

Piquero, A. R., Jennings, W. G., Jemison, E., Kaukinen, C., & Knaul, F. M. (2021). Domestic violence during the COVID-19 pandemic: Evidence from a systematic review and meta-analysis. *Journal of Criminal Justice*, 74, 101806. https://doi.org/10.1016/j.jcrimjus.2021.101806.

Pokharel, B., Hegadoren, K., & Papathanassoglou, E. (2020). Factors influencing silencing of women who experience intimate partner violence: An integrative review. *Aggression and Violent Behavior*, 52, 101422. https://doi.org/10.1016/j.avb.2020.101422.

Purtle, J. (2020). Systematic review of evaluations of trauma-informed organizational interventions that include staff trainings. *Trauma, Violence, & Abuse*, 21(4), 725–740. https://doi.org/10.1177/1524838018791304.

Purtle, J., & Lewis, M. (2017). Mapping "trauma-informed" legislative proposals in U.S. Congress. *Administration and Policy in Mental Health and Mental Health Services Research*, 44(6), 867–876. https://doi.org/10.1007/s10488-017-0799-9.

Quintas, J., & Sousa, P. (2021). Does a coordinated program between the police and prosecution services matter?: The impacts on satisfaction and safety of domestic violence victims. *Criminal Justice Policy Review*, 32(4), 331–351. https://doi.org/10.1177/0887403420920331.

Ragavan, M. I., Thomas, K. A., Fulambarker, A., Zaricor, J., Goodman, L. A., & Bair-Merritt, M. H. (2020). Exploring the needs and lived experiences of racial and ethnic minority domestic violence survivors through community-based participatory research: A systematic review. *Trauma, Violence & Abuse*, 21(5), 946–963. https://doi.org/10.1177/1524838018813204.

Richards, T. N., Schwartz, J. A., & Wright, E. (2021). Examining adverse childhood experiences among Native American persons in a nationally representative sample: Differences among racial/ethnic groups and race/ethnicity-sex dyads. *Child Abuse & Neglect*, 111, 104812. https://doi.org/10.1016/j.chiabu.2020.104812.

Roesch, P. T., Velonis, A. J., Sant, S. M., Habermann, L. E., & Hirschtick, J. L. (2021). Implications of interpersonal violence on population mental health status in a low-income urban community-based sample of adults. *Journal of Interpersonal Violence*, 36 (19–20), 8891–8914. https://doi.org/10.1177/0886260519862365.

Ross, M. C., Sartin-Tarm, A. S., Letkiewicz, A. M., Crombie, K. M., & Cisler, J. M. (2021). Distinct cortical thickness correlates of early life trauma exposure and post-traumatic stress disorder are shared among adolescent and adult females with interpersonal violence exposure. *Neuropsychopharmacology*, 46(4), 741–749. https://doi.org/10.1038/s41386-020-00918-y.

Russell, J. D., Keding, T. J., He, Q., Li, J. J., & Herringa, R. J. (2020). Childhood exposure to interpersonal violence is associated with greater transdiagnostic integration of psychiatric symptoms. *Psychological Medicine*, 52(10), 1883–1891. https://doi.org/10.1017/S0033291720003712.

Sayrs, L. W., Ortiz, J. B., Notrica, D. M., Kirsch, L., Kelly, C., Stottlemyre, R., Cohen, A., Misra, S., Green, T. R., Adelson, P. D., Lifshitz, J., & Rowe, R. K. (2022). Intimate partner violence, clinical indications, and other family risk factors associated with pediatric abusive head trauma. *Journal of Interpersonal Violence*, 37(9–10), NP6785–NP6812. https://doi.org/10.1177/0886260520967151.

Serrano-Montilla, C., Lozano, L. M., Bender, M., & Padilla, J. L. (2020). Individual and societal risk factors of attitudes justifying intimate partner violence against women: A multilevel cross-sectional study. *BMJ Open*, 10(12), e037993. https://doi.org/10.1136/bmjopen-2020-037993.

Setién-Suero, E., Suárez-Pinilla, P., Ferro, A., Tabarés-Seisdedos, R., Crespo-Facorro, B., & Ayesa-Arriola, R. (2020). Childhood trauma and substance use underlying psychosis: A systematic review. *European Journal of Psychotraumatology*, 11(1), 1748342. https://doi.org/10.1080/20008198.2020.1748342.

Scheer, J. R., & Poteat, V. P. (2021). Trauma-informed care and health among LGBTQ intimate partner violence survivors. *Journal of Interpersonal Violence*, 36(13–14), 6670–6692. https://doi.org/10.1177/0886260518820688.

Sherin, J. E., & Nemeroff, C. B. (2022). Post-traumatic stress disorder: The neurobiological impact of psychological trauma. *Dialogues in Clinical Neuroscience*, 13(3), 263–278. https://doi.org/10.31887/DCNS.2011.13.2/jsherin.

Sikweyiya, Y., Addo-Lartey, A. A., Alangea, D. O., Dako-Gyeke, P., Chirwa, E. D., Coker-Appiah, D., Adanu, R.M.K., & Jewkes, R. (2020). Patriarchy and gender-inequitable attitudes as drivers of intimate partner violence against women in the central region of Ghana. *BMC Public Health*, 20(1), 1–11. https://doi.org/10.1186/s12889-020-08825-z.

Song, Y., Zhang, J., & Zhang, X. (2021). Cultural or institutional?: Contextual effects on domestic violence against women in rural China. *Journal of Family Violence*, 36(6), 643–655. https://doi.org/10.1007/s10896-020-00198-6.

Speranza, A. M., Farina, B., Bossa, C., Fortunato, A., Maggiora Vergano, C., Palmiero, L., Quintigliano, M., & Liotti, M. (2022). The role of complex trauma and attachment patterns in intimate partner violence. *Frontiers in Psychology*, 12, 769584. https://doi.org/10.3389/fpsyg.2021.769584.

Spinazzola, J., van der Kolk, B., & Ford, J. D. (2018). When nowhere is safe: Interpersonal trauma and attachment adversity as antecedents of posttraumatic stress disorder and developmental trauma disorder. *Journal of Traumatic Stress*, 31(5), 631–642. https://doi.org/10.1002/jts.22320.

Spinazzola, J., van der Kolk, B., & Ford, J. D. (2021). Developmental trauma disorder: A legacy of attachment trauma in victimized children. *Journal of Traumatic Stress*, 34(4), 711–720. https://doi.org/10.1002/jts.22697.

Stempel, H., Cox-Martin, M., Bronsert, M., Dickinson, L. M., & Allison, M. A. (2017). Chronic school absenteeism and the role of adverse childhood experiences. *Academic Pediatrics*, 17(8), 837–843. https://doi.org/10.1016/j.acap.2017.09.013.

Stephens, D., & Eaton, A. (2020). Cultural factors influencing young adult Indian women's beliefs about disclosing domestic violence victimization. *Journal of Social Issues*, 76(2), 416–446. https://doi.org/10.1111/josi.12385.

Stoffel, B. C. M. M., Henrique, P. K. F., Flavio, P., Olivier, S. M. F., Tatiana, H. L., Group, B. C., & Marcelo, S. C. (2019). Crack users and violence: What is the relationship between trauma, antisocial personality disorder and posttraumatic stress disorder? *Addictive Behaviors*, 98, 106012. https://doi.org/10.1016/j.addbeh.2019.06.001.

Sullivan, C. M., Goodman, L. A., Virden, T., Strom, J., & Ramirez, R. (2018). Evaluation of the effects of receiving trauma-informed practices on domestic violence shelter residents. *American Journal of Orthopsychiatry*, 88(5), 563–570. https://doi.org/10.1037/ort0000286.

Sullivan, T. P., Weiss, N. H., Woerner, J., & Belliveau, D. (2021). Criminal protection orders: Implications of requested versus issued orders on domestic violence revictimization and mental health among women. *Journal of Interpersonal Violence*, 37(19–20), NP18445–NP18464. https://doi.org/10.1177/08862605211035875.

Tache, R. M., Lambert, S. F., & Ialongo, N. S. (2020). The role of depressive symptoms in substance use among African American boys exposed to community violence. *Journal of Traumatic Stress*, 33(6), 1039–1047. https://doi.org/10.1002/jts.22566.

Talevi, D., Pacitti, F., Costa, M., Rossi, A., Collazzoni, A., Crescini, C., & Rossi, R. (2019). Further exploration of personal and social functioning: The role of interpersonal violence, service engagement, and social network. *The Journal of Nervous and Mental Disease*, 207(10), 832–837. https://doi.org/10.1097/NMD.0000000000001036.

Tekkas Kerman, K., & Betrus, P. (2020). Violence against women in Turkey: A social ecological framework of determinants and prevention strategies. *Trauma, Violence, & Abuse*, 21(3), 510–526. https://doi.org/10.1177/1524838018781104.

Teva, I., Hidalgo-Ruzzante, N., Pérez-García, M., & Bueso-Izquierdo, N. (2021). Characteristics of childhood family violence experiences in Spanish batterers. *Journal of Interpersonal Violence*, 36(23–24), 11212–11235. https://doi.org/10.1177/0886260519898436.

Theall, K. P., Shirtcliff, E. A., Dismukes, A. R., Wallace, M., & Drury, S. S. (2017). Association between neighborhood violence and biological stress in children. *JAMA Pediatrics*, 171(1), 53–60. https://doi.org/10.1001/jamapediatrics.2016.2321.

Travers, Á., McDonagh, T., McLafferty, M., Armour, C., Cunningham, T., & Hansen, M. (2022). Adverse experiences and mental health problems in perpetrators of intimate partner violence in Northern Ireland: A latent class analysis. *Child Abuse & Neglect*, 125, 105455. https://doi.org/10.1016/j.chiabu.2021.105455.

Tussey, B. E., Tyler, K. A., & Simons, L. G. (2021). Poor parenting, attachment style, and dating violence perpetration among college students. *Journal of Interpersonal Violence*, 36(5–6), 2097–2116. https://doi.org/10.1177/0886260518760017.

Wamser-Nanney, R., Cherry, K. E., Campbell, C., & Trombetta, E. (2021). Racial differences in children's trauma symptoms following complex trauma exposure. *Journal of Interpersonal Violence*, 36(5–6), 2498–2520. https://doi.org/10.1177/0886260518760019.

Watt, T. T., Hartfield, K., Kim, S., & Ceballos, N. (2021). Adverse childhood experiences contribute to race/ethnic differences in post-secondary academic performance among college students. *Journal of American College Health*, 1–9. Advance online publication. https://doi.org/10.1080/07448481.2021.1947838.

Woodhall-Melnik, J., Dunn, J. R., Svenson, S., Patterson, C., & Matheson, F. I. (2018). Men's experiences of early life trauma and pathways into long-term homelessness. *Child Abuse & Neglect*, 80, 216–225. https://doi.org/10.1016/j.chiabu.2018.03.027.

Yalley, A. A., & Olutayo, M. S. (2020). Gender, masculinity and policing: An analysis of the implications of police masculinised culture on policing domestic violence in southern Ghana and Lagos, Nigeria. *Social Sciences & Humanities Open*, 2(1), 100077. https://doi.org/10.1016/j.ssaho.2020.100077.

Yearwood, K., Vliegen, N., Chau, C., Corveleyn, J., & Luyten, P. (2019). When do peers matter?: The moderating role of peer support in the relationship between environmental adversity, complex trauma, and adolescent psychopathology in socially disadvantaged adolescents. *Journal of Adolescence*, 72, 14–22. https://doi.org/10.1016/j.adolescence.2019.02.001.

Yearwood, K., Vliegen, N., Chau, C., Corveleyn, J., & Luyten, P. (2021). Prevalence of exposure to complex trauma and community violence and their associations with internalizing and externalizing symptoms. *Journal of Interpersonal Violence*, 36(1–2), 843–861. https://doi.org/10.1177/0886260517731788.

Zeoli, A. M., Frattaroli, S., Roskam, K., & Herrera, A. K. (2019). Removing firearms from those prohibited from possession by domestic violence restraining orders: A survey and analysis of state laws. *Trauma, Violence, & Abuse*, 20(1), 114–125. https://doi.org/10.1177/1524838017692384.

6

CONCEPTUALIZATION OF DEVELOPMENTAL TRAUMA FROM A STRENGTHS AND RESILIENCY PERSPECTIVE

Do you love yourself? Can you accept yourself for who you are regardless of your short-comings? How is your self-esteem, and what influences how you feel about yourself? Do you feel generally positive or negative about yourself? What helps you to feel good about yourself? What do you value in yourself and others? Also, how do these values influence your decisions, life choices, and relationships? Who do you love, feel most connected to, and trust enough to see you at your best and worst?

Carl Rogers – the originator of Humanistic and Person-Centered Psychology – believed that people are born with all the personal capital (resources) needed to survive, solve problems, and, more importantly, flourish and contribute positively to the lives of others (Rogers, 1980). Rogers postulated that people are inherently kind, strong, and capable of living what he referred to as "the good life." The good life, according to Rogers, is a life that is genuine, present-centered, and compatible with one's core values, beliefs, and strengths.

Rogers also viewed as vital to well-being the presence of supportive environments, including developing genuine/authentic relationships with others characterized by unconditional positive regard. For DTD children, this would mean that we would care for them regardless of their psychological and behavioral disturbances, avoid stigmatizing them, and convey that their extreme displays of anger and aggression are likely because they are fearful and need validation, acceptance, love, and support from others. When we respond negatively to individuals affected by early traumas, we are likely to re-traumatize them because we may mirror the types of negative interactions they once had with caregivers. If we focus only on their negative behaviors, we also miss opportunities to get to know them beyond their diagnoses, symptoms, and challenges.

Carl Rogers believed that referring to people by their diagnoses or referring to people as patients undermines their identity, diversity, individuality, value,

DOI: 10.4324/9781003304715-6

and intersubjective experiences, all of which are key to understanding and treating individuals who come to the attention of healthcare providers. According to Rogers, our ideas are *socially constructed*, meaning they are inextricably linked to social and cultural norms, values, stereotypes, and expectations, which, in turn, influence how individuals understand themselves and others (and how healthcare providers understand and work with clients; Nowakowski et al., 2019; Street & Dardis, 2018).

To illustrate the concept of social constructionism in more detail, I invite you to consider the following reflection exercise.

Case in Point

Are you good or evil? Do you consider yourself talented, outgoing, and extroverted, or do you prefer to stay home, watch television, and avoid crowds and social gatherings at all costs? How have others described you? As artistic? Bossy? Anxious? Funny? Lazy?

The questions raised here illustrate that many of the terms we use to describe ourselves and others (including the diagnostic labels we use to describe psychological disorders) are not easily defined or measured because they are psychological and social ideas that are inextricably linked to social and cultural norms. Researchers use social constructivism to describe how we use our personal experiences and beliefs (cognitive schemas and assumptions) to classify information (into categories and groups) and to interpret concepts such as intelligence, personality, anxiety, spirituality, trauma, and resilience (Fried, 2017; Hayden, 2022; Hirschberger, 2018; Knight et al., 2018). I raise these ideas because they will inevitably influence how we think about individuals who have experienced trauma, including how we come to understand and evaluate their strengths. Our ideas also change (sometimes dramatically) over time, and different cultures respond differently to stress and trauma as well as in the ways they express positive adaptions and well-being.

Introduction to Positive Psychology

Advances in theory, research, and practice (e.g., Achenbach and Cicchetti's developmental psychopathology model; transdiagnostic mechanisms – risk and protective factors evident across psychological and medical adaptations to ACEs, stress, and trauma; and Mark Seligman's positive psychology and neuroscience framework; See detailed reviews by Chaplin et al., 2018; Eme, 2017; Lai et al., 2019; Oppenheimer et al., 2022; Snyder et al., 2019; Waters et al., 2021b; Weissman et al., 2019) have delineated broad positive influences associated with stress that have the potential to enhance children's social, cognitive, physiological, and emotional development. Scholars have asserted that an exclusive focus on ACEs and traumatic stress disorders limits opportunities for balanced evaluation and treatment as well as advances in research that can inform the development of positive, strengths-based prevention and interventions (Bethell et al., 2019; Crandall et al., 2019; Ross et al., 2020). Although ACEs and developmental trauma positively correlate with trauma–related symptoms, studies have shown that this relationship is mediated and moderated by family/social support, positive coping, mindfulness, resilience and enculturation, acculturation, and assimilation to multiple cultures, including with one's family of origin (Bravo et al., 2022; Clements-Nolle & Waddington, 2019; Goldenson et al., 2021; Kuhar & Zager Kocjan, 2021, 2022; McKeen et al., 2021).

Contemporary research and practice in humanistic and positive psychology and neuroscience has resulted in an upsurge of scientific scholarship, evidence-based practice models, and strengths-based approaches that recognize and assess individual and community capacities (rather than deficiencies). From this perspective, concepts such as salutogenesis (i.e., the scientific study of positive health and well-being), stress–related growth (SRG), resiliency, human capital, and positive childhood experiences (PCEs) have been identified and studied (Antebi-Gruszka et al., 2022; Figley & Burnette, 2017; Höltge et al., 2018; Huss & Samson, 2018; Liu et al., 2017; Rabenu et al., 2017). Likewise, these approaches have been extended to mainstream practice models, such as the collaborative/therapeutic assessment and neuropsychological assessment model (Durosini et al., 2017; Gorske, 2017; Kamphuis & Finn, 2019; Waldron-Perrine et al., 2021) and the character strengths and virtues assessment framework (Martínez-Martí & Ruch, 2017, Niemiec, 2020; Ruch et al., 2021; Snow, 2019), which exclusively focuses on strengths and assets. The possible range of positive and resilient adaptations to stress and trauma raised here will be discussed in more detail in this chapter, including how to measure individual strengths in assessment and evaluation procedures for children, adolescents, and adults affected by developmental trauma.

Positive Physiological Stress Response

The stress response system has been linked to longstanding psychological and physiological problems, such as those that adversely affect individuals who have experienced DTD. At the same time, the stress response has also evolved to enhance positive growth-promoting physiological changes. Recognition that stress can result in positive and protective "buffering" effects has also led to advances in theory, research, and practice (i.e., heart-rate variability and poly-vagal theory, which emphasize the brain-gut connection in the development of adaptive [and maladaptive] responses to stress and trauma, such as improving safety and attachment security, interpersonal communication, body awareness, resilience, and self-regulation capacities) (Conroy & Perryman, 2022; Liu et al., 2018; Ord et al. 2020; Kolacz et al., 2019). Positive physiological mechanisms associated with stress have been shown to offset the adverse effects of allostasis and toxic stress, giving rise to a more comprehensive understanding of the diverse outcomes linked to trauma, PTSD, and DTD. Scholars have described these strengths in a number of ways, including stress resistance and resilience, physiological compensation, stress-related growth, and posttraumatic growth (PTG).

As part of the stress-related growth process, monoamine neurotransmitters, such as serotonin and dopamine, as well as hormones, such as oxytocin released by the paraventricular nucleus, help individuals return to a state of equanimity and refocus their attention on safe, positive, and rewarding experiences (e.g., music, positive memories, and relationships, including their trust in a higher power; Averill et al., 2018; Maul et al., 2020; Sack et al., 2017). Oxytocin has been found to enhance self-soothing, promote well-being (by coupling with neurotransmitters, such as dopamine), counter-act the hypothalamic-pituitary-adrenal axis stress response, and decrease pain sensitivity by increasing the release of natural opioids in the periaqueductal gray area, which mediates subjective experiences of pain (Saito et al., 2021; Xin et al., 2017; Zheng et al., 2021). Dopamine is linked to the pleasure centers of the brain (i.e., the ventral tegmental area and nucleus accumbens), enhancing positive emotional experiences and social and cognitive capacities (Ferreri et al., 2019; Gold et al., 2018; Worley, 2017)

Research suggests that physiological mechanisms linked to positive neurotransmitters can prevent traumatic stress symptoms from overriding an individual's ability to function (Alexander et al., 2021; Hunter et al., 2018; Wang et al., 2020). Experimental studies have found that high oxytocin levels can lower activity in the limbic system (e.g., amygdala) and lessen the measurable adverse effects of ACEs and trauma (Frijling, 2017; Matsushita et al., 2019; Yoon & Kim, 2022). Researchers have also found that these and other positive neurotransmitters may reverse epigenetic changes associated with developmental trauma and enhance resilience. For example, stress-related changes in protein and glucocorticoid signaling (protein binding and nuclear receptor activities linked to cortisol; Mehta et al., 2020; Miller et al., 2020; Wolf et al., 2018) have been shown to correlate with PTSD, stress-related growth, and resiliency. Researchers using sophisticated neuroimaging technology (e.g., diffusion tensor imaging, brain mapping) have uncovered strengths-based neural networks exclusively dedicated to resilience, hope, kindness and generosity, motivation, and creativity (Alexander et al., 2021; Deshayes et al., 2021; Kim et al., 2021; Regev-Tsur et al., 2020; Roeckner et al., 2021).

We now understand that not all children, adolescents, and adults who experience trauma develop symptoms of PTSD or DTD. Research exploring individual differences in responses to trauma, including differentiated risks of exposure to developmental trauma, has highlighted protective factors that mitigate adverse childhood experiences, trauma, and impairments in functional capacities. They include resilience (i.e., the resilient stress response), compensatory mechanisms (i.e., buffering effects from individual coping resources and social supports), social support, cultural resources, and personal values and beliefs, such as self-transcendence, connection to nature and conservation, and a positive outlook on life, which correlate with and buffer the adverse effects of developmental trauma; Gallagher et al., 2020; Garland, 2021; Hatch et al., 2020; Johnson et al., 2021; Kira et al., 2020; Kramer et al., 2020; Oh et al., 2022).

Stress-Related Growth (SRG)

Contemporary theories of stress, toxic stress, and trauma have demonstrated that traumatic experiences can be deleterious while, at the same time, underscoring the potential observable and measurable benefits that may develop from these very same experiences. Research suggests, for example, that psychological resources, such as spirituality, self-efficacy, resilience, and problem solving, can serve as foundational coping strategies to deal with developmental traumas, but they also may develop as a result (Ben-Zur & Michael, 2020; Ferris & O'Brien, 2022; Kira et al., 2020; Laslo-Roth et al., 2022; Lee et al., 2020; Vazquez et al., 2021). This latter finding is mediated by several processes, such as how an individual appraises (or later reappraises) the perceived stressor(s) (e.g., as overwhelming and uncontrollable or as manageable and possibly growth-promoting) and the availability of social and emotional support from friends, family, and mental health providers.

SRG refers to individuals' personal growth experiences in response to highly stressful life experiences. While SRG is not necessarily associated with a decrease in the adverse reactions or suffering individuals experience in response to traumatic events (which is important to acknowledge so that we don't invalidate the traumatic experiences of others), it effectively broadens one's perspectives (i.e., positive reappraisal) and, in turn, promotes healing and recovery and ultimately leads to a more positive and fulfilling experience in life (David et al., 2022; Kim et al., 2021). Traumatic experiences often challenge one's worldview (e.g., fairness and justice, safety, and security) and prompt existential reflection (e.g., meaning and purpose in life), which are fundamental to the development of SRG (Park, 2022; Lee et al., 2022; Waters et al., 2021a).

Scholars have described positive adaptations to stress and trauma characteristic of SRG for decades, some of which I have discussed previously. However, they have used several other terms, such as perceived benefits, negative growth, transformational coping, growth from experience, or benevolent childhood experiences (BCEs) (Brooks et al., 2019; Karatzias et al., 2020). In fact, SRG is derived from scholars in stress and coping, including Lazarus and Folkman (1984), who proposed the cognitive appraisal theory, which suggests that cognitive appraisals and coping resources mediate reactions to stress and trauma.

Researchers have found that SRG correlates with diverse positive outcomes from traumatic life stressors or events. The results of several cross-sectional studies suggest that SRG mitigates responses to developmental trauma at multiple levels, including individual and family (e.g., polyvictimization, multigenerational trauma) as well as society-level responses to discrimination, bullying, and violence (Alessi et al., 2021; Howell et al., 2021; Shevell & Denov, 2021). Indeed, scholars have applied the concept of SRG to racial and ethnic minorities, low-income children and families, and individuals who have experienced sexual-minority stress and trauma. Studies have found that gay, lesbian, bisexual, and transgender individuals who have experienced multiple traumas often have relatively high scores of SRG, which also correspond to positive attachments (including to their racial and sexual minority groups) and a greater sense of purpose in life (Jones et al., 2022; Ratcliff et al., 2022; Tineo et al., 2021). In the same vein, studies examining factors correlated with SRG in diverse multinational samples have also discerned several strengths-based characteristics – such as hope, positive reappraisal, spirituality, self-efficacy, and acceptance – that protect against the adverse effects of intersectional traumas from violence, discrimination, and neglect (Cénat et al., 2018; Foka et al., 2021; Gatt et al., 2020).

Mindfulness

Children and adults who have experienced trauma and violence often benefit from mindfulness by recognizing their own dispositional mindfulness or through carefully designed psychological and spiritual interventions. Mindfulness refers to a state of reflective experiential awareness characterized by a non-judgmental, unbiased, objective (non-reactive) acceptance of one's experiences as they arise in the present moment. The concept of mindfulness is rooted in non-Western belief systems that prioritize minimalist values, religious and spiritual practices, and an appreciation for the lack of separateness that exists across all aspects of nature (e.g., emphasis on shared experiences, connection to nature and the living, and higher levels of consciousnesses that extend beyond socially constructed ideas). Higher levels of mindfulness correlate with self-acceptance and compassion, insight, introspection, self-regulation, problem-solving, and positive emotions and negatively correlate with psychological distress, anxiety, depression, and trauma (Barcaccia et al., 2020; Faustino et al., 2020; Liu et al., 2022).

Mindfulness and mindfulness-based interventions (e.g., acceptance and commitment therapy, yoga, mindfulness-based stress reduction, meta-cognitive therapy; Jansen et al., 2020; Johannsen et al., 2022; Taylor et al., 2020) may also exert a positive influence over ACEs and early traumatic events by (1) engendering broader views about the ontology and meaning of those events (i.e., decentering, which refers to the immediate awareness of, and disengagement from, automatic schemas about experiences and events in one's immediate environment; Bennett et al., 2021); (2) challenging core assumptions about oneself and the world, thereby leading to reflection about meaning and purpose in life (Chu et al., 2020); (3) increasing mental flexibility and decreasing state anxiety, traumatic rumination, and negative referential thoughts and feelings (Zou et al., 2020); and (4) reversing physiological regulation impaired by stress and trauma (e.g., heart rate variability, cortisol, blood pressure, and neurocognitive capacities; Bergen-Cico et al., 2021). This is in line with the mindfulness to meaning theory (MMT) (Garland et al., 2017; Hanley et al., 2021; Klussman et al., 2020), which proposes that attention to novel aspects of highly stressful, possibly traumatic circumstances enhances positive reappraisal and existential awareness and, in turn, benefits problem-solving, well-being, perspective-taking capacities, and recovery from trauma.

Several physical and emotional health benefits associated with resilient outcomes among DTD children, adolescents, and adults have been described in the literature, many of which correspond to characteristics of SRG and mindfulness (Agin-Liebes et al., 2021; Huang et al., 2022). For example, Williams et al. (2021) found that mindfulness positively predicts SRG for individuals who have experienced traumatic grief. This finding was enhanced by meaning-making, or the extent to which an individual has developed a meaningful, cohesive narrative about their traumatic experiences (e.g., finding a new purpose in life, such as to help other victims of trauma). Scholars assert that SRG, spirituality, and mindfulness correspond to psychological well-being because they mitigate the negative emotions and unhealthy automatic reactions often associated with early traumas. Moreover, mindfulness and spirituality correlate with positive reappraisals of stress, less cognitive rumination, positive emotion, and resiliency, suggesting that individuals can thrive after trauma if provided with the right resources and support to help them foster self-acceptance, compassion, integrity, efficacy, and competency.

Positive Emotions

Mindfulness, stress-related growth, and the DMN also mediate eudemonic and hedonic emotional experiences and physiological processes, including the experience of positive emotions (Du et al., 2019; Lindsay et al., 2018a) and gratitude (Duprey et al., 2018; Swickert et al., 2019). Positive emotions refer to reactions to experiences that are positively reinforcing, meaningful, and fulfilling and that enhance interest and engagement and acknowledge personal strengths and assets. According to Frederickson's broaden-and-build theory, positive emotions, such as love, happiness, forgiveness, hope, and inspiration, expand people's self-awareness, including those who have experienced long-standing abuse and neglect, which in turn reinforces the development of enduring positive psychological resources, including mindfulness, gratitude, positive reappraisal, resilience, and healthy relationships (Ballew & Omoto, 2018; Du et al., 2019; Kiken et al., 2018; Lindsay et al., 2018b; Song et al., 2019; Tranter et al., 2021).

Gratitude

Gratitude has been described as a general state of being thankful – an awareness of, as well as a natural propensity for or disposition to appreciate, positive experiences and to positively reappraise adversity. Gratitude is associated with higher levels of empathy, kindness, positive emotions (e.g., happiness, joy) and cognitive reappraisals, and self-acceptance as well as lower levels of depression, loneliness, and anxiety (Kong et al., 2021; Portocarrero et al., 2020). Likewise, research suggests that gratitude negatively correlates with alcohol and drug abuse, depression, anxiety, and eating disturbances. Individuals who have experienced trauma and who report high levels of gratitude also report greater levels of life satisfaction and personal growth experiences in response to ACEs and interpersonal traumas (Greene & McGovern, 2017; Vieselmeyer et al., 2017).

Strengths-Based Assessment and Treatment

A humanistic, strengths-based view of trauma-informed care is primarily influenced by contemporary research in positive psychology and neuroscience as well as minority (and multiple minorities) resilience frameworks, which emphasize positive reappraisal, mixed-methods evaluation procedures (qualitative and quantitative), and objective measurement standards (e.g., individual assets, assessment of coping resources, positive attachments, and role models, strengths-based parent- and teacher-report questionnaires).

Strengths-based approaches to understanding children, adolescents, and adults who have experienced trauma require us to shift our framework from a deficit-oriented focus to an evaluation and treatment protocol rooted in humanistic and positive psychology. A strengths-based approach is applicable to multiple levels of analysis, such as individual interventions, organizational policies and practices, and state and federal responses to trauma-informed care (including the development and enforcement of strengths-based policies and practices).

According to humanistic and positive psychology scholars, thriving in the face of all odds, even the most devastating traumatic experiences, such as those commonly seen in developmental trauma survivors, is far from inconceivable, particularly given the increasing focus and recognition of positive outcomes. In this regard, scholars have advanced strengths-based diagnostic frameworks, similar to the APA's DSM, but that focus on measuring strengths across various objective dimensions, such as capacities, strengths, interests, resources, well-being and life satisfaction, future orientation, situational benefits, and values.

Positive trauma-informed measures are often multidimensional and compatible with a socioecological framework. They include the Benevolent Childhood Experiences (BCEs) and Positive Childhood Experiences (PCEs)

(Narayan et al., 2020) questionnaires designed with strengths and assets in mind and evaluation procedures that elucidate individual and family supports (e.g., optimism, self-efficacy, parenting, parental warmth, family cohesion) and broader social support from friends, religious communities, and teachers. Focusing on positive life experiences, including strengths-based measurement and evaluation procedures, may help highlight protective factors that may counteract the adverse effects of developmental trauma.

A strengths-based evaluation also includes an appreciation for an individual's unique ideas and behavioral expressions of anger, fear and anxiety, problem-solving, empathy, optimism, and coping, as these adaptations were likely considered to be strengths and assets when they originated from early adversity and can now be used (with reframing techniques) to help apply them effectively and in different contexts. The evaluation of positive traits, emotional and behavioral competencies, and characteristics that enhance problem-solving and decision-making, such as positive and supportive relationships, talents, and interests (e.g., art, music, sports), academic and vocational skills, and the reframing of weaknesses as strengths given the circumstances or contexts (e.g., expressing anger and behaving aggressively to protect a parent who is being victimized by violence).

Individual strengths, including character strengths, promote growth and flourishing and do not diminish with adversity. These types of strengths and assets are considered in detail in the *Oxford Handbook of Positive Psychology* and in *Character Strengths and Virtues: A Handbook and Classification*, which are available for use by clinicians who wish to integrate a strengths-based assessment and treatment with diverse populations (Snyder et al., 2020; Peterson & Seligman, 2004). Values assessed by VIA measures (e.g., the VIA Inventory of Strengths for Youth) include, for example, creativity, perseverance, justice sensitivity, forgiveness, meaning and purpose in life, and authenticity/transparency (Peterson & Seligman, 2004).

Treatment

In therapy, providers working with individuals who have experienced developmental trauma often help them distinguish between who they are (core identity, values, and beliefs) and who they have become (in response to ACEs and DTD). This is a central goal in humanistic, trauma-informed therapies, including trauma-focused CBT (TF-CBT), narrative therapy, and acceptance and commitment therapy (ACT). These therapies often use moment-to-moment interactions between the client and therapist to process emotions, reflect on observations (e.g., to reframe negative or self-deprecating language and replace it with logical and positive ideas), and practice new skills through thoughtful therapy exercises and experiments designed to promote self-discovery.

Research has shown that psychological health assets (e.g., positive emotions, life satisfaction, optimism, life purpose, social support) are associated with various measures of health (Gomez-Baya et al., 2022; Pérez-Wilson et al., 2021). Positive psychology interventions (PPIs) have been empirically validated for addiction (substance abuse and internet addiction), anxiety and depression (including social anxiety and phobia), chronic pain, and PTSD/DTD in multinational samples with diverse individuals (Carr et al., 2021; Chakhssi et al., 2018; Zacchaeus, 2020). PPIs have also been shown to enhance positive emotions, such as happiness, spirituality, hope, search for meaning in life, psychological grit, and hedonic and eudemonic well-being (Hendriks et al., 2020; Jankowski et al., 2020; Kotera et al., 2022; Koydemir et al., 2021).

Concluding Thoughts

Maladaptive responses to trauma are not deterministic; they do not seal an individual's fate and render them helpless or incapable of living a meaningful and fulfilling life. Our ideas about resilience, achievement, and growth are often influenced by mainstream values and norms that vary across scientific disciplines, cultures, and levels of analysis. Children affected by trauma often depend on their caregivers and others for their healthy development, including strengthening their capacity to live a mindful life that is filled with peace, positive and fulfilling experiences, and meaningful relationships, which build resiliency at the individual, family, community, and systems levels. The shift to consider strengths and resiliency in DTD survivors must include research, practice, and policy perspectives. However, children have a broad range of physiological resources that protect them from adversity, including neuroplasticity, specific neurotransmitters, and neural networks linked to positive psychological constructs. Individuals who have experienced developmental trauma may cope through whatever means they have available to them at the time, which are likely to be limited given children's lack of cognitive capacities (at least compared to adults). As such, they will require support from adolescents and adults and from social systems and institutions to help them find their value and realize their potential. They need this support to help them learn to love and accept themselves for who they are and not for the symptoms they display, which are often precipitated by experiences of fear, insecurity, or invalidation as well as by harsh adults who fail to recognize their needs and fail to provide them with corrective/supportive experiences. Circumstances linked to the experience of love, support, validation and acceptance, positive relationships, and caring adults, who stand by these children regardless of their disruptive behaviors, can plant a seed that, over time, can make all the difference in the ways these children respond to stress, cope with adversity, and discover new reasons to live, love, and connect with others.

References

Agin-Liebes, G., Ekman, E., Anderson, B., Malloy, M., Haas, A., & Woolley, J. (2021). Participant reports of mindfulness, posttraumatic growth, and social connectedness in psilocybin-assisted group therapy: An interpretive phenomenological analysis. *Journal of Humanistic Psychology*, 00221678211022949. https://doi.org/10.1177/00221678211022949.

Alessi, E. J., Cheung, S., Kahn, S., & Yu, M. (2021). A scoping review of the experiences of violence and abuse among sexual and gender minority migrants across the migration trajectory. *Trauma, Violence, & Abuse*, 22(5), 1339–1355. https://doi.org/10.1177/15248380211043892.

Alexander, R., Aragón, O. R., Bookwala, J., Cherbuin, N., Gatt, J. M., Kahrilas, I. J., Kästner, N., Lawrence, A., Lowe, L., Morrison, R. G., Mueller, S. C., Nusslock, R., Papadelis, C., Polnaszek, K. L., Helene Richter, S., Silton, R. L., & Styliadis, C. (2021). The neuroscience of positive emotions and affect: Implications for cultivating happiness and wellbeing. *Neuroscience and Biobehavioral Reviews*, 121, 220–249. https://doi.org/10.1016/j.neubiorev.2020.12.002.

Antebi-Gruszka, N., Cain, D., Millar, B. M., Parsons, J. T., & Rendina, H. J. (2022). Stress-related growth among transgender women: Measurement, correlates, and insights for clinical interventions. *Journal of Homosexuality*, 69(10), 1679–1702. https://doi.org/10.1080/00918369.2021.1921511.

Averill, L. A., Averill, C. L., Kelmendi, B., Abdallah, C. G., & Southwick, S. M. (2018). Stress response modulation underlying the psychobiology of resilience. *Current Psychiatry Reports*, 20(4), 27. https://doi.org/10.1007/s11920-018-0887-x.

Ballew, M. T., & Omoto, A. M. (2018). Absorption: How nature experiences promote awe and other positive emotions. *Ecopsychology*, 10(1), 26–35. https://doi.org/10.1089/eco.2017.0044.

Barcaccia, B., Cervin, M., Pozza, A., Medvedev, O. N., Baiocco, R., & Pallini, S. (2020). Mindfulness, self-compassion and attachment: A network analysis of psychopathology symptoms in adolescents. *Mindfulness*, 11(11), 2531–2541. https://doi.org/10.1007/s12671-020-01466-8.

Bennett, M. P., Knight, R., Patel, S., So, T., Dunning, D., Barnhofer, T., Smith, P., Kuyken, W., Ford, T., & Dalgleish, T. (2021). Decentering as a core component in the psychological treatment and prevention of youth anxiety and depression: A narrative review and insight report. *Translational Psychiatry*, 11(1), 288. https://doi.org/10.1038/s41398-021-01397-5.

Ben-Zur, H., & Michael, K. (2020). Positivity and growth following stressful life events: Associations with psychosocial, health, and economic resources. *International Journal of Stress Management*, 27(2), 126–134. https://doi.org/10.1037/str0000142.

Bergen-Cico, D., Grant, T., Hirshfield, L., Razza, R., Costa, M. R., & Kilaru, P. (2021). Using fNIRS to examine neural mechanisms of change associated with mindfulness-based interventions for stress and trauma: Results of a pilot study for women. *Mindfulness*, 12(9), 2295–2310. https://doi.org/10.1007/s12671-021-01705-6.

Bethell, C., Jones, J., Gombojav, N., Linkenbach, J., & Sege, R. (2019). Positive childhood experiences and adult mental and relational health in a statewide sample: Associations across adverse childhood experiences levels. *JAMA Pediatrics*, 173(11), e193007. https://doi.org/10.1001/jamapediatrics.2019.3007.

Bravo, L. G., Nagy, G. A., Stafford, A. M., McCabe, B. E., & Gonzalez-Guarda, R. M. (2022). Adverse childhood experiences and depressive symptoms among young adult

Hispanic immigrants: Moderating and mediating effects of distinct facets of accul-turation stress. *Issues in Mental Health Nursing*, 43(3), 209–219. https://doi.org/10.1080/01612840.2021.1972190.

Brooks, M., Graham-Kevan, N., Robinson, S., & Lowe, M. (2019). Trauma character-istics and posttraumatic growth: The mediating role of avoidance coping, intrusive thoughts, and social support. *Psychological Trauma: Theory, Research, Practice, and Policy*, 11(2), 232–238. https://doi.org/10.1037/tra0000372.

Carr, A., Cullen, K., Keeney, C., Canning, C., Mooney, O., Chinseallaigh, E., & O'Dowd, A. (2021). Effectiveness of positive psychology interventions: A systematic review and meta-analysis. *The Journal of Positive Psychology*, 16(6), 749–769. https://doi.org/10.1080/17439760.2020.1818807.

Cénat, J. M., Derivois, D., Hébert, M., Amédée, L. M., & Karray, A. (2018). Multiple traumas and resilience among street children in Haiti: Psychopathology of survival. *Child Abuse & Neglect*, 79, 85–97. https://doi.org/10.1016/j.chiabu.2018.01.024.

Chakhssi, F., Kraiss, J. T., Sommers-Spijkerman, M., & Bohlmeijer, E. T. (2018). The effect of positive psychology interventions on well-being and distress in clinical sam-ples with psychiatric or somatic disorders: A systematic review and meta-analysis. *BMC Psychiatry*, 18(1), 211. https://doi.org/10.1186/s12888-018-1739-2.

Chaplin, T. M., Niehaus, C., & Gonçalves, S. F. (2018). Stress reactivity and the developmental psychopathology of adolescent substance use. *Neurobiology of Stress*, 9, 133–139. https://doi.org/10.1016/j.ynstr.2018.09.002.

Chu, S. T. W., & Mak, W. W. (2020). How mindfulness enhances meaning in life: A meta-analysis of correlational studies and randomized controlled trials. *Mindfulness*, 11 (1), 177–193. https://doi.org/10.1007/s12671-019-01258-9.

Clements-Nolle, K., & Waddington, R. (2019). Adverse childhood experiences and psychological distress in juvenile offenders: The protective influence of resilience and youth assets. *Journal of Adolescent Health*, 64(1), 49–55. https://doi.org/10.1016/j.jadohealth.2018.09.025.

Conroy, J., & Perryman, K. (2022). Treating trauma with child-centred play therapy through the SECURE lens of polyvagal theory. *International Journal of Play Therapy*, 31 (3), 143–152. https://doi.org/10.1037/pla0000172.

Crandall, A., Miller, J. R., Cheung, A., Novilla, L. K., Glade, R., Novilla, M. L. B., Magnusson, B. M., Leavitt, B. L., Barnes, M. D., & Hanson, C. L. (2019). ACEs and counter-ACEs: How positive and negative childhood experiences influence adult health. *Child Abuse & Neglect*, 96, 104089. https://doi.org/10.1016/j.chiabu.2019.104089.

David, G., Shakespeare-Finch, J., & Krosch, D. (2022). Testing theoretical predictors of posttraumatic growth and posttraumatic stress symptoms. *Psychological Trauma: Theory, Research, Practice, and Policy*, 14(3), 399–409. https://doi.org/10.1037/tra0000777.

Deshayes, C., Paban, V., Ferrer, M. H., Alescio-Lautier, B., & Chambon, C. (2021). A comprehensive approach to study the resting-state brain network related to creative potential. *Brain Structure & Function*, 226(6), 1743–1753. https://doi.org/10.1007/s00429-021-02286-9.

Du, J., An, Y., Ding, X., Zhang, Q., & Xu, W. (2019). State mindfulness and positive emotions in daily life: An upward spiral process. *Personality and Individual Differences*, 141, 57–561. https://doi.org/10.1016/j.paid.2018.11.037.

Duprey, E. B., McKee, L. G., O'Neal, C. W., & Algoe, S. B. (2018). Stressful life events and internalising symptoms in emerging adults: The roles of mindfulness and gratitude. *Mental Health & Prevention*, 12, 1–9. https://doi.org/10.1016/j.mhp.2018.08.003.

Durosini, I., Tarocchi, A., & Aschieri, F. (2017). Therapeutic assessment with a client with persistent complex bereavement disorder: A single-case time-series design. *Clinical Case Studies*, 16(4), 295–312. https://doi.org/10.1177/1534650117693942.

Eme, R. (2017). Developmental psychopathology: A primer for clinical pediatrics. *World Journal of Psychiatry*, 7(3), 159–162. https://doi.org/10.5498/wjp.v7.i3.159.

Faustino, B., Vasco, A. B., Silva, A. N., & Marques, T. (2020). Relationships between emotional schemas, mindfulness, self-compassion and unconditional self-acceptance on the regulation of psychological needs. *Research in Psychotherapy*, 23(2), 442. https://doi.org/10.4081/ripppo.2020.442.

Ferreri, L., Mas-Herrero, E., Zatorre, R. J., Ripollés, P., Gomez-Andres, A., Alicart, H., Olivé, G., Marco-Pallarés, J., Antonijoan, R. M., Valle, M., Riba, J., & Rodriguez-Fornells, A. (2019). Dopamine modulates the reward experiences elicited by music. *Proceedings of the National Academy of Sciences of the United States of America*, 116(9), 3793–3798. https://doi.org/10.1073/pnas.1811878116.

Ferris, C., & O'Brien, K. (2022). The ins and outs of posttraumatic growth in children and adolescents: A systematic review of factors that matter. *Journal of Traumatic Stress*, 35, 1305–1317. https://doi.org/10.1002/jts.22845.

Figley, C. R., & Burnette, C. E. (2017). Building bridges: Connecting systemic trauma and family resilience in the study and treatment of diverse traumatized families. *Traumatology*, 23(1), 95. https://doi.org/10.1037/trm0000089.

Foka, S., Hadfield, K., Pluess, M., & Mareschal, I. (2021). Promoting well-being in refugee children: An exploratory controlled trial of a positive psychology intervention delivered in Greek refugee camps. *Development and Psychopathology*, 33(1), 87–95. https://doi.org/10.1017/S0954579419001585.

Fried, E. I. (2017). What are psychological constructs?: On the nature and statistical modelling of emotions, intelligence, personality traits and mental disorders. *Health Psychology Review*, 11(2), 130–134. https://doi.org/10.1080/17437199.2017.1306718.

Frijling, J. L. (2017). Preventing PTSD with oxytocin: Effects of oxytocin administration on fear neurocircuitry and PTSD symptom development in recently trauma-exposed individuals. *European Journal of Psychotraumatology*, 8(1), 1302652. https://doi.org/10.1080/20008198.2017.1302652.

Gallagher, M. W., Long, L. J., & Phillips, C. A. (2020). Hope, optimism, self-efficacy, and posttraumatic stress disorder: A meta-analytic review of the protective effects of positive expectancies. *Journal of Clinical Psychology*, 76(3), 329–355. https://doi.org/10.1002/jclp.22882.

Garland, E. L. (2021). Mindful positive emotion regulation as a treatment for addiction: From hedonic pleasure to self-transcendent meaning. *Current Opinion in Behavioral Sciences*, 39, 168–177. https://doi.org/10.1016/j.cobeha.2021.03.019.

Garland, E. L., Hanley, A. W., Goldin, P. R., & Gross, J. J. (2017). Testing the mindfulness-to-meaning theory: Evidence for mindful positive emotion regulation from a reanalysis of longitudinal data. *PloS One*, 12(12), e0187727. https://doi.org/10.1371/journal.pone.0187727.

Gatt, J. M., Alexander, R., Emond, A., Foster, K., Hadfield, K., Mason-Jones, A., Reid, S., Theron, L., Ungar, M., Wouldes, T. A., & Wu, Q. (2020). Trauma, resilience, and mental health in migrant and non-migrant youth: An international cross-sectional study across six countries. *Frontiers in Psychiatry*, 10, 997. https://doi.org/10.3389/fp syt.2019.00997.

Gold, M. S., Blum, K., Febo, M., Baron, D., Modestino, E. J., Elman, I., & Badgaiyan, R. D. (2018). Molecular role of dopamine in anhedonia linked to reward deficiency syndrome (RDS) and anti-reward systems. *Frontiers in Bioscience*, 10(2), 309–325. https://doi.org/10.2741/s518.

Goldenson, J., Kitollari, I., & Lehman, F. (2021). The relationship between ACEs, trauma-related psychopathology and resilience in vulnerable youth: Implications for screening and treatment. *Journal of Child & Adolescent Trauma*, 14(1), 151–160. https://doi.org/10.1007/s40653-020-00308-y.

Gomez-Baya, D., Santos, T., & Gaspar de Matos, M. (2022). Developmental assets and positive youth development: An examination of gender differences in Spain. *Applied Developmental Science*, 26(3), 516–531. https://doi.org/10.1080/10888691.2021. 1906676.

Gorske, T. T. (2017). Collaborative therapeutic neuropsychological assessment. In J. E. Morgan & J. H. Ricker (Eds.), *Textbook of Clinical Neuropsychology* (pp. 1068–1077). New York: Taylor & Francis.

Green, N., & McGovern, K. (2017). Gratitude, psychological well-being, and perceptions of post traumatic growth in adults who lost a parent in childhood. *Death Studies*, 41(7), 436–446. https://doi.org/10.1080/07481187.2017.1296505.

Hanley, A. W., de Vibe, M., Solhaug, I., Farb, N., Goldin, P. R., Gross, J. J., & Garland, E. L. (2021). Modeling the mindfulness-to-meaning theory's mindful reappraisal hypothesis: Replication with longitudinal data from a randomized controlled study. *Stress and Health*, 37(4), 778–789. https://doi.org/10.1002/smi.3035.

Hatch, V., Swerbenski, H., & Gray, S. A. O. (2020). Family social support buffers the intergenerational association of maternal adverse childhood experiences and preschoolers' externalizing behavior. *American Journal of Orthopsychiatry*, 90(4), 489–501. https://doi.org/10.1037/ort0000451.

Hayden, E. P. (2022). A call for renewed attention to construct validity and measurement in psychopathology research. *Psychological Medicine*, 52(14), 2930–2936. https://doi.org/10.1017/S0033291722003221.

Hendriks, T., Schotanus-Dijkstra, M., Hassankhan, A., De Jong, J., & Bohlmeijer, E. (2020). The efficacy of multi-component positive psychology interventions: A systematic review and meta-analysis of randomized controlled trials. *Journal of Happiness Studies*, 21(1), 357–390. https://doi.org/10.1007/s10902-019-00082-1.

Hirschberger, G. (2018). Collective trauma and the social construction of meaning. *Frontiers in Psychology*, 9, 1441. https://doi.org/10.3389/fpsyg.2018.01441.

Höltge, J., Mc Gee, S. L., Maercker, A., & Thoma, M. V. (2018). A salutogenic perspective on adverse experiences. *European Journal of Health Psychology*, 25(2), 53–69. https://doi.org/10.1027/2512-8442/a000011.

Howell, K. H., Miller-Graff, L. E., Martinez-Torteya, C., Napier, T. R., & Carney, J. R. (2021). Charting a course towards resilience following adverse childhood experiences: Addressing intergenerational trauma via strengths-based intervention. *Children*, 8(10), 844. https://doi.org/10.3390/children8100844.

Huang, Y. L., Li, Z. W., Kung, Y. W., & Su, Y. J. (2022). The facilitating role of dispositional mindfulness in the process of posttraumatic growth: A prospective investigation. *Psychological Trauma: Theory, Research, Practice, and Policy*, 14(S1), S174. https://doi.org/10.1037/tra0001163.

Hunter, R. G., Gray, J. D., & McEwen, B. S. (2018). The neuroscience of resilience. *Journal of the Society for Social Work and Research*, 9(2), 305–339. https://doi.org/10. 1086/697956.

Huss, E., & Samson, T. (2018). Drawing on the arts to enhance salutogenic coping with health-related stress and loss. *Frontiers in Psychology*, 9, 1612. https://doi.org/10.3389/ fpsyg.2018.01612.

Jankowski, P. J., Sandage, S. J., Bell, C. A., Davis, D. E., Porter, E., Jessen, M., Motzny, C. L., Ross, K. V., & Owen, J. (2020). Virtue, flourishing, and positive psychology in psychotherapy: An overview and research prospectus. *Psychotherapy*, 57(3), 291–309. https://doi.org/10.1037/pst0000285.

Jansen, J. E., Gleeson, J., Bendall, S., Rice, S., & Alvarez-Jimenez, M. (2020). Acceptance-and mindfulness-based interventions for persons with psychosis: A systematic review and meta-analysis. *Schizophrenia Research*, 215, 25–37. https://doi.org/10. 1016/j.schres.2019.11.016.

Johannsen, M., Nissen, E. R., Lundorff, M., & O'Toole, M. S. (2022). Mediators of acceptance and mindfulness-based therapies for anxiety and depression: A systematic review and meta-analysis. *Clinical Psychology Review*, 94, 102156. https://doi.org/10. 1016/j.cpr.2022.102156.

Johnson, E. E. H., Wilder, S. M. J., Andersen, C. V. S., Horvath, S. A., Kolp, H. M., Gidycz, C. A., & Shorey, R. C. (2021). Trauma and alcohol use among transgender and gender diverse women: An examination of the stress-buffering hypothesis of social support. *The Journal of Primary Prevention*, 42(6), 567–581. https://doi.org/10. 1007/s10935-021-00646-z.

Jones, A. K., Wehner, C. L., Andrade, I. M., Jones, E. M., Wooten, L. H., & Wilson, L. C. (2022). Minority stress and posttraumatic growth in the transgender and nonbinary community. *Psychology of Sexual Orientation and Gender Diversity*. Advance online publication. https://doi.org/10.1037/sgd0000610.

Kamphuis, J. H., & Finn, S. E. (2019). Therapeutic assessment in personality disorders: Toward the restoration of epistemic trust. *Journal of Personality Assessment*, 101(6), 662–674. https://doi.org/10.1080/00223891.2018.1476360.

Karatzias, T., Shevlin, M., Fyvie, C., Grandison, G., Garozi, M., Latham, E., Sinclair, M., Ho, G. W. K., McAnee, G., Ford, J. D., & Hyland, P. (2020). Adverse and benevolent childhood experiences in Posttraumatic Stress Disorder (PTSD) and Complex PTSD (CPTSD): Implications for trauma-focused therapies. *European Journal of Psychotraumatology*, 11(1), 1793599. https://doi.org/10.1080/20008198.2020.1793599.

Kiken, L. G., Shook, N. J., Robins, J. L., & Clore, J. N. (2019). Association between mindfulness and interoceptive accuracy in patients with diabetes: Preliminary evidence from blood glucose samples. *Complementary Therapies in Medicine*, 36, 90–92. https:// doi.org/10.1016/j.ctim.2017.12.003.

Kim, W. J., Park, K. M., Park, J. T., Seo, E., Bang, M., An, S. K., Park, H. Y., & Lee, E. (2021). Effect of childhood trauma on the association between stress-related psychological factors and hair cortisol level in young adults. *Psychiatry Investigation*, 18(11), 1131–1136. https://doi.org/10.30773/pi.2021.0256.

Kira, I. A., Arıcı Özcan, N., Shuwiekh, H., Kucharska, J., Al-Huwailah, A. H., & Kanaan, A. (2020). The compelling dynamics of "will to exist, live, and survive" on effecting posttraumatic growth upon exposure to adversities: Is it mediated, in part, by emotional regulation, resilience, and spirituality? *Traumatology*, 26(4), 405. https://doi. org/10.1037/trm0000263.

Kong, F., Yang, K., Yan, W., & Li, X. (2021). How does trait gratitude relate to subjective well-being in Chinese adolescents?: The mediating role of resilience and social support. *Journal of Happiness Studies*, 22, 1611–1622. https://doi.org/10.1007/s10902-020-00286-w.

Klussman, K., Nichols, A. L., & Langer, J. (2020). The role of self-connection in the relationship between mindfulness and meaning: A longitudinal examination. *Applied Psychology: Health and Well-Being*, 12(3), 636–659. https://doi.org/10.1111/aphw.12200.

Knight, G. P., Safa, M. D., & White, R. M. B. (2018). Advancing the assessment of cultural orientation: A developmental and contextual framework of multiple psychological dimensions and social identities. *Development and Psychopathology*, 30(5), 1867–1888. https://doi.org/10.1017/S095457941800113X.

Kolacz, J., Kovacic, K. K., & Porges, S. W. (2019). Traumatic stress and the autonomic brain-gut connection in development: Polyvagal Theory as an integrative framework for psychosocial and gastrointestinal pathology. *Developmental Psychology*, 61(5), 796–809. https://doi.org/10.1002/dev.21852.

Kotera, Y., Green, P., & Sheffield, D. (2022). Positive psychology for mental wellbeing of UK therapeutic students: Relationships with engagement, motivation, resilience and self-compassion. *International Journal of Mental Health and Addiction*, 20(3), 1611–1626. https://doi.org/10.1007/s11469-020-00466-y.

Koydemir, S., Sökmez, A. B., & Schütz, A. (2021). A meta-analysis of the effectiveness of randomized controlled positive psychological interventions on subjective and psychological well-being. *Applied Research in Quality of Life*, 16(3), 1145–1185. https://doi.org/10.1007/s11482-019-09788-z.

Kramer, L. B., Whiteman, S. E., Witte, T. K., Silverstein, M. W., & Weathers, F. W. (2020). From trauma to growth: The roles of event centrality, posttraumatic stress symptoms, and deliberate rumination. *Traumatology*, 26(2), 152. https://doi.org/10.1037/trm0000214.

Kuhar, M., & Zager Kocjan, G. (2021). Associations of adverse and positive childhood experiences with adult physical and mental health and risk behaviours in Slovenia. *European Journal of Psychotraumatology*, 12(1), 1924953. https://doi.org/10.1080/20008198.2021.1924953.

Kuhar, M., & Zager Kocjan, G. (2022). Adverse childhood experiences and somatic symptoms in adulthood: A moderated mediation effects of disturbed self-organization and resilient coping. *Psychological Trauma: Theory, Research, Practice, and Policy*, 14(8), 1288–1298. https://doi.org/10.1037/tra0001040.

Lai, S. T., Lim, K. S., Low, W. Y., & Tang, V. (2019). Positive psychological interventions for neurological disorders: A systematic review. *The Clinical Neuropsychologist*, 33(3), 490–518. https://doi.org/10.1080/13854046.2018.1489562.

Laslo-Roth, R., George-Levi, S., & Margalit, M. (2022). Social participation and posttraumatic growth: The serial mediation of hope, social support, and reappraisal. *Journal of Community Psychology*, 50(1), 47–63. https://doi.org/10.1002/jcop.22490.

Lazarus, R. S., & Folkman, S. (1984). Coping and Adaptation. In W. D. Gentry (Ed.), *The Handbook of Behavioral Medicine* (pp. 282–325.). New York: Guilford.

Lee, D., Yu, E. S., & Kim, N. H. (2020). Resilience as a mediator in the relationship between posttraumatic stress and posttraumatic growth among adult accident or crime victims: The moderated mediating effect of childhood trauma. *European Journal of Psychotraumatology*, 11(1), 1704563. https://doi.org/10.1080/20008198.2019.1704563.

Lee, S. Y., Park, C. L., & Laflash, S. (2022). Perceived posttraumatic growth in cardiac patients: A systematic scoping review. *Journal of Traumatic Stress*, 35(3), 791–803. http s://doi.org/10.1002/jts.22799.

Lindsay, E. K., Chin, B., Greco, C. M., Young, S., Brown, K. W., Wright, A. G. C., Smyth, J. M., Burkett, D., & Creswell, J. D. (2018a). How mindfulness training promotes positive emotions: Dismantling acceptance skills training in two randomized controlled trials. *Journal of Personality and Social Psychology*, 115(6), 944–973. https://doi.org/10.1037/pspa0000134.

Lindsay, E. K., Young, S., Smyth, J. M., Brown, K. W., & Creswell, J. D. (2018b). Acceptance lowers stress reactivity: Dismantling mindfulness training in a randomised controlled trial. *Psychoneuroendocrinology*, 87, 63–73. https://doi.org/10.1016/j.psy neuen.2017.09.015.

Liu, A. N., Wang, L. L., Li, H. P., Gong, J., & Liu, X. H. (2017). Correlation between posttraumatic growth and posttraumatic stress disorder symptoms based on Pearson correlation coefficient: A meta-analysis. *The Journal of Nervous and Mental Disease*, 205 (5), 380–389. https://doi.org/10.1097/NMD.0000000000000605.

Liu, H., Zhang, C., Ji, Y., & Yang, L. (2018). Biological and psychological perspectives of resilience: Is it possible to improve stress resistance? *Frontiers in Human Neuroscience*, 12, 326. https://doi.org/10.3389/fnhum.2018.00326.

Liu, Q., Zhu, J., & Zhang, W. (2022). The efficacy of mindfulness-based stress reduction intervention 3 for post-traumatic stress disorder (PTSD) symptoms in patients with PTSD: A meta-analysis of four randomized controlled trials. *Stress and Health: Journal of the International Society for the Investigation of Stress*, 38(4), 626–636. https://doi.org/ 10.1002/smi.3138.

Martínez-Martí, M. L., & Ruch, W. (2017). Character strengths predict resilience over and above positive affect, self-efficacy, optimism, social support, self-esteem, and life satisfaction. *The Journal of Positive Psychology*, 12(2), 110–119. https://doi.org/10.1080/ 17439760.2016.1163403.

Matsushita, H., Latt, H. M., Koga, Y., Nishiki, T., & Matsui, H. (2019). Oxytocin and stress: Neural mechanisms, stress-related disorders, and therapeutic approaches. *Neuroscience*, 417, 1–10. https://doi.org/10.1016/j.neuroscience.2019.07.046.

Maul, S., Giegling, I., Fabbri, C., Corponi, F., Serretti, A., & Rujescu, D. (2020). Genetics of resilience: Implications from genome-wide association studies and candidate genes of the stress response system in posttraumatic stress disorder and depression. *American Journal of Medical Genetics Part B: Neuropsychiatric Genetics*, 183(2), 77–94. http s://doi.org/10.1002/ajmg.b.32763.

McKeen, H., Hook, M., Podduturi, P., Beitzell, E., Jones, A., & Liss, M. (2021). Mindfulness as a mediator and moderator in the relationship between adverse childhood experiences and depression. *Current Psychology*, 1–11. https://doi.org/10.1007/ s12144-021-02003-z.

Mehta, D., Miller, O., Bruenig, D., David, G., & Shakespeare-Finch, J. (2020). A Systematic Review of DNA Methylation and Gene Expression Studies in Posttraumatic Stress Disorder, Posttraumatic Growth, and Resilience. *Journal of Traumatic Stress*, 33 (2), 171–180. https://doi.org/10.1002/jts.22472.

Miller, O., Shakespeare-Finch, J., Bruenig, D., & Mehta, D. (2020). DNA methylation of NR3C1 and FKBP5 is associated with posttraumatic stress disorder, posttraumatic growth, and resilience. *Psychological Trauma: Theory, Research, Practice, and Policy*, 12(7), 750–755. https://doi.org/10.1037/tra0000574.

Narayan, A. J., Atal, V. M., Merck, J. M., Harris, W. W., & Lieberman, A. F. (2020). Developmental origins of ghosts and angels in the nursery: Adverse and benevolent childhood experiences. *Adversity and Resilience Science*, 1, 121–134. https://doi.org/10.1007/s42844-020-00008-4.

Niemiec, R. M. (2020). Six functions of character strengths for thriving at times of adversity and opportunity: A theoretical perspective. *Applied Research in Quality of Life*, 15(2), 551–572. https://doi.org/10.1007/s11482-018-9692-2.

Nowakowski, A. C. H., & Sumerau, J. E. (2019). Reframing health and illness: A collaborative autoethnography on the experience of health and illness transformations in the life course. *Sociology of Health & Illness*, 41(4), 723–739. https://doi.org/10.1111/1467-9566.12849.

Oh, S., Litam, S. D. A., & Chang, C. Y. (2022). Racism and stress-related growth among Asian internationals: Ethnic identity, resilience, and coping during COVID-19. *International Journal for the Advancement of Counselling*, 1–23. https://doi.org/10.1007/s10447-022-09494-w.

Oppenheimer, C. W., Glenn, C. R., & Miller, A. B. (2022). Future directions in suicide and self-injury revisited: Integrating a developmental psychopathology perspective. *Journal of Clinical Child & Adolescent Psychology*, 51(2), 242–260. https://doi.org/10.1080/15374416.2022.2051526.

Ord, A. S., Stranahan, K. R., Hurley, R. A., & Taber, K. H. (2020). Stress-related growth: Building a more resilient brain. *The Journal of Neuropsychiatry and Clinical Neurosciences*, 32(3), A4–212. https://doi.org/10.1176/appi.neuropsych.20050111.

Park, C. L. (2022). Meaning Making Following Trauma. *Frontiers in Psychology*, 13, 844891. https://doi.org/10.3389/fpsyg.2022.844891.

Pérez-Wilson, P., Marcos-Marcos, J., Morgan, A., Eriksson, M., Lindström, B., & Álvarez-Dardet, C. (2021). 'A synergy model of health': An integration of salutogenesis and the health assets model. *Health Promotion International*, 36(3), 884–894. https://doi.org/10.1093/heapro/daaa084.

Peterson, C., & Seligman, M. E. P. (2004). *Character strengths and virtues: A handbook and classification*, vol. 1. Oxford: Oxford University Press.

Portocarrero, F. F., Gonzalez, K., & Ekema-Agbaw, M. (2020). A meta-analytic review of the relationship between dispositional gratitude and well-being. *Personality and Individual Differences*, 164, 110101. https://doi.org/10.1016/j.paid.2020.110101.

Rabenu, E., Yaniv, E., & Elizur, D. (2017). The relationship between psychological capital, coping with stress, well-being, and performance. *Current Psychology*, 36(4), 875–887. https://doi.org/10.1007/s12144-016-9477-4.

Ratcliff, J. J., Tombari, J. M., Miller, A. K., Brand, P. F., & Witnauer, J. E. (2022). Factors promoting posttraumatic growth in sexual minority adults following adolescent bullying experiences. *Journal of Interpersonal Violence*, 37(7–8), NP5419–NP5441. https://doi.org/10.1177/0886260520961.

Regev-Tsur, S., Demiray, Y. E., Tripathi, K., Stork, O., Richter-Levin, G., & Albrecht, A. (2020). Region-specific involvement of interneuron subpopulations in trauma-related pathology and resilience. *Neurobiology of Disease*, 143, 104974. https://doi.org/10.1016/j.nbd.2020.104974.

Roeckner, A. R., Oliver, K. I., Lebois, L. A., van Rooij, S. J., & Stevens, J. S. (2021). Neural contributors to trauma resilience: A review of longitudinal neuroimaging studies. *Translational Psychiatry*, 11(1), 1–17. https://doi.org/10.1038/s41398-021-01633-y.

Rogers, C. R. (1980). *Way of being*. Boston, MA: Houghton Mifflin.

Ross, N., Gilbert, R., Torres, S., Dugas, K., Jefferies, P., McDonald, S., Savage, S., & Ungar, M. (2020). Adverse childhood experiences: Assessing the impact on physical and psychosocial health in adulthood and the mitigating role of resilience. *Child Abuse & Neglect*, 103, 104440. https://doi.org/10.1016/j.chiabu.2020.104440.

Ruch, W., Gander, F., Wagner, L., & Giuliani, F. (2021). The structure of character: On the relationships between character strengths and virtues. *The Journal of Positive Psychology*, 16(1), 116–128. https://doi.org/10.1080/17439760.2019.1689418.

Sack, M., Spieler, D., Wizelman, L., Epple, G., Stich, J., Zaba, M., & Schmidt, U. (2017). Intranasal oxytocin reduces provoked symptoms in female patients with posttraumatic stress disorder despite exerting sympathomimetic and positive chronotropic effects in a randomized controlled trial. *BMC Medicine*, 15(1), 1–11. https://doi.org/10.1186/s12916-017-0801-0.

Saito, H., Hidema, S., Otsuka, A., Suzuki, J., Kumagai, M., Kanaya, A., Murakami, T., Takei, Y., Saito, K., Sugino, S., Toyama, H., Saito, R., Tominaga, T., Nishimori, K., & Yamauchi, M. (2021). Effects of oxytocin on responses to nociceptive and non-nociceptive stimulation in the upper central nervous system. *Biochemical and Biophysical Research Communications*, 574, 8–13. https://doi.org/10.1016/j.bbrc.2021.08.042.

Shevell, M. C., & Denov, M. S. (2021). A multidimensional model of resilience: Family, community, national, global and intergenerational resilience. *Child Abuse & Neglect*, 119, 105035. https://doi.org/10.1016/j.chiabu.2021.105035.

Snow, N. E. (2019). Positive psychology, the classification of character strengths and virtues, and issues of measurement. *The Journal of Positive Psychology*, 14(1), 20–31. https://doi.org/10.1080/17439760.2018.1528376.

Snyder, C. R., Lopez, S. J., Edwards, L. M., & Marques, S. C. (Eds.). (2020). *The Oxford handbook of positive psychology*. 2nd ed. Oxford: Oxford University Press.

Snyder, H. R., Friedman, N. P., & Hankin, B. L. (2019). Transdiagnostic mechanisms of psychopathology in youth: Executive functions, dependent stress, and rumination. *Cognitive Therapy and Research*, 43(5), 834–851. https://doi.org/10.1007/s10608-019-10016-z.

Song, R., Sun, N., & Song, X. (2019). The efficacy of psychological capital intervention (PCI) for depression from the perspective of positive psychology: A pilot study. *Frontiers in Psychology*, 10, 1816. https://doi.org/10.3389/fpsyg.2019.01816.

Street, A. E., & Dardis, C. M. (2018). Using a social construction of gender lens to understand gender differences in posttraumatic stress disorder. *Clinical Psychology Review*, 66, 97–105. https://doi.org/10.1016/j.cpr.2018.03.001.

Swickert, R., Bailey, E., Hittner, J., Spector, A., Benson-Townsend, B., & Silver, N. C. (2019). The meditational roles of gratitude and perceived support in explaining the relationship between mindfulness and mood. *Journal of Happiness Studies*, 20, 815–828. https://doi.org/10.1007/s10902-017-9952-0.

Taylor, J., McLean, L., Korner, A., Stratton, E., & Glozier, N. (2020). Mindfulness and yoga for psychological trauma: Systematic review and meta-analysis. *Journal of Trauma & Dissociation*, 21(5), 536–573. https://doi.org/10.1080/15299732.2020.1760167.

Tineo, P., Bonumwezi, J. L., & Lowe, S. R. (2021). Discrimination and posttraumatic growth among Muslim American youth: Mediation via posttraumatic stress disorder symptoms. *Journal of Trauma & Dissociation*, 22(2), 188–201. https://doi.org/10.1080/15299732.2020.1869086.

Tranter, H., Brooks, M., & Khan, R. (2021). Emotional resilience and event centrality mediate post traumatic growth following adverse childhood experiences. *Psychological*

Trauma: Research, Practice, and Policy, 13(2), 165–173. https://doi.org/10.1037/tra 0000953.

Vazquez, C., Valiente, C., García, F. E., Contreras, A., Peinado, V., Trucharte, A., & Bentall, R. P. (2021). Post-traumatic growth and stress-related responses during the COVID-19 pandemic in a national representative sample: The role of positive core beliefs about the world and others. *Journal of Happiness Studies*, 22(7), 2915–2935. https://doi.org/10.1007/s10902-020-00352-3.

Viselmeyer, J., Holguin, J., & Mezulis, A. (2017). The role of resilience and gratitude in posttraumatic stress and growth following a campus shooting. *Psychological Trauma*, 9 (1), 62–69. https://doi.org/10.1037/tra0000149.

Waldron-Perrine, B., Rai, J. K., & Chao, D. (2021). Therapeutic assessment and the art of feedback: A model for integrating evidence-based assessment and therapy techniques in neurological rehabilitation. *NeuroRehabilitation*, 49(2), 293–306. https://doi.org/10.3233/NRE-218027.

Wang, S., Zhao, Y., Li, J., Lai, H., Qiu, C., Pan, N., & Gong, Q. (2020). Neurostructural correlates of hope: Dispositional hope mediates the impact of the SMA gray matter volume on subjective well-being in late adolescence. *Social Cognitive and Affective Neuroscience*, 15(4), 395–404. https://doi.org/10.1093/scan/nsaa046.

Waters, L., Allen, K. A., & Arslan, G. (2021a). Stress-related growth in adolescents returning to school after COVID-19 school closure. *Frontiers in Psychology*, 12, 643443. https://doi.org/10.3389/fpsyg.2021.643443.

Waters, L., Cameron, K., Nelson-Coffey, S. K., Crone, D. L., Kern, M. L., Lomas, T., Oades, L., Owens, R. L., Pawelski, J. O., Rashid, T., Warren, M. A., White, M. A., & Williams, P. (2021b). Collective wellbeing and posttraumatic growth during COVID-19: How positive psychology can help families, schools, workplaces and marginalized communities. *The Journal of Positive Psychology*, 17(6), 761–789. https://doi.org/10.1080/17439760.2021.1940251.

Weissman, D. G., Bitran, D., Miller, A. B., Schaefer, J. D., Sheridan, M. A., & McLaughlin, K. A. (2019). Difficulties with emotion regulation as a transdiagnostic mechanism linking child maltreatment with the emergence of psychopathology . *Development and Psychopathology*, 31(3), 899–915. https://doi.org/10.1017/S0954579419000348.

Williams, H., Skalisky, J., Erickson, T. M., & Thoburn, J. (2021). Posttraumatic growth in the context of grief: Testing the mindfulness-to-meaning theory. *Journal of Loss and Trauma*, 26(7), 611–623. https://doi.org/10.1080/15325024.2020.1855048.

Wolf, E. J., Miller, M. W., Sullivan, D. R., Amstadter, A. B., Mitchell, K. S., Goldberg, J., & Magruder, K. M. (2018). A classical twin study of PTSD symptoms and resilience: Evidence for a single spectrum of vulnerability to traumatic stress. *Depression and Anxiety*, 35(2), 132–139. https://doi.org/10.1002/da.22712.

Worley, J. (2017). The role of pleasure neurobiology and dopamine in mental health disorders. *Journal of Psychosocial Nursing and Mental Health Services*, 55(9), 17–21. https://doi.org/10.3928/02793695-20170818-09.

Xin, Q., Bai, B., & Liu, W. (2017). The analgesic effects of oxytocin in the peripheral and central nervous system. *Neurochemistry International*, 103, 57–64. https://doi.org/10.1016/j.neuint.2016.12.021.

Yoon, S., & Kim, Y. K. (2022). Possible oxytocin-related biomarkers in anxiety and mood disorders. *Progress in Neuro-Psychopharmacology & Biological Psychiatry*, 116, 110531. https://doi.org/10.1016/j.pnpbp.2022.110531.

Zacchaeus, E. A. (2020). Post-traumatic growth: A positive angle to psychological trauma. *International Journal of Science and Research*, 9(10), 1053–1061.

Zheng, H., Lim, J. Y., Kim, Y., Jung, S. T., & Hwang, S. W. (2021). The role of oxytocin, vasopressin, and their receptors at nociceptors in peripheral pain modulation. *Frontiers in Neuroendocrinology*, 63, 100942. https://doi.org/10.1016/j.yfrne.2021.100942.

Zou, Y., Li, P., Hofmann, S. G., & Liu, X. (2020). The mediating role of non-reactivity to mindfulness training and cognitive flexibility: A randomized controlled trial. *Frontiers in Psychology*, 11, 1053. https://doi.org/10.3389/fpsyg.2020.01053.

7

DEVELOPMENTAL TRAUMA IN SCHOOLS

Educational Assessment and Intervention

Many children experience ACEs and repeated traumas throughout their development, possibly resulting from repeated separation from caregivers or placements in foster care systems and juvenile detention centers, which cause them to experience problems with learning, self-regulating, and trusting or emotionally connecting to peers and teachers (Blake et al., 2022; O'Higgins et al., 2017; Koslouski & Stark, 2021; Loomis, 2021; Prince et al., 2022). Children exposed to trauma and interpersonal violence are likely to react with fear, anger, and cognitive/behavioral disorganization (e.g., dissociation, psychosis, reactive aggression, self-injury) in classrooms in ways that mirror their traumatic circumstances at home (Bloomfield et al., 2020; Blose et al., 2022; Farina et al., 2019; Luoni et al., 2018).

Regrettably, the severity of DTD children's behavioral problems is likely to result in punitive, often exclusionary consequences, particularly as they escalate in severity, disrupt the learning environment, and fail to respond to interventions from teachers and counselors. For example, a study of over 500 students (Báez et al., 2019) found that standard academic interventions failed to meet the needs of traumatized students and that additional supports were unsuccessful for individuals who had experienced severe traumas. Children who experience trauma and behavioral disturbances in schools often require individualized care plans, special education services, academic accommodations, and placement in alternative schools (Diggins, 2021; Hahnefeld et al., 2022; Michna et al., 2022; Ravi & Black, 2022; Rodgers & Hassan, 2021).

Trauma often causes children to have difficulty learning either because of poor self-regulation capacities or physiological and cognitive impairments resulting from toxic stress, repeated abuse and neglect, and unsafe school conditions – for example, experiencing additional traumas at school, including

DOI: 10.4324/9781003304715-7

verbal and physical assaults by peers. Research suggests that multiple repeated ACEs negatively correlate with student attendance and participation, and they place children at higher risk for grade retention (Crouch et al., 2019; McDoniel & Bierman, 2022; Stempel et al., 2017).

Children who experience developmental traumas at school – in addition to exposure in the home and in their communities – lose their only possible safe haven. Ideally, schools would offer safety and security, teach about self-regulating and coping with stress, and provide healthy models of relationships (via interactions with peers, teachers, and school counselors) that have the potential to mitigate the adverse effects of trauma and enhance resilience.

Unfortunately, schools have become unsafe for many children, given the high rates of school violence, including bullying and mass shootings, which have regrettably become all too familiar (Idsoe et al., 2021; Mundy et al., 2017; Polanin et al., 2021). Violence leading to fatalities, such as those at Sandy Hook, Columbine, and the Robb Elementary School massacre in Uvalde, Texas, have considerable adverse effects on children exposed to them and, more broadly, on the mental health and well-being of all individuals and families (Curran et al., 2020; Livingston et al., 2019; Peterson et al., 2021). Children and adolescents exposed to such devastating events, either by personally witnessing the loss of their teachers and peers or observing similar tragedies in the media, experience high rates of anxiety, fear, and academic problems that make it difficult to self-regulate and learn effectively (Bharadwaj et al., 2021; Cimolai et al., 2021; Stene et al., 2019). The lasting effects of such traumatic experiences have been reported in studies linking school violence to increasing levels of aggressive and disruptive behaviors in the classroom and lower math and reading proficiency rates, especially among racial and ethnic minorities and socioeconomically disadvantaged students (Gershenson & Tekin, 2018; Stevens et al., 2020).

Introduction to Developmental Trauma in Schools

Contemporary theoretical and empirical observations of developmental trauma have dramatically improved our understanding of the adverse impacts of trauma on children's learning and academic achievement. For example, self-determination theory posits that individuals who experience trauma learn more effectively with age-appropriate autonomy, connection to teachers and peers, and when they have opportunities to demonstrate their skills, competencies, and resiliency (e.g., Blakeslee et al., 2020; Herrick et al., 2022; Ntoumanis et al., 2021). Numerous studies link repeated abuse and neglect to severe impairments in learning and memory, which are worsened by negative schemas (e.g., *"Teachers don't care about me," "Why should I care about school when I keep failing?"* and *"I'm not smart like the other kids at school"*), and low academic engagement and efficacy, referring to an individual's attitudes and beliefs about accomplishing academic tasks effectively and succeeding academically (Dannehl et al., 2017; Malarbi et al., 2017; Mullins & Panlilio, 2021; van Os et al., 2017).

Children who experience trauma, including sexual, physical, and emotional abuse as well as neglect and violence, often experience shame, low self-esteem, anxiety, and aggression that adversely affect their adjustment to school and increase their risk for grade retention, learning problems, and school failure or dropout (Crouch et al., 2019; Fry et al., 2018; McGuire & Jackson, 2018; Pelcovitz et al., 2017). High absenteeism rates and low GPAs, poor school engagement, less student-teacher connectedness than peers, and low standardized achievement test scores have been linked to trauma (Larson et al., 2017; McGuire & Jackson, 2018; Mullins & Panlilio, 2021; Ryan et al., 2018; Stempel et al., 2017). The adverse effects of trauma often give rise to cognitive and emotional problems due to insecure attachment, poor self-regulation (high emotional reactivity and low distress tolerance associated with challenges engaging physiological resources underlying planned, goal-directed behaviors), and attention and concentration disturbances.

As such, children who experience trauma often have to work harder to show their full cognitive and academic potential because they tend to direct most of their mental energy on continually surveilling the environment for their physical and emotional safety and preparing for immediate action. Children with trauma also tend to avoid outward expressions of vulnerability (Baugh et al., 2019; Chung & Chen, 2021; Wermuth et al., 2021; Woodward et al., 2020). As such, they may avoid reading aloud and responding to questions because they may struggle academically and experience additional rejection by peers and teachers if they provide incorrect responses to questions or make errors in front of others. As a result, they may prioritize immediacy (i.e., safety) over delayed foresight and action (i.e., evaluating different responses to stress, self-regulating for learning), fall behind in class, and often stigmatize themselves (and are recognized by others) as failing themselves, their loved ones, and the school system.

Children who have experienced trauma often display a broad range of behavioral problems that may suggest they are disinterested in learning and succeeding at school. They often want to succeed academically and develop relationships with others; however, they lack the skills and experiences to do so effectively. In addition, they may have been manipulated, coerced, and revictimized in previous attempts to trust others. DTD children have limited exposure to healthy relationship models, structured (predictable and safe) environments, and opportunities to take healthy risks in relationships, such as approaching teachers and peers for help and guidance. As such, they are likely to withdraw from others or attempt to push them away or even hurt them, responding in ways that have helped them survive in previous circumstances (i. e., fight-flight adaptation).

DTD children are likely to demonstrate longstanding interpersonal, academic, and behavioral problems at school, given the broad impacts of trauma on children's behavior, psychological and physical health, and academic competencies, including foundational skills in reading and math literacy (Berber Çelik & Odacı, 2020; Kim et al., 2017; Mwakanyamale et al., 2018; Rumsey & Milsom, 2019). These children may experience high rates of aggression, resulting in suspension and expulsion (as early as preschool) and extreme internalizing and externalizing behaviors, such as avoiding school or continuously fighting with peers and teachers (e.g., throwing objects at others, acting out sexually, and defying authority due to fear and avoidance; Hsieh et al., 2021; Jackson et al., 2021; Pierce et al., 2022; Thompson et al., 2021). Some children with DTD may appear to function like their peers while they are actually experiencing troubling reminders of their traumas, helplessness, and recurrent thoughts of suicide, oftentimes hoping that a peer/teacher will recognize their felt psychological distress and, in turn, provide them with the support and interventions they need to recover. It is noteworthy that children with trauma often have impaired mentalization/theory of mind capacities and may assume that others are aware of their suffering and possibly ignoring their needs intentionally (Heleniak & McLaughlin, 2020; Simon et al., 2019; Turner et al., 2022; Vaskinn et al., 2020).

Some children resort to high-risk lifestyles to cope with stress and assert power and control. They may decide to avoid relying on their caregivers, who may be struggling with poverty, homelessness, and/or addictions (Abate et al., 2017; Dileo et al., 2017). As such, children who experience trauma often have different needs than their peers, which should be addressed by schools, preferably through evidence-based, trauma-informed practices. For example, research suggests that insecurely attached girls who experience sexual abuse by a family member (i.e., incest or intrafamilial child sexual abuse) are less likely to rely on fight-flight adaptations to cope with fear, stress, and anxiety (Katz et al., 2020, 2021; Katz & Nicolet, 2022; Levy et al., 2019).

Trauma and Learning

Trauma is pervasive among schoolchildren, and educators are likely to have frequent interactions with students exposed to traumatic events, including those characteristic of complex developmental trauma. As we have been discussing, trauma undermines children's ability to learn in school or demonstrate what they have learned to others, in part because they experience heightened physiological stress and cognitive interference during learning, which are precipitated by heightened levels of stress (i.e., repeated fight-flight-freeze responses in anticipation of revictimization at school) and compromise their ability to focus, self-regulate, connect with others, and learn/process new information effectively.

Nevertheless, developing academic competencies, including proficiency in reading, writing, and math, is inextricably linked to self-regulation and other cognitive capacities, such as auditory and visual attention, concentration, and short- and long-term memory (Fletcher & Grigorenko, 2017; Raghubar & Barnes, 2017). Decades of research suggest that trauma contributes to measurable and persistent cognitive disturbances, including working memory, processing speed, language (expressive and receptive language and verbal learning and memory), and executive control resulting from the trauma-mediated reorganization of the nervous system to adapt to short-term, highly stressful (and life-threatening) circumstances (Alvarado et al., 2022; Nikulina & Widom, 2019; Quidé et al., 2017; van Os et al., 2017; Winter et al. 2022; Xu et al., 2020a). Physiological stress responses compete for cognitive resources needed to engage higher-order thinking (e.g., there is an inverse relationship between the amygdala and prefrontal cortex, which mediates working memory, attentional and behavioral control, and complex problem solving; Hawkins et al., 2021; Ousdal et al., 2019; Stevens & Jovanovic, 2019; Williams et al., 2020). These changes interrupt children's progress in school, often giving rise to challenges, such as depression, anxiety, and frustration/anger, all of which diminish cognitive resources to devote to learning and lead to underperformance on academic outcome measures.

Mainstream teaching practices and assessment methods may underappreciate DTD children's full potential. In particular, the high curricular focus in schools, including verbal justification, high levels of inference, and increasingly complex reading, writing, and math assignments, may be frustrating to children with trauma, especially DTD children, who also frequently experience comorbid medical, psychological, and learning disorders. Repeated abuse and neglect result in physiological and epigenetic changes in areas needed for learning and higher-order problem-solving, most notably the prefrontal cortex, which mediates self-regulation and working memory, and the hippocampus, which is responsible for learning and memory.

Trauma, Executive Functioning, and Academic Achievement

Executive functioning refers to cognitive processes that support an individual's ability to focus, self-regulate, learn, and solve complex problems (Austin et al., 2020; Theodoraki et al., 2020; Zink et al., 2021). More specifically, three cognitive processes – response inhibition, working memory, and cognitive flexibility – comprise executive functions. Executive functioning is inextricably linked to children's emotion and behavior regulation capacities and academic achievement. Sustaining attention for extended periods of time, taking notes in class, solving multistep math problems effectively, and adapting to different school activities, content areas, and problem-solving approaches are examples of the neurocognitive processes underlying executive functioning (Allen et al., 2019, 2020; Johann et al., 2020).

Research suggests that executive functioning capacities correlate with several academic outcomes, including GPA, and are adversely affected by psychological and neurodevelopmental disturbances, including anxiety, ADHD, autism, and trauma (Bloemen et al., 2018; Otterman et al., 2019; Purpura et al., 2017; Waters et al., 2021; Zainal & Newman, 2021). Children who have been exposed to trauma often have problems with working memory, self-regulation, and mental flexibility, which adversely affect their academic performance, including their ability to attend to classroom tasks and instructions, organize and remember information, and understand abstract concepts needed for the development of independent thinking and problem-solving (Goodman et al., 2019; Horn et al., 2018; Kavanaugh et al., 2017; Lawson & Farah, 2017; Peters et al., 2019).

Scholars have reported on the adverse functional impacts of executive functioning challenges on the academic achievement of children who have experienced trauma. In one study (Nooner et al., 2018), abused and neglected children performed more poorly on measures of intelligence, attention, language, memory, executive function, and academic achievement in reading and math compared to children who did not have these traumatic experiences. These findings are consistent with previous empirical studies that also suggest mediating effects on learning from trauma-induced executive dysfunction (Chafouleas et al., 2019; Ensink et al., 2017; Fisher & Widom, 2021; Op den Kelder et al., 2017; Sheridan et al., 2017; Tan et al., 2017; Tyrell et al., 2019; Young-Southward et al., 2020).

Trauma, Verbal Learning and Memory, and Academic Achievement

Developmental trauma makes it difficult for children to learn, assimilate, and accommodate new information; perform well on tests; and respond to questions in the classroom. They may be overwhelmed by reminders of their trauma or by the thought of having to return to such circumstances at the end of the school day. Trauma often makes these children dissociate from reality and experience fear and terror, regardless of the circumstances. Memory activities and the ability to retrieve and utilize short- and long-term information are often impaired and interrupted by reminders of trauma. Because information cannot be easily processed or generalized by children who have experienced trauma, they tend to have more difficulty with short- and long-term memory. For example, whereas most children can rest, self-regulate, and recover from stress at home, those with developmental trauma are often unable to do so. Since these children experience repeated stress and trauma, DTD children may become overwhelmed and preoccupied with fear, often leading to chronic and debilitating sleep disturbances, which make learning more challenging given that memories form (i.e., consolidate) with sleep.

Experiences of abuse and neglect have been linked to more severe disturbances in verbal comprehension and long-term memory regardless of trauma/PTSD diagnosis (Biedermann et al., 2018; Dodaj et al., 2017; Scharpf et al., 2021; Su et al., 2019). Children who have experienced abuse and neglect are likely to misunderstand instructions, including homework requirements, and may provide inaccurate and incomplete work or fail to hand in assignments. Research suggests that physiological disturbances in the hippocampus mediate the adverse effects of trauma on learning and memory. The academic challenges associated with these impairments differentially affect boys and girls and racial and ethnic minorities, and they are often worsened by peer bullying, depression, re-experiencing symptoms, neuroticism, emotion dysregulation, and substance abuse (Brown et al., 2022; Huang, 2022; Lansing et al., 2019; Lin et al., 2017; Moyano & del Mar Sánchez-Fuentes, 2020; Nooner et al., 2018; Riffle et al., 2021; Xu et al., 2020b).

Trauma and Learning Disorders

Characterizing the link between developmental trauma and neurocognitive capacities adversely affected by early abuse and neglect is crucial for accurately understanding, evaluating, and treating individuals who have experienced ACEs and trauma and who have experienced broad psychological and learning deficits. Children who have experienced trauma often demonstrate impaired performance on measures of executive functioning, verbal learning, and memory (Motsan et al., 2022; Peters et al., 2019; Subbie-Saenz de Viteri et al., 2020). However, these findings may not generalize to all children who have experienced trauma, particularly those who demonstrate symptoms characteristic of DTD and who experience broad and severe interpersonal, cognitive, and physiological disturbances and high rates of psychological and medical comorbidities. Unfortunately, most school systems do not recognize DTD symptoms as such, and, regrettably, these children often do not receive the type of attention and treatment they need to thrive. As a result, these children often experience disciplinary actions and other responses that can distract them from uncovering and responding appropriately to their early traumas and DTD challenges. Learning disabilities have been linked to trauma, and scholars posit that those with learning disabilities and psychiatric disorders like trauma experience additional stress and risks, such as social skill deficits, anxiety/phobia, loneliness/isolation, and low self-efficacy, which can heighten their vulnerability to victimization (and re-victimization) and impede academic engagement, learning, and responses to interventions (Franklin & Smeaton, 2017; Haft et al., 2019; Helton et al., 2018; Seppälä et al., 2021).

DTD children may meet diagnostic criteria for neurodevelopmental learning disorders, characterized by persistent measurable impairments in reading (e.g., low reading speed/fluency and comprehension), writing (clarity and organization of written text, flow of ideas, grammar, and punctuation), and mathematics, including understanding and applying math facts and rules effectively to solve complex problems (Altay & Görker, 2017; Larson et al., 2017; Ryan et al., 2018). Learning disabilities indicate that achievements in reading, writing, and math are substantially lower than expected for an individual's age and grade level. Schools often use terms like dyslexia, dysgraphia, and dyscalculia to describe (and classify) children with measurable impairments in reading, writing, and math. Classifying students with a learning disability often allows them to receive specialized social, emotional, and academic supports (i.e., students with physical, psychological, cognitive, and learning disorders often qualify for a federally mandated Individualized Education Plan [IEP], which includes an interdisciplinary evaluation from a school social worker, psychologist, speech and language pathologist, and learning disabilities consultant as well as individualized academic accommodations to help these students succeed; Buxton, 2018; Fletcher & Grigorenko, 2017; Hurless & Kong, 2021; Maddox et al. 2022). Schools use these guidelines to determine whether a child's learning challenges are severe enough to warrant one or more classifications under the Americans with Disabilities Act.

Research suggests that individuals who have experienced trauma and other comorbid conditions have significantly more developmental, social, emotional, and academic needs than children who have not experienced complex traumas. For example, polyvictimized children who failed to meet grade-level standards in mathematics, reading, and writing, and standardized cognitive assessments reveal demonstrable impairments in several areas, including general intelligence, working memory, as well as verbal and nonverbal cognitive capacities (e.g., receptive and expressive language, visual and spatial problem-solving, information processing speed; Blodgett & Lanigan, 2018; Malarbi et al., 2017; Spiegel et al., 2021). In addition, children who have experienced developmental traumas and ADHD, autism, and learning disabilities have additional risks associated with low levels of fetal attachment, prematurity, low birth weight, lack of prenatal care, and exposure to alcohol and drugs.

Perfect et al. (2016) conducted a meta-analysis on trauma and learning impairments among schoolchildren. They reported widespread impacts of trauma exposure and traumatic stress symptoms on students' cognitive, academic, and social-emotional-behavioral outcomes. For example, children who experienced trauma were more likely to have multiple psychiatric comorbidities, higher rates of IEPs, lower school engagement, and more grade retentions. Several other studies have corroborated these findings, in addition to suggesting cumulative adverse effects from poverty, caregiver incarceration, and interpersonal violence exposure (Hinojosa et al., 2019; McKelvey et al., 2018; Tessier et al., 2018). Children who experience learning challenges and are diagnosed with multiple comorbidities, such as trauma, ADHD, motor/mobility impairments and autism, often have difficulty adjusting to mainstream schools and may require special education accommodations, including placement in alternative school settings (Chan et al., 2018; Tessier et al., 2018).

You can see how the cumulative effects of trauma, including abuse, poverty, and violence, can be devastating for children, who may also be experiencing bullying, school failure, and isolation. These children develop low academic efficacy, which puts them at high risk for dropout and low-wage jobs that undermine their strengths. These reactions are likely to be worsened by learning disabilities, whereby children may experience stigma, shame, and hopelessness, mainly as they receive multiple disability classifications.

College Students

When individuals with DTD move into young adulthood, they may struggle to manage independently and experience difficulty adjusting to new settings. If they attend college or university, they may need help self-regulating and mapping out the steps to complete assignments and tasks successfully. Research suggests that adolescents not only entered college with lower high school GPAs but also demonstrated poor college academic outcomes as assessed by GPA and self-report measures for academic adjustment and attachment to the college or university (Welsh et al., 2017).

Some individuals with DTD may drop out of school, experience inconsistent employment, or hold employment positions that could be more satisfying. A recent study of adults who experienced developmental traumas as children (Maercker et al., 2022) found lower educational attainment, poorer financial status, and low life satisfaction compared to adults who had not experienced developmental traumas as children. Adults who experienced developmental traumas as children may also lack confidence and have low self-esteem, both of which can lead to further increased anxiety and job instability. They may feel worried about re-traumatization or being stigmatized because of their challenges. As a result, some will choose not to disclose personal information to others who might be able to help them, believing that the vulnerability could put them at a disadvantage for recruitment or advancement.

College students with DTD may also have unique needs that may evolve for the first time in their adult lives. They may be transitioning from relying on parents and teachers to establishing an internal locus, developing autonomy, and self-regulating and managing their academic habits (e.g., managing their time, developing regular reading and writing practices). Moreover, years of negative feedback, poor performance on school assignments, high levels of peer and teacher rejection, depression, isolation, and perfectionistic anxiety all likely contribute to stress, avoidance, catastrophizing, and, ultimately, academic challenges in college.

Trauma Informed Schools

Trauma-informed schools (TISs) are designed to meet the social, emotional, and academic needs of all students (and staff), including those adversely affected by ACEs, polyvictimization, and developmental trauma (Berger, 2019; Collier et al., 2020; Myat Zaw et al., 2022; Thomas et al., 2019). The impetus for TIS approaches includes national calls to action by government leaders and policy-makers in response to growing research demonstrating broad and lasting effects associated with ACEs and early trauma. Research suggests that trauma-informed practices are linked to reductions in student behavior problems, suspensions, and expulsions as well as increases in resilience (Herrenkohl et al., 2019; Kataoka et al., 2018; Lai et al., 2018; McIntyre et al., 2019; Pataky et al., 2019).

TISs are differentiated by evidence-based, trauma-sensitive policies and practices, including widespread training on the impact of, and appropriate responses to, vulnerable students affected by ACEs and trauma. Students who experience trauma often require cognitive, psychological, and emotional sup-port in addition to academic interventions. For example, children who have experienced trauma may feel fear and psychological distress, causing them to behave in ways that lead to punishment and exclusionary practices, including detention and suspension, which only reinforce their attachment disturbances, interfere with self-regulation, and increase their risk for school failure. These experiences will also reinforce for DTD children that they are damaged and unlovable. In addition, traditional interventions for disruptive behaviors may include behavioral plans to reduce the frequency and intensity of problem behaviors, which undermine children's social and emotional needs as well as exacerbate their insecure attachment and the fear and anxiety from which these disturbances originate. As such, mainstream practices that are not trauma-informed may fail to address the needs of children with trauma and could instead result in traumatic re-victimization from harsh, punitive, or dismissive responses, which likely mirror negative responses from caregivers.

A TIS also considers prevention, de-escalation, and positive and restorative responses to disruptive behavior by implementing strengths-based, social-jus-tice-informed, culturally responsive procedures, including interdisciplinary eva-luation, teacher and staff professional development, positive psychology principles, and collaboration between school staff, community agencies, and mental health professionals (Chafouleas et al., 2019; Rishel et al., 2019; Thomas et al., 2019). Examples of effective trauma-informed practices linked to mea-surable positive outcomes in children and adolescents affected by trauma include providing classroom trauma specialists and coaches to support teachers in recognizing and responding to trauma effectively; enhancing social-emo-tional learning (SEL); addressing vicarious trauma, offering patterned activities, such as daily mindfulness and yoga exercises; identifying and reinforcing strengths; and reframing undesirable behaviors as behavioral expressions of fear, anxiety, and attachment insecurity (Brunzell et al., 2019; Crosby et al., 2018; Joseph et al., 2020; Tabone et al., 2020).

Studies have shown that building a positive relationship with teachers can mitigate the effects of trauma and improve self-regulation capacities and aca-demic competencies (Keane & Evans, 2022; Kibriya et al., 2017). Children who have experienced trauma may be suspicious and distrustful of teachers and can react aggressively to protect themselves from being re-victimized. They may reject peers to avoid further pain and suffering. Thus, understanding attachment concepts will also assist teachers in understanding and responding to behavioral disturbances effectively.

Trauma-Informed Assessment

Trauma-informed assessments consider the impact of trauma throughout the entire process from referral to interpretation, regardless of the primary referral concern. Assessment and treatment of children who have experienced multiple traumas must address psychological symptoms, emotion and behavior disturbances, and functional impairments in multiple areas, including self-regulation, physical health/somatic stress, cognitive problems in attention and concentration, and academic efficacy, engagement, and performance (Charak et al., 2019; Kottenstette et al., 2020; Tyler et al., 2019). School assessment findings can help students identify their strengths and develop coping skills and compensatory learning strategies. School assessments can also help to determine if academic accommodations are needed so that students who experience trauma can show their potential and succeed at the same rate as their peers. TISs often recognize that children with trauma can learn effectively and succeed academically with the support of their teachers, peers, and counselors, particularly if they are evaluated appropriately and provided with meaningful academic accommodations.

A comprehensive assessment should include measures to assess executive functioning; memory; learning; and physical and psychological health and well-being, including symptoms and comorbidities associated with trauma/PTSD, polyvictimization, attachment, dissociation, interpersonal sensitivity, ADHD, and autism (Choi & Graham-Bermann, 2018; John et al., 2019; Karatzias et al., 2022; Malarbi et al., 2017; Spinazzola et al., 2021). Comprehensive multi-informant interviews, validated psychometric instruments, and historical data may help confirm the diagnosis of trauma and associated comorbidities and learning disorders. One approach to measuring cognitive and learning disturbances in traumatized children, especially if academic accommodations are warranted, is to use objective cognitive and academic assessment measures, such as the Wechsler Intelligence Scale for Children (WISC-V) (Wechsler, 2014) and the Woodcock-Johnson Tests of Achievement (WJ-IV Ach) (Schrank et al., 2014), which schools commonly use to evaluate children for cognitive and learning disorders. These measures provide meaningful data on children's functioning, including verbal and nonverbal reasoning, processing speed, and expressive/receptive language, as well as working memory, reading, writing, and math competencies (van Os et al., 2017). Consider the following case of DJ (Mainwaring, 2015).

DJ is a 13-year-old girl referred for a school evaluation. She had been removed from her family of origin when she was four years old and experienced developmental trauma due to abuse and neglect, including drug dealing, multiple foster care placements, separation from siblings, and domestic violence exposure. She experienced longstanding problems with her learning, resulting in repeating the 5th grade, although she had not been evaluated by school personnel, resulting in different experiences of neglect. Teacher observations revealed that DJ often appeared sad and depressed and that she struggled with peer relationships. DJ reportedly shared with peers and teachers that several of her foster care placements had been unsuccessful, prompting concerns by school officials about DJ's interpersonal boundaries. An evaluation revealed that DJ had speech and language difficulties, measurable learning challenges, disorganized attachment, and low cognitive capacities (IQ fell within the low average range).

DJ was also administered a broad range of social and emotional well-being measures, including hobbies and interests as well as strengths and resiliencies. Results revealed low self-efficacy, feelings of isolation, a sense of not belonging, poor psychological distress tolerance, and difficulty asking for help and support from others. DJ reported adequate social skills; however, these findings were inconsistent with multiple reports and behavioral observations from staff. DJ was provided with several interventions, including the Cognitive Behavioral Intervention for Trauma in Schools (CBITS) (Jaycox, 2004), a group-based treatment for children who have experienced PTSD, complex PTSD, and DTD. Staff also received specialized training on trauma and attachment as well as specific strategies to help DJ thrive. Interventions included scaffolding academic tasks (breaking them down into smaller steps to reduce the cognitive demands), social skills training, assertiveness and conflict resolution, and relaxation techniques.

DTD children experience diverse symptoms, broad neurocognitive disturbances, and social and academic challenges. For victims of repeated abuse and neglect, separation from caregivers is often compounded by other stressors, including being displaced and separated from siblings and extended family. Children may also experience additional abuse and neglect in foster-care systems or schools, particularly if they are ostracized and bullied by peers. With regard to learning, the physiological resources needed to learn effectively are compromised (and continuously compromised) by repeated adversities, such as those described in DJ's circumstances.

Conclusions

Adverse childhood experiences, polyvictimization, and neglect, including by teachers and, more broadly, school systems, can damage children and adolescents, who depend on adults for guidance and support. At the same time, trauma causes significant disturbances in attachment and self-regulation, which can lead children to reject the love and support of others, sometimes in highly disruptive ways. They may have difficulty deferring to authority figures given their negative internal working models of adults as untrustworthy, which will take considerable time to repair. Low grades, poor self-esteem, confusion/cognitive disturbances, high rates of learning disorders, and negative interactions with peers and teachers put DTD children at high risk for school dropout and, eventually, underemployment or unemployment. As school systems increase their understanding of trauma, including complex developmental trauma, children will have more opportunities to develop positive, lasting relationships as well as cognitive and academic competencies. As such, we encourage schools to adopt a trauma-informed framework that includes universal screening for ACEs and trauma; building partnerships with families and community agencies; reframing negative behaviors as indications of fear, helplessness, and emotional crisis; and building social networks that help students, teachers, and staff reach their potential and thrive as a collective community.

References

Abate, A., Marshall, K., Sharp, C., & Venta, A. (2017). Trauma and aggression: Investigating the mediating role of mentalizing in female and male inpatient adolescents. *Child Psychiatry and Human Development*, 48(6), 881–890. https://doi.org/10.1007/s10578-017-0711-6.

Allen, K., Giofrè, D., Higgins, S., & Adams, J. (2020). Working memory predictors of written mathematics in 7-to 8-year-old children. *Quarterly Journal of Experimental Psychology*, 73(2), 239–248. https://doi.org/10.1177/1747021819871243.

Allen, K., Higgins, S., & Adams, J. (2019). The relationship between visuospatial working memory and mathematical performance in school-aged children: A systematic review. *Educational Psychology Review*, 31(3), 509–531. https://doi.org/10.1007/s10648-019-09470-8.

Altay, M. A., & Görker, I. (2017). Assessment of psychiatric comorbidity and WISC-R profiles in cases diagnosed with specific learning disorder according to DSM-5 criteria. *Noro Psikiyatri arsivi*, 55(2), 127–134. https://doi.org/10.5152/npa.2017.18123.

Alvarado, C., Selin, C., Herman, E. A., Ellner, S., & Jackson, Y. (2022). Methodological inconsistencies confound understanding of language measurement in the child maltreatment population: A systematic review. *Child Abuse & Neglect*, 105928. https://doi.org/10.1016/j.chiabu.2022.105928.

Austin, G., Bondü, R., & Elsner, B. (2020). Executive function, theory of mind, and conduct-problem symptoms in middle childhood. *Frontiers in Psychology*, 11, 539. https://doi.org/10.3389/fpsyg.2020.00539.

Báez, J. C., Renshaw, K. J., Bachman, L. E., Kim, D., Smith, V. D., & Stafford, R. E. (2019). Understanding the necessity of trauma-informed care in community schools: A mixed-methods program evaluation. *Children & Schools*, 41(2), 101–110. https://doi.org/10.1093/cs/cdz007.

Baugh, L. M., Cox, D. W., Young, R. A., & Kealy, D. (2019). Partner trust and childhood emotional maltreatment: The mediating and moderating roles of maladaptive schemas and psychological flexibility. *Journal of Contextual Behavioral Science*, 12, 66–73. https://doi.org/10.1016/j.jcbs.2019.02.001.

Berber Çelik, Ç., & Odacı, H. (2020). Does child abuse have an impact on self-esteem, depression, anxiety and stress conditions of individuals? *The International Journal of Social Psychiatry*, 66(2), 171–178. https://doi.org/10.1177/0020764019894618.

Berger, E. (2019). Multi-tiered approaches to trauma-informed care in schools: A systematic review. *School Mental Health*, 11(4), 650–664. https://doi.org/10.1007/s12310-019-09326-0.

Bharadwaj, P., Bhuller, M., Løken, K. V., & Wentzel, M. (2021). Surviving a mass shooting. *Journal of Public Economics*, 201, 104469. https://doi.org/10.1016/j.jpubeco.2021.104469.

Biedermann, S. V., Meliss, S., Simmons, C., Nöthling, J., Suliman, S., & Seedat, S. (2018). Sexual abuse but not posttraumatic stress disorder is associated with neurocognitive deficits in South African traumatized adolescents. *Child Abuse & Neglect*, 80, 257–267. https://doi.org/10.1016/j.chiabu.2018.04.003.

Blake, A. J., Ruderman, M., Waterman, J. M., & Langley, A. K. (2022). Long-term effects of pre-adoptive risk on emotional and behavioral functioning in children adopted from foster care. *Child Abuse & Neglect*, 130(Pt 2), 105031. https://doi.org/10.1016/j.chiabu.2021.105031.

Blakeslee, J. E., Powers, L. E., Geenen, S., Schmidt, J., Nelson, M., Fullerton, A., George, K., McHugh, E., & Bryant, M. (2020). Evaluating the My Life self-determination model for older youth in foster care: Establishing efficacy and exploring moderation of response to intervention. *Children and Youth Services Review*, 119, 105419. https://doi.org/10.1016/j.childyouth.2020.105419.

Blodgett, C., & Lanigan, J. D. (2018). The association between adverse childhood experience (ACE) and school success in elementary school children. *School Psychology Quarterly*, 33(1), 137–146. https://doi.org/10.1037/spq0000256.

Bloemen, A. J. P., Oldehinkel, A. J., Laceulle, O. M., Ormel, J., Rommelse, N. N. J., & Hartman, C. A. (2018). The association between executive functioning and psychopathology: General or specific? *Psychological Medicine*, 48(11), 1787–1794. https://doi.org/10.1017/S0033291717003269.

Bloomfield, M. A., Yusuf, F. N., Srinivasan, R., Kelleher, I., Bell, V., & Pitman, A. (2020). Trauma-informed care for adult survivors of developmental trauma with psychotic and dissociative symptoms: a systematic review of intervention studies. *The Lancet Psychiatry*, 7(5), 449–462. https://doi.org/10.1016/S2215-0366(20)30041–30049.

Blose, B. A., Godleski, S. A., Houston, R. J., & Schenkel, L. S. (2022). The indirect effect of peritraumatic dissociation on the relationship between childhood maltreatment and schizotypy. *Journal of Interpersonal Violence*, 38(5–6), 5282–5304. Advance online publication. https://doi.org/10.1177/08862605221122832.

Brown, M. J., Jiang, Y., Hung, P., Haider, M. R., & Crouch, E. (2022). Disparities by gender and race/ethnicity in child maltreatment and memory performance. *Journal of Interpersonal Violence*, 37(15–16), NP14633–NP14655. https://doi.org/10.1177/08862605211015222.

Brunzell, T., Stokes, H., & Waters, L. (2019). Shifting teacher practice in trauma-affected classrooms: Practice pedagogy strategies within a trauma-informed positive education model. *School Mental Health*, 11(3), 600–614. https://doi.org/10.1007/s12310-018-09308-8.

Buxton, P. S. (2018). Viewing the behavioral responses of ED children from a trauma-informed perspective. *Educational Research Quarterly*, 41(4), 30–49.

Chafouleas, S. M., Koriakin, T. A., Roundfield, K. D., & Overstreet, S. (2019). Addressing childhood trauma in school settings: A framework for evidence-based practice. *School Mental Health: A Multidisciplinary Research and Practice Journal*, 11(1), 40–53. https://doi.org/10.1007/s12310-018-9256-5.

Chan, K. L., Lo, C., & Ip, P. (2018). Associating disabilities, school environments, and child victimization. *Child Abuse & Neglect*, 83, 21–30. https://doi.org/10.1016/j.chiabu.2018.07.001.

Charak, R., Ford, J. D., Modrowski, C. A., & Kerig, P. K. (2019). Polyvictimization, emotion dysregulation, symptoms of posttraumatic stress disorder, and behavioral health problems among justice-involved youth: A latent class analysis. *Journal of Abnormal Child Psychology*, 47(2), 287–298.

Choi, K. R., & Graham-Bermann, S. A. (2018). Developmental considerations for assessment of trauma symptoms in preschoolers: A review of measures and diagnoses. *Journal of Child and Family Studies*, 27(11), 3427–3439. https://doi.org/10.1007/s10826-018-1177-2.

Chung, M. C., & Chen, Z. S. (2021). The interrelationship between child abuse, emotional processing difficulties, alexithymia and psychological symptoms among Chinese adolescents. *Journal of Trauma & Dissociation*, 22(1), 107–121. https://doi.org/10.1080/15299732.2020.1788689.

Cimolai, V., Schmitz, J., & Sood, A. B. (2021). Effects of mass shootings on the mental health of children and adolescents. *Current Psychiatry Reports*, 23(3), 1–10. https://doi.org/10.1007/s11920-021-01241-z.

Collier, S., Bryce, I., Trimmer, K., & Krishnamoorthy, G. (2020). Evaluating frameworks for practice in mainstream primary school classrooms catering for children with developmental trauma: An analysis of the literature. *Children Australia*, 45(4), 258–265. https://doi.org/10.1017/cha.2020.53.

Crosby, S. D., Howell, P., & Thomas, S. (2018). Social justice education through trauma-informed teaching. *Middle School Journal*, 49(4), 15–23. https://doi.org/10.1080/00940771.2018.1488470.

Crouch, E., Radcliff, E., Hung, P., & Bennett, K. (2019). Challenges to school success and the role of adverse childhood experiences. *Academic Pediatrics*, 19(8), 899–907. https://doi.org/10.1016/j.acap.2019.08.006.

Curran, F. C., Fisher, B. W., & Viano, S. L. (2020). Mass school shootings and the short-run impacts on use of school security measures and practices: national evidence from the Columbine tragedy. *Journal of School Violence*, 19(1), 6–19. https://doi.org/10.1080/15388220.2019.1703713.

Dannehl, K., Rief, W., & Euteneuer, F. (2017). Childhood adversity and cognitive functioning in patients with major depression. *Child Abuse & Neglect*, 70, 247–254. https://doi.org/10.1016/j.chiabu.2017.06.013.

Diggins, J. (2021). Reductions in behavioural and emotional difficulties from a specialist, trauma-informed school. *Educational and Developmental Psychologist*, 38(2), 194–205. https://doi.org/10.1080/20590776.2021.1923131.

Dileo, J. F., Brewer, W., Northam, E., Yucel, M., & Anderson, V. (2017). Investigating the neurodevelopmental mediators of aggression in children with a history of child maltreatment: An exploratory field study. *Child Neuropsychology*, 23(6), 655–677. https://doi.org/10.1080/09297049.2016.1186159.

Dodaj, A., Krajina, M., Sesar, K., & Šimić, N. (2017). The effects of maltreatment in childhood on working memory capacity in adulthood. *Europe's Journal of Psychology*, 13(4), 618–632. https://doi.org/10.5964/ejop.v13i4.1373.

Ensink, K., Bégin, M., Normandin, L., Godbout, N., & Fonagy, P. (2017). Mentalization and dissociation in the context of trauma: Implications for child psychopathology. *Journal of Trauma & Dissociation*, 18(1), 11–30. https://doi.org/10.1080/15299732.2016.1172536.

Farina, B., Liotti, M., & Imperatori, C. (2019). The role of attachment trauma and disintegrative pathogenic processes in the traumatic-dissociative dimension. *Frontiers in Psychology*, 10, 933. https://doi.org/10.3389/fpsyg.2019.00933.

Fisher, J. H., & Widom, C. S. (2021). Child maltreatment and cognitive and academic functioning in two generations. *Child Abuse & Neglect*, 115, 105011. https://doi.org/10.1016/j.chiabu.2021.105011.

Fletcher, J. M., & Grigorenko, E. L. (2017). Neuropsychology of learning disabilities: The past and the future. *Journal of the International Neuropsychological Society*, 23(9–10), 930–940. https://doi.org/10.1017/S1355617717001084.

Franklin, A., & Smeaton, E. (2017). Recognising and responding to young people with learning disabilities who experience, or are at risk of, child sexual exploitation in the UK. *Children and Youth Services Review*, 73, 474–481. https://doi.org/10.1016/j.childyouth.2016.11.009.

Fry, D., Fang, X., Elliott, S., Casey, T., Zheng, X., Li, J., Florian, L., & McCluskey, G. (2018). The relationships between violence in childhood and educational outcomes: A global systematic review and meta-analysis. *Child Abuse & Neglect*, 75, 6–28. https://doi.org/10.1016/j.chiabu.2017.06.021.

Gershenson, S., & Tekin, E. (2018). The effect of community traumatic events on student achievement: Evidence from the beltway sniper attacks. *Education Finance and Policy*, 13(4), 513–544. https://doi.org/10.1162/edfp_a_00234.

Goodman, J. B., Freeman, E. E., & Chalmers, K. A. (2019). The relationship between early life stress and working memory in adulthood: A systematic review and meta-analysis. *Memory*, 27(6), 868–880. https://doi.org/10.1080/09658211.2018.1561897.

Haft, S. L., Duong, P. H., Ho, T. C., Hendren, R. L., & Hoeft, F. (2019). Anxiety and attentional bias in children with specific learning disorders. *Journal of Abnormal Child Psychology*, 47(3), 487–497. https://doi.org/10.1007/s10802-018-0458-y.

Hahnefeld, A., Sukale, T., Weigand, E., Dudek, V., Münch, K., Aberl, S., Eckler, L. V., Nehring, I., Friedmann, A., Plener, P. L., Fegert, J. M., & Mall, V. (2022). Non-verbal cognitive development, learning, and symptoms of PTSD in 3- to 6-year-old refugee children. *European Journal of Pediatrics*, 181(3), 1205–1212. https://doi.org/10.1007/s00431-021-04312-8.

Hawkins, M. A. W., Layman, H. M., Ganson, K. T., Tabler, J., Ciciolla, L., Tsotsoros, C. E., & Nagata, J. M. (2021). Adverse childhood events and cognitive function among young adults: Prospective results from the national longitudinal study of adolescent to adult health. *Child Abuse & Neglect*, 115, 105008. https://doi.org/10.1016/j.chiabu.2021.105008.

Heleniak, C., & McLaughlin, K. A. (2020). Social-cognitive mechanisms in the cycle of violence: Cognitive and affective theory of mind, and externalizing psychopathology in children and adolescents. *Development and Psychopathology*, 32(2), 735–750. https://doi.org/10.1017/S0954579419000725.

Helton, J. J., Gochez-Kerr, T., & Gruber, E. (2018). Sexual abuse of children with learning disabilities. *Child Maltreatment*, 23(2), 157–165. https://doi.org/10.1177/1077559517733814.

Herrenkohl, T. I., Hong, S., & Verbrugge, B. (2019). Trauma-informed programs based in schools: Linking concepts to practices and assessing the evidence. *American Journal of Community Psychology*, 64(3–4), 373–388. https://doi.org/10.1002/ajcp.12362.

Herrick, S. S. C., Rocchi, M. A., Sweet, S. N., & Duncan, L. R. (2022). Exploring proximal LGBTQ+ minority stressors within physical activity contexts from a self-determination theory perspective. *Annals of Behavioral Medicine*, 56(6), 551–561. https://doi.org/10.1093/abm/kaab052.

Hinojosa, M. S., Hinojosa, R., Bright, M., & Nguyen, J. (2019). Adverse childhood experiences and grade retention in a national sample of US children. *Sociological Inquiry*, 89(3), 401–426. https://doi.org/10.1111/soin.12272.

Horn, S. R., Roos, L. E., Beauchamp, K. G., Flannery, J. E., & Fisher, P. A. (2018). Polyvictimization and externalizing symptoms in foster care children: The moderating role of executive function. *Journal of Trauma & Dissociation*, 19(3), 307–324. https://doi.org/10.1080/15299732.2018.1441353.

Hsieh, Y. P., Shen, A. C. T., Hwa, H. L., Wei, H. S., Feng, J. Y., & Huang, S. C. Y. (2021). Associations between child maltreatment, dysfunctional family environment, post-traumatic stress disorder and children's bullying perpetration in a national representative sample in Taiwan. *Journal of Family Violence*, 36(1), 27–36. https://doi.org/10.1007/s10896-020-00144-6.

Huang, L. (2022). Exploring the relationship between school bullying and academic performance: The mediating role of students' sense of belonging at school. *Educational Studies*, 48(2), 216–232. https://doi.org/10.1080/03055698.2020.1749032.

Hurless, N., & Kong, N. Y. (2021). Trauma-informed strategies for culturally diverse students diagnosed with emotional and behavioral disorders. *Intervention in School and Clinic*, 57(1), 56–61. https://doi.org/10.1177/1053451221994814.

Idsoe, T., Vaillancourt, T., Dyregrov, A., Hagen, K. A., Ogden, T., & Nærde, A. (2021). Bullying victimization and trauma. *Frontiers in Psychiatry*, 11, 480353. https://doi.org/10.3389/fpsyt.2020.480353.

Jackson, D. B., Testa, A., & Vaughn, M. G. (2021). Adverse childhood experiences and school readiness among preschool-aged children. *The Journal of Pediatrics*, 230, 191–197. https://doi.org/10.1016/j.jpeds.2020.11.023.

Jaycox, L. (2004). *Cognitive-behavioural intervention for trauma in schools: Training manual.* Longmont, CO: Sopris West Educational Services.

Johann, V., Könen, T., & Karbach, J. (2020). The unique contribution of working memory, inhibition, cognitive flexibility, and intelligence to reading comprehension and reading speed. *Child Neuropsychology*, 26(3), 324–344. https://doi.org/10.1080/09297049.2019.1649381.

John, S. G., Brandt, T. W., Secrist, M. E., Mesman, G. R., Sigel, B. A., & Kramer, T. L. (2019). Empirically-guided assessment of complex trauma for children in foster care: A focus on appropriate diagnosis of attachment concerns. *Psychological Services*, 16(1), 120–133. https://doi.org/10.1037/ser0000263.

Joseph, A. A., Wilcox, S. M., Hnilica, R. J., & Hansen, M. C. (2020). Keeping race at the center of school discipline practices and trauma-informed care: An interprofessional framework. *Children & Schools*, 42(3), 161–170. https://doi.org/10.1093/cs/cdaa013.

Karatzias, T., Shevlin, M., Ford, J. D., Fyvie, C., Grandison, G., Hyland, P., & Cloitre, M. (2022). Childhood trauma, attachment orientation, and complex PTSD (CPTSD) symptoms in a clinical sample: Implications for treatment. *Development and Psychopathology*, 34(3), 1192–1197. https://doi.org/10.1017/S0954579420001509.

Kataoka, S. H., Vona, P., Acuna, A., Jaycox, L., Escudero, P., Rojas, C., Ramirez, E., Langley, A., & Stein, B. D. (2018). Applying a trauma informed school systems approach: Examples from school community-academic partnerships. *Ethnicity & Disease*, 28(Suppl 2), 417–426. https://doi.org/10.18865/ed.28.S2.417.

Katz, C., & Nicolet, R. (2022). "If only I could have stopped it": Reflections of adult child sexual abuse survivors on their responses during the abuse. *Journal of Interpersonal Violence*, 37(3–4), NP2076–NP2100. https://doi.org/10.1177/0886260520935485.

Katz, C., Tsur, N., Nicolet, R., Klebanov, B., & Carmel, N. (2020). No way to run or hide: Children's perceptions of their responses during intrafamilial child sexual abuse. *Child Abuse & Neglect*, 106, 104541. https://doi.org/10.1016/j.chiabu.2020.104541.

Katz, C., Tsur, N., Talmon, A., & Nicolet, R. (2021). Beyond fight, flight, and freeze: Towards a new conceptualization of peritraumatic responses to child sexual abuse based on retrospective accounts of adult survivors. *Child Abuse & Neglect*, 112, 104905. https://doi.org/10.1016/j.chiabu.2020.104905.

Kavanaugh, B. C., Dupont-Frechette, J. A., Jerskey, B. A., & Holler, K. A. (2017). Neurocognitive deficits in children and adolescents following maltreatment: Neurodevelopmental consequences and neuropsychological implications of traumatic stress. *Applied Neuropsychology: Child*, 6(1), 64–78. https://doi.org/10.1080/21622965.2015.1079712.

Keane, K., & Evans, R. R. (2022). The potential for teacher-student relationships and the whole school, whole community, whole child model to mitigate adverse childhood experiences. *Journal of School Health*, 92(5), 504–513. https://doi.org/10.1111/josh.13154.

Kibriya, S., Xu, Z. P., & Zhang, Y, (2017). The negative consequences of school bullying on academic performance and mitigation through female teacher participation: Evidence from Ghana. *Applied Economics*, 49(25), 2480–2490. https://doi.org/10.1080/00036846.2016.1240350.

Kim, B. N., Park, S., & Park, M. H. (2017). The relationship of sexual abuse with self-esteem, depression, and problematic internet use in Korean adolescents. *Psychiatry Investigation*, 14(3), 372. https://doi.org/10.4306/pi.2017.14.3.372.

Koslouski, J. B., & Stark, K. (2021). Promoting learning for students experiencing adversity and trauma: The everyday, yet profound, actions of teachers. *The Elementary School Journal*, 121(3), 430–453. https://doi.org/10.1086/712606.

Kottenstette, S., Segal, R., Roeder, V., Rochford, H., Schnieders, E., Bayman, L., McKissic, D. A., Dahlberg, G. J., Krewer, R., Chambliss, J., Theurer, J. L., & Oral, R. (2020). Two-generational trauma-informed assessment improves documentation and service referral frequency in a child protection program. *Child Abuse & Neglect*, 101, 104327. https://doi.org/10.1016/j.chiabu.2019.104327.

Lai, B. S., Osborne, M. C., Lee, N., Self-Brown, S., Esnard, A. M., & Kelley, M. L. (2018). Trauma-informed schools: Child disaster exposure, community violence and somatic symptoms. *Journal of Affective Disorders*, 238, 586–592. https://doi.org/10.1016/j.jad.2018.05.062.

Lansing, A. E., Plante, W. Y., Golshan, S., Fennema-Notestine, C., & Thuret, S. (2019). Emotion regulation mediates the relationship between verbal learning and internalizing, trauma-related and externalizing symptoms among early-onset, persistently delinquent adolescents. *Learning and Individual Differences*, 70, 201–215. https://doi.org/10.1016/j.lindif.2017.01.014.

Larson, S., Chapman, S., Spetz, J., & Brindis, C. D. (2017). Chronic childhood trauma, mental health, academic achievement, and school-based health center mental health services. *Journal of School Health*, 87(9), 675–686. https://doi.org/10.1111/josh.12541.

Lawson, G. M., & Farah, M. J. (2017). Executive function as a mediator between SES and academic achievement throughout childhood. *International Journal of Behavioral Development*, 41(1), 94–104. https://doi.org/10.1177/0165025415603489.

Levy, K. N., Hlay, J. K., Johnson, B. N., & Witmer, C. P. (2019). An attachment theoretical perspective on tend-and-befriend stress reactions. *Evolutionary Psychological Science*, 5(4), 426–439. https://doi.org/10.1007/s40806-019-00197-x.

Lin, P. Z., Bai, H. Y., Sun, J. W., Guo, W., Zhang, H. H., & Cao, F. L. (2017). Association between child maltreatment and prospective and retrospective memory in adolescents: The mediatory effect of neuroticism. *Child Abuse & Neglect*, 65, 58–67. https://doi.org/10.1016/j.chiabu.2017.01.010.

Livingston, M. D., Rossheim, M. E., & Hall, K. S. (2019). A descriptive analysis of school and school shooter characteristics and the severity of school shootings in the United States, 1999–2018. *The Journal of Adolescent Health*, 64(6), 797–799. https://doi.org/10.1016/j.jadohealth.2018.12.006.

Loomis, A. M. (2021). Effects of household and environmental adversity on indices of self-regulation for Latino and African American preschool children: Closing the school readiness gap. *Early Education and Development*, 32(2), 228–248. https://doi.org/10.1080/10409289.2020.1745513.

Luoni, C., Agosti, M., Crugnola, S., Rossi, G., & Termine, C. (2018). Psychopathology, dissociation and somatic symptoms in adolescents who were exposed to traumatic experiences. *Frontiers in Psychology*, 9, 2390. https://doi.org/10.3389/fpsyg.2018.02390.

Maddox, R. P., Rujimora, J., Nichols, L. M., Williams, M. K., Hunt, T., & Carter Jr, R. A. (2022). Trauma-Informed Schools: Implications for Special Education and School Counseling. *TEACHING Exceptional Children*, 00400599221107142. https://doi.org/10.1177/00400599221107142.

Maercker, A., Bernays, F., Rohner, S. L., & Thoma, M. V. (2022). A cascade model of complex posttraumatic stress disorder centered on childhood trauma and maltreatment, attachment, and socio-interpersonal factors. *Journal of Traumatic Stress*, 35(2), 446–460. https://doi.org/10.1002/jts.22756.

Mainwaring, D. (2015). Creating a safe space: A case study of complex trauma and a call for proactive comprehensive psychoeducational assessments and reviews. *Journal of Psychologists and Counsellors in Schools*, 25(1), 87–103. https://doi.org/10.1017/jgc.2014.24.

Malarbi, S., Abu-Rayya, H. M., Muscara, F., & Stargatt, R. (2017). Neuropsychological functioning of childhood trauma and post-traumatic stress disorder: A meta-analysis. *Neuroscience and Biobehavioral Reviews*, 72, 68–86. https://doi.org/10.1016/j.neubiorev.2016.11.004.

McDoniel, M. E., & Bierman, K. L. (2022). Exploring pathways linking early childhood adverse experiences to reduced preadolescent school engagement. *Child Abuse & Neglect*, 105572. Advance online publication. https://doi.org/10.1016/j.chiabu.2022.105572.

McGuire, A., & Jackson, Y. (2018). A multilevel meta-analysis on academic achievement among maltreated youth. *Clinical Child and Family Psychology Review*, 21(4), 450–465. https://doi.org/10.1007/s10567-018-0265-6.

McIntyre, E. M., Baker, C. N., Overstreet, S., & The New Orleans Trauma-Informed Schools Learning Collaborative. (2019). Evaluating foundational professional development training for trauma-informed approaches in schools. *Psychological Services*, 16 (1), 95–102. https://doi.org/10.1037/ser0000312.

McKelvey, L. M., Edge, N. C., Mesman, G. R., Whiteside-Mansell, L., & Bradley, R. H. (2018). Adverse experiences in infancy and toddlerhood: Relations to adaptive behavior and academic status in middle childhood. *Child Abuse & Neglect*, 82, 168–177. https://doi.org/10.1016/j.chiabu.2018.05.026.

Michna, G. A., Trudel, S. M., Bray, M. A., Reinhardt, J., Dirsmith, J., Theodore, L., Zhou, Z., Patel, I., Jones, P., & Gilbert, M. L. (2022). Best practices and emerging trends in assessment of trauma in students with autism spectrum disorder. *Psychology in the Schools*, 1–16. https://doi.org/10.1002/pits.22769.

Motsan, S., Yirmiya, K., & Feldman, R. (2022). Chronic early trauma impairs emotion recognition and executive functions in youth; specifying biobehavioral precursors of risk and resilience. *Development and Psychopathology*, 34(4), 1339–1352. https://doi.org/10.1017/S0954579421000067.

Moyano, N., & del Mar Sánchez-Fuentes, M. (2020). Homophobic bullying at schools: A systematic review of research, prevalence, school-related predictors and consequences. *Aggression and Violent Behavior*, 53, s101441. https://doi.org/10.1016/j.avb.2020.101441.

Mullins, C. A., & Panlilio, C. C. (2021). Exploring the mediating effect of academic engagement on math and reading achievement for students who have experienced maltreatment. *Child Abuse & Neglect*, 117, 105048. https://doi.org/10.1016/j.chiabu.2021.105048.

Mundy, L. K., Canterford, L., Kosola, S., Degenhardt, L., Allen, N. B., & Patton, G. C. (2017). Peer victimization and academic performance in primary school children. *Academic Pediatrics*, 17(8), 830–836. https://doi.org/10.1016/j.acap.2017.06.012.

Mwakanyamale, A. A., Wande, D. P., & Yizhen, Y. (2018). Multi-type child maltreatment: Prevalence and its relationship with self-esteem among secondary school students in Tanzania. *BMC Psychology*, 6(1), 1–8. https://doi.org/10.1186/s40359-018-0244-1.

Myat Zaw, A. M., Win, N. Z., & Thepthien, B. (2022). Adolescents' academic achievement, mental health, and adverse behaviors: Understanding the role of resilience and adverse childhood experiences. *School Psychology International*, 43(5), 516–536. https://doi.org/10.1177/01430343221107114.

Nikulina, V., & Widom, C. S. (2019). Higher levels of intelligence and executive functioning protect maltreated children against adult arrests: a prospective study. *Child Maltreatment*, 24(1), 3–16. https://doi.org/10.1177/1077559518808218.

Nooner, K. B., Hooper, S. R., & De Bellis, M. D. (2018). An examination of sex differences on neurocognitive functioning and behavior problems in maltreated youth. *Psychological Trauma: Theory, Research, Practice, and Policy*, 10(4), 435–443. https://doi.org/10.1037/tra0000356.

Ntoumanis, N., Ng, J. Y. Y., Prestwich, A., Quested, E., Hancox, J. E., Thøgersen-Ntoumani, C., Deci, E. L., Ryan, R. M., Lonsdale, C., & Williams, G. C. (2021). A meta-analysis of self-determination theory-informed intervention studies in the health domain: Effects on motivation, health behavior, physical, and psychological health. *Health Psychology Review*, 15(2), 214–244. https://doi.org/10.1080/17437199.2020.1718529.

O'Higgins, A., Sebba, J., & Gardner, F. (2017). What are the factors associated with educational achievement for children in kinship or foster care: A systematic review. *Children and Youth Services Review*, 79, 198–220. https://doi.org/10.1016/j.childyouth. 2017.06.004.

Op den Kelder, R., Ensink, J., Overbeek, G., Maric, M., & Lindauer, R. (2017). Executive function as a mediator in the link between single or complex trauma and posttraumatic stress in children and adolescents. *Quality of Life Research*, 26(7), 1687–1696. https://doi.org/10.1007/s11136-017-1535-3.

Otterman, D. L., Koopman-Verhoeff, M. E., White, T. J., Tiemeier, H., Bolhuis, K., & Jansen, P. W. (2019). Executive functioning and neurodevelopmental disorders in early childhood: A prospective population-based study. *Child and Adolescent Psychiatry and Mental Health*, 13(1), 1–12. https://doi.org/10.1186/s13034-019-0299-7.

Ousdal, O. T., Milde, A. M., Craven, A. R., Ersland, L., Endestad, T., Melinder, A., Huys, Q. J., & Hugdahl, K. (2019). Prefrontal glutamate levels predict altered amygdala-prefrontal connectivity in traumatized youths. *Psychological Medicine*, 49(11), 1822–1830. https://doi.org/10.1017/S0033291718002519.

Pataky, M. G., Báez, J. C., & Renshaw, K. J. (2019). Making schools trauma informed: Using the ACE study and implementation science to screen for trauma. *Social Work in Mental Health*, 17(6), 639–661. https://doi.org/10.1080/15332985. 2019.1625476.

Pelcovitz, D., Pelcovitz, M., Sunday, S., Labrunad, V., Lehrman, D., Kline, M., Salzingerg, S., & Kaplan, S. (2017). Academic achievement in young adults with a history of adolescent physical abuse. *Adolescent Psychiatry*, 7(4), 286–299. https://doi.org/ 10.2174/2210676608666180222124009.

Perfect, M. M., Turley, M. R., Carlson, J. S., Yohanna, J., & Saint Gilles, M. P. (2016). School-related outcomes of traumatic event exposure and traumatic stress symptoms in students: A systematic review of research from 1990 to 2015. *School Mental Health*, 8(1), 7–43. https://doi.org/10.1007/s12310-016-9175-2.

Peters, A. T., Ren, X., Bessette, K. L., Goldstein, B. I., West, A. E., Langenecker, S. A., & Pandey, G. N. (2019). Interplay between pro-inflammatory cytokines, childhood trauma, and executive function in depressed adolescents. *Journal of Psychiatric Research*, 114, 1–10. https://doi.org/10.1016/j.jpsychires.2019.03.030.

Peterson, J., Densley, J., & Erickson, G. (2021). Presence of armed school officials and fatal and nonfatal gunshot injuries during mass school shootings, United States, 1980–2019. *JAMA Network Open*, 4(2), e2037394. https://doi.org/10.1001/jamanetworkop en.2020.37394.

Pierce, H., Jones, M. S., & Gibbs, B. G. (2022). Early adverse childhood experiences and exclusionary discipline in high school. *Social Science Research*, 101, 102621. https://doi. org/10.1016/j.ssresearch.2021.102621.

Polanin, J. R., Espelage, D. L., Grotpeter, J. K., Spinney, E., Ingram, K. M., Valido, A., El Sheikh, A., Torgal, C., & Robinson, L. (2021). A meta-analysis of longitudinal partial correlations between school violence and mental health, school performance, and criminal or delinquent acts. *Psychological Bulletin*, 147(2), 115–133. https://doi. org/10.1037/bul0000314.

Prince, D. M., Ray-Novak, M., Gillani, B., & Peterson, E. (2022). Sexual and gender minority youth in foster care: An evidence-based theoretical conceptual model of disproportionality and psychological comorbidities. *Trauma, Violence & Abuse*, 23(5), 1643–1657. https://doi.org/10.1177/15248380211013129.

Purpura, D. J., Schmitt, S. A., & Ganley, C. M. (2017). Foundations of mathematics and literacy: The role of executive functioning components. *Journal of Experimental Child Psychology*, 153, 15–34. https://doi.org/10.1016/j.jecp.2016.08.010.

Quidé, Y., O'Reilly, N., Rowland, J. E., Carr, V. J., Elzinga, B. M., & Green, M. J. (2017). Effects of childhood trauma on working memory in affective and non-affective psychotic disorders. *Brain Imaging and Behavior*, 11(3), 722–735. https://doi.org/10.1007/s11682-016-9548-z.

Raghubar, K. P., & Barnes, M. A. (2017). Early numeracy skills in preschool-aged children: A review of neurocognitive findings and implications for assessment and intervention. *The Clinical Neuropsychologist*, 31(2), 329–351. https://doi.org/10.1080/13854046.2016.1259387.

Ravi, K. E., & Black, B. M. (2022). The relationship between children's exposure to intimate partner violence and an emotional-behavioral disability: A scoping review. *Trauma, Violence & Abuse*, 23(3), 868–876. https://doi.org/10.1177/1524838020979846.

Riffle, L. N., Kelly, K. M., Demaray, M. L., Malecki, C. E., Santuzzi, A. M., Rodriguez-Harris, D. J., & Emmons, J. D. (2021). Associations among bullying role behaviors and academic performance over the course of an academic year for boys and girls. *Journal of School Psychology*, 86, 49–63. https://doi.org/10.1016/j.jsp.2021.03.002.

Rishel, C. W., Tabone, J. K., Hartnett, H. P., & Szafran, K. F. (2019). Trauma-informed elementary schools: Evaluation of school-based early intervention for young children. *Children & Schools*, 41(4), 239–248. https://doi.org/10.1093/cs/cdz017.

Rodgers, S., & Hassan, S. (2021). Therapeutic Crisis Intervention in Schools (TCI-S): An international exploration of a therapeutic framework to reduce critical incidents and improve teacher and student emotional competence in schools. *Journal of Psychologists and Counsellors in Schools*, 31(2), 238–245. https://doi.org/10.1017/jgc.2021.2.

Rumsey, A. D., & Milsom, A. (2019). Supporting school engagement and high school completion through trauma-informed school counseling. *Professional School Counseling*, 22(1). https://doi.org/10.1177/2156759X19867254.

Ryan, J. P., Jacob, B. A., Gross, M., Perron, B. E., Moore, A., & Ferguson, S. (2018). Early exposure to child maltreatment and academic outcomes. *Child Maltreatment*, 23(4), 365–375. https://doi.org/10.1177/1077559518786815.

Scharpf, F., Mueller, S. C., Masath, F. B., Nkuba, M., & Hecker, T. (2021). Psychopathology mediates between maltreatment and memory functioning in Burundian refugee youth. *Child Abuse & Neglect*, 118, 105165. https://doi.org/10.1016/j.chiabu.2021.105165.

Schrank, F. A., Mather, N., & McGrew, K. S. (2014). *Woodcock-Johnson IV Tests of Achievement*. Rolling Meadows, IL: Riverside.

Seppälä, P., Vornanen, R., & Toikko, T. (2021). Multimorbidity and polyvictimization in children: An analysis on the association of children's disabilities and long-term illnesses with mental violence and physical violence. *Child Abuse & Neglect*, 122, 105350. https://doi.org/10.1016/j.chiabu.2021.105350.

Sheridan, M. A., Peverill, M., Finn, A. S., & McLaughlin, K. A. (2017). Dimensions of childhood adversity have distinct associations with neural systems underlying executive functioning. *Development and Psychopathology*, 29(5), 1777–1794. https://doi.org/10.1017/S0954579417001390.

Simon, M., Németh, N., Gálber, M., Lakner, E., Csernela, E., Tényi, T., & Czéh, B. (2019). Childhood adversity impairs theory of mind abilities in adult patients with major depressive disorder. *Frontiers in Psychiatry*, 10, 867. https://doi.org/10.3389/fp syt.2019.00867.

Spiegel, J. A., Goodrich, J. M., Morris, B. M., Osborne, C. M., & Lonigan, C. J. (2021). Relations between executive functions and academic outcomes in elementary school children: A meta-analysis. *Psychological Bulletin*, 147(4), 329–351. https://doi.org/10. 1037/bul0000322.

Spinazzola, J., Van der Kolk, B., & Ford, J. D. (2021). Developmental trauma disorder: A legacy of attachment trauma in victimized children. *Journal of Traumatic Stress*, 34(4), 711–720. https://doi.org/10.1002/jts.22697.

Stempel, H., Cox-Martin, M., Bronsert, M., Dickinson, L. M., & Allison, M. A. (2017). Chronic school absenteeism and the role of adverse childhood experiences. *Academic Pediatrics*, 17(8), 837–843. https://doi.org/10.1016/j.acap.2017.09.013.

Stene, L. E., Schultz, J. H., & Dyb, G. (2019). Returning to school after a terror attack: A longitudinal study of school functioning and health in terror-exposed youth. *European Child & Adolescent Psychiatry*, 28(3), 319–328. https://doi.org/10.1007/ s00787-018-1196-y.

Stevens, J. S., & Jovanovic, T. (2019). Role of social cognition in post-traumatic stress disorder: A review and meta-analysis. *Genes, Brain, and Behavior*, 18(1), e12518. http s://doi.org/10.1111/gbb.12518.

Stevens, T., Barnard-Brak, L., Roberts, B., Acosta, R., & Wilburn, S. (2020). Aggression toward teachers, interaction with school shooting media, and secondary trauma: Lockdown drills as moderator. *Psychology in the Schools*, 57(4), 583–605. https://doi. org/10.1002/pits.22329.

Su, Y., D'Arcy, C., Yuan, S., & Meng, X. (2019). How does childhood maltreatment influence ensuing cognitive functioning among people with the exposure of child-hood maltreatment?: A systematic review of prospective cohort studies. *Journal of Affective Disorders*, 252, 278–293. https://doi.org/10.1016/j.jad.2019.04.026.

Subbie-Saenz de Viteri, S., Pandey, A., Pandey, G., Kamarajan, C., Smith, R., Anokhin, A., Bauer, L., Bender, A., Chan, G., Dick, D., Edenberg, H., Kinreich, S., Kramer, J., Schuckit, M., Zang, Y., McCutcheon, V., Bucholz, K., Porjesz, B., & Meyers, J. L. (2020). Pathways to post-traumatic stress disorder and alcohol dependence: Trauma, executive functioning, and family history of alcoholism in adolescents and young adults. *Brain and Behavior*, 10(11), e01789. https://doi.org/10.1002/brb3.1789.

Tabone, J. K., Rishel, C. W., Hartnett, H. P., & Szafran, K. F. (2020). Examining the effectiveness of early intervention to create trauma-informed school environments. *Children and Youth Services Review*, 113, 104998. https://doi.org/10.1016/j.childyouth. 2020.104998.

Tan, T. X., Wang, Y., & Ruggerio, A. D. (2017). Childhood adversity and chil-dren's academic functioning: Roles of parenting stress and neighborhood support. *Journal of Child and Family Studies*, 26(10), 2742–2752. https://doi.org/10.1007/ s10826-017-0775-8.

Tessier, N. G., O'Higgins, A., & Flynn, R. J. (2018). Neglect, educational success, and young people in out-of-home care: Cross-sectional and longitudinal analyses. *Child Abuse & Neglect*, 75, 115–129. https://doi.org/10.1016/j.chiabu.2017.06.005.

Theodoraki, T. E., McGeown, S. P., Rhodes, S. M., & MacPherson, S. E. (2020). Developmental changes in executive functions during adolescence: A study of inhibition, shifting, and working memory. *British Journal of Developmental Psychology*, 38(1), 74–89. https://doi.org/10.1111/bjdp.12307.

Thomas, M. S., Crosby, S., & Vanderhaar, J. (2019). Trauma-informed practices in schools across two decades: An interdisciplinary review of research. *Review of Research in Education*, 43(1), 422–452. https://doi.org/10.3102/0091732X18821123.

Thompson, E. L., O'Connor, K. E., & Farrell, A. D. (2021). Childhood adversity and co-occurring post-traumatic stress and externalizing symptoms among a pre-dominantly low-income, African American sample of early adolescents. *Development and Psychopathology*, 1–13. https://doi.org/10.1017/S0954579421001383.

Turner, R., Louie, K., Parvez, A., Modaffar, M., Rezaie, R., Greene, T., Bisby, J., Fonagy, P., & Bloomfield, M. (2022). The effects of developmental trauma on theory of mind and its relationship to psychotic experiences: A behavioural study. *Psychiatry Research*, 312, 114544. https://doi.org/10.1016/j.psychres.2022.114544.

Tyler, P. M., Patwardan, I., Ringle, J. L., Chmelka, M. B., & Mason, W. A. (2019). Youth needs at intake into trauma-informed group homes and response to services: An examination of trauma exposure, symptoms, and clinical impression. *American Journal of Community Psychology*, 64(3–4), 321–332. https://doi.org/10.1002/ajcp.12364.

Tyrell, F. A., Marcelo, A. K., Trang, D. T., & Yates, T. M. (2019). Prospective asso-ciations between trauma, placement disruption, and ethnic-racial identity among newly emancipated foster youth. *Journal of Adolescence*, 76, 88–98. https://doi.org/10.1016/j.adolescence.2019.08.010.

van Os, J., Marsman, A., van Dam, D., Simons, C. J., & GROUP Investigators. (2017). Evidence that the impact of childhood trauma on IQ is substantial in controls, mod-erate in siblings, and absent in patients with psychotic disorder. *Schizophrenia Bulletin*, 43(2), 316–324. https://doi.org/10.1093/schbul/sbw177.

Vaskinn, A., Melle, I., Aas, M., & Berg, A. O. (2020). Sexual abuse and physical neglect in childhood are associated with affective theory of mind in adults with schizophrenia. *Schizophrenia Research: Cognition*, 23, 100189. https://doi.org/10.1016/j.scog.2020.100189.

Waters, N. E., Ahmed, S. F., Tang, S., Morrison, F. J., & Davis-Kean, P. E. (2021). Pathways from socioeconomic status to early academic achievement: The role of specific executive functions. *Early Childhood Research Quarterly*, 54, 321–331. https://doi.org/10.1016/j.ecresq.2020.09.008.

Wechsler, D. (2014). *Wechsler Intelligence Scale for Children–Fifth Edition*. San Antonio, TX: NCS Pearson.

Welsh, M. C., Peterson, E., & Jameson, M. M. (2017). History of childhood maltreat-ment and college academic outcomes: Indirect effects of hot execution function. *Frontiers in Psychology*, 8, 1091. https://doi.org/10.3389/fpsyg.2017.01091.

Wermuth, K., Ülsmann, D., Borngräber, J., Gallinat, J., Schulte-Herbrüggen, O., & Kühn, S. (2021). Structural signature of trauma: White matter volume in right inferior frontal gyrus is positively associated with use of expressive suppression in recently traumatized individuals. *European Journal of Psychotraumatology*, 12(1), 1837512. https://doi.org/10.1080/20008198.2020.1837512.

Williams, J. R., Cole, V., Girdler, S., & Cromeens, M. G. (2020). Exploring stress, cognitive, and affective mechanisms of the relationship between interpersonal trauma and opioid misuse. *PloS One*, 15(5), e0233185. https://doi.org/10.1371/journal.pone.0233185.

Winter, S. M., Dittrich, K., Dörr, P., Overfeld, J., Moebus, I., Murray, E., Karaboycheva, G., Zimmermann, C., Knop, A., Voelkle, M., Entringer, S., Buss, C., Haynes, J. D., Binder, E. B., & Heim, C. (2022). Immediate impact of child maltreatment on mental, developmental, and physical health trajectories. *Journal of Child Psychology and Psychiatry, and Allied Disciplines,* 63(9), 1027–1045. https://doi.org/10.1111/jcpp.13550.

Woodward, E. C., Viana, A. G., Trent, E. S., Raines, E. M., Zvolensky, M. J., & Storch, E. A. (2020). Emotional nonacceptance, distraction coping and PTSD symptoms in a trauma-exposed adolescent inpatient sample. *Cognitive Therapy and Research,* 44(2), 412–419. https://doi.org/10.1007/s10608-019-10065-4.

Xu, J., Guan, X., Li, H., Zhang, M., & Xu, X. (2020a). The effect of early life stress on memory is mediated by anterior hippocampal network. *Neuroscience,* 451, 137–148. https://doi.org/10.1016/j.neuroscience.2020.10.018.

Xu, M., Macrynikola, N., Waseem, M., & Miranda, R. (2020b). Racial and ethnic differences in bullying: Review and implications for intervention. *Aggression and Violent Behavior,* 50, 101340. https://doi.org/10.1016/j.avb.2019.101340.

Young-Southward, G., Eaton, C., O'Connor, R., & Minnis, H. (2020). Investigating the causal relationship between maltreatment and cognition in children: A systematic review. *Child Abuse & Neglect,* 107, 104603. https://doi.org/10.1016/j.chiabu.2020.104603.

Zainal, N. H., & Newman, M. G. (2021). Within-person increase in pathological worry predicts future depletion of unique executive functioning domains. *Psychological Medicine,* 51(10), 1676–1686. https://doi.org/10.1017/S0033291720000422.

Zink, N., Lenartowicz, A., & Markett, S. (2021). A new era for executive function research: On the transition from centralized to distributed executive functioning. *Neuroscience and Biobehavioral Reviews,* 124, 235–244. https://doi.org/10.1016/j.neubiorev.2021.02.011.

8

VOCATIONAL DEVELOPMENT AND DEVELOPMENTAL TRAUMA IN THE WORKPLACE

What did you want to be when you were young? Did you want to be an artist, teacher, builder, police officer, professional athlete, or veterinarian? Did those interests and goals come to fruition, or did life take you in a different direction? Do you (and others) have a good sense of your career interests, values, skills, talents, and preferences? Can you use your strengths at work effectively, or are there stressors or barriers getting in the way? What changes can you make to do meaningful, satisfying, and fulfilling work for you and your loved ones?

Career counselors, social workers, and psychologists explore these questions to help individuals assess their interests, values, and skills and find work that is aligned with these. Researchers and practitioners now understand that work can make all the difference in helping people who have experienced trauma feel connected, valued, and supported. These individuals may use alcohol and drugs, displace their anger and frustration on loved ones, or live in constant fear, anxiety, and depression as they reconcile their experiences in the workplace, including challenging (stressful) interactions with peers and supervisors. Stress experienced at work can result in chronic illness, and the effects are likely to be more severe for individuals who have experienced developmental trauma. Before we consider the adverse effects of trauma on workplace adjustment, behaviors, and employment outcomes, I want to devote space here to discussing career development more broadly, because it is critical to establishing a good understanding of how early experiences, needs, and learning opportunities (or lack thereof) cause individuals to re-enact traumas in the workplace or re-experience abusive and neglectful circumstances that mirror early interactions with caregivers.

DOI: 10.4324/9781003304715-8

Super's Career Development Theory

Career development is a continuous, lifelong process. Developmental scholars often frame the process as originating from early childhood experiences with caregivers and peers and as unfolding in ways that mirror psychological, cognitive, and moral/spiritual models of development (e.g., Erikson's theory of psychosocial development and Piaget's and Kohlberg's conceptualizations of cognitive and moral development; Creed et al., 2020; Gbeleyi, et al., 2022; Howard & Ferrari, 2022; Hu et al., 2022; Li et al., 2021a; Xu, 2021). One of the most influential thinkers on the process of career development is Donald Super (1980, 1990), who asserted that an individual's career development, vocational identity, and career choices and preferences develop (and change) in the context of one's age or phase of life and social, cognitive, interpersonal, and cultural experiences. Super provided a detailed account of career development throughout the lifespan and intersections with identity, self-esteem, mental health, well-being, and vocational self-concept, referring to a multifaceted construct that underscores how individuals understand and evaluate themselves (Abdinoor & Ibrahim, 2019; Cordeiro et al., 2018; Creed et al., 2020; Kim & Wickrama, 2021; Kvitkovičová et al., 2017; Watson & McMahon, 2022).

In the earliest stage, *growth*, career development is influenced by attachment, peer relationships, and psychological and cognitive capacities, such as attitudes and beliefs, self-efficacy, and academic engagement/achievement (Bolat & Odacı, 2017; Green, 2020; Kim & Wickrama, 2021; Pulliam & Bartek, 2018). Individuals develop increasing levels of autonomy and industry, academic identity, competency, vocational skills, and interests, all of which are influenced by self-awareness, emotion and behavior regulation, self-esteem, and interpersonal communication capacities (Negru-Subtirica & Pop, 2018). Early positive experiences, such as caring and supportive home and school environments, help children transition to adolescence effectively, where they may accumulate work-related experience and competencies and increasingly participate in real-world training opportunities (e.g., volunteering, shadowing, internships, and apprenticeships).

Growth is followed by *exploration*, where adolescents and young adults develop more specific career goals and interests (i.e., crystallization), choices and preferences (i.e., specification), and independent work experiences (i.e., implementation). Studies suggest that career exploration correlates with self-efficacy, family values and expectations, media exposure, hobbies and interests, and academic achievement and competencies (Abdinoor & Ibrahim, 2019; Chung et al., 2017; Lent et al., 2019). More specifically, Super's conceptualization of career development underscores influences from multiple factors in shaping career choices and decisions, such as gender roles and norms, ethnic and racial identity, socioeconomic status, family values and expectations, and individual and collectivist worldviews. Contemporary research investigations have indeed linked these factors to career development and outcomes in line with Super's vocational development framework (Akosah-Twumasi et al., 2018; Bolat & Odacı, 2017; Garriott et al., 2017; Lewis et al., 2018; McWhirter et al., 2018; Rogers et al., 2018; Sawitri & Creed, 2017). For example, research suggests that gender-role norms and expectations strongly influence career development growth and exploration (i.e., Bem's gender schema theory suggests that children and adolescents are socialized to pursue careers that are consistent with stereotyped gender norms; Buckley, 2018; Dray et al., 2020; Weisgram & Bruun, 2018). Boys are often encouraged (and sometimes pressured) to explore stereotypically masculine careers, such as carpentry, engineering, mechanics, and law enforcement. Girls are often pressured to consider careers in nursing, cosmetology, interior design, and teaching. Consequently, social norms may limit individuals' career interests and options and give rise to stress and additional traumas if they choose careers that are not considered gender congruent by mainstream standards.

According to Super's career development framework, adults are in the *establishment* stage. The establishment stage is characterized by stable work and, at the same time, efforts focused on career achievement and advancement, which solidify job-related preferences, skills, and responsibilities. In this stage, individuals form a clear role and identity within the career context. In the final stages, *maintenance* and *disengagement*, individuals experience vocational maturity (i.e., realistic appraisals and logical decisions related to their needs, strengths, weaknesses, and job options; Li et al., 2022; Lim & You, 2019), maintain long-term employment, adjust to changing circumstances (job/role transitions), and eventually shift their priorities to transitioning out of the workforce and into retirement.

Super's theory is compatible with contemporary research in counseling and psychology (Bocciardi et al., 2017; Bolat & Odacı, 2017; Lee & Lee, 2018; Peila-Shuster, 2018; Zacher et al., 2019) as well as with APA's Professional Practice Guidelines for Integrating the Role of Work and Career into Psychological Practice. APA's Professional Practice Guidelines state, in part, that healthcare providers, career counselors, and vocational psychologists should strive to

> have an awareness of the pervasive impact of work on an individual's identity and quality of life, ... [the] influence work has on behavioral, emotional and physical health, as well as the influence of health on work, ... [and] understand how cultural, individual, and role differences, including those based on age, gender, gender identity, geographic location, race, ethnicity, culture, national origin, socioeconomic status, religion, sexual orientation, disability, and language, may influence the pursuit and experience of work.
>
> *(American Psychological Association, 2016, p. 9)*

Developmental Trauma and Career Development

Individuals who have endured significant adversity in their lives, especially during early childhood, are at increased risk of experiencing avoidance, anger, frustration, and anxiety as primary ways of responding to psychological distress, including in the workplace (DeCou et al., 2019; Zheng et al., 2022). In their original proposal of the DTD diagnostic framework, van der Kolk and colleagues (2009) describe the impact of early trauma on employee satisfaction, stability, and success. Specifically, the authors assert that these individuals often demonstrate "disinterest in work/vocation, inability to get or keep jobs, persistent conflict with co-workers or supervisors, under-employment in relation to abilities, [and] failure to achieve expectable advancements" (van der Kolk et al., 2009, p. 8).

DTD is linked to low self-confidence and self-esteem, which can lead to increased anxiety, behavior dysregulation, and housing/job instability (Copeland et al., 2018; Hardcastle et al., 2018; Macia et al., 2021). Individuals who have experienced trauma (including repeated trauma) may feel worried about re-traumatization or being stigmatized at work because of their challenges. As a result, some will choose not to disclose personal information to others, including human resources and employee-health staff who might be able to help them, believing that the vulnerability could put them at a disadvantage for recruitment or advancement.

Adults with indications of DTD have difficulty focusing, processing information, self-regulating, and modulating their thoughts and feelings at work and are at increased risk of experiencing interpersonal challenges and workplace behavior problems (Robson et al., 2020; Steine et al., 2017). The types of responses to stress reported among individuals who have experienced trauma can be damaging to their career development, including for adolescents who may be entering the workforce for the first time. Career development and job stability for adolescents who experience developmental traumas are challenging, given the high rates of cognitive, behavioral, interpersonal, and physiological disturbances associated with early trauma and the high rates of medical and psychiatric comorbidities (Chung et al., 2017; Samuelson et al., 2017). A recent study (Ulusoy & Akcan, 2022) reported that higher ACEs, including early psychological/physical abuse and neglect, differentiated unemployed from employed adolescents. These findings suggest that trauma is likely to complicate the school-to-work transition for emerging adults. Scholars have referred to this process as an individual's career adaptability.

Career adaptability refers to an individual's readiness and resource availability to effectively transition from school to work (Hou et al., 2019; Ramos & Lopez, 2018; Šverko & Babarović, 2019). It includes an individual's ability to cope with vocational roles and responsibilities, life transitions, and work-related challenges. Studies have demonstrated that early experiences of trauma adversely affect one's career adaptability by contributing to maladaptive work habits, unhealthy relationships (e.g., heightened risk for teen dating violence), and unemployment (Jouriles et al., 2017; Kim & Smith, 2021; Koçtürk et al., 2019; Lin & Chiao, 2022). These challenges are likely worsened by other risk factors associated with trauma, including a heightened risk of school dropout, lack of vocational engagement, insecure attachment, criminal behavior, and incarceration (Ahn et al., 2022; Parola & Marcionetti, 2022; Ramos & Lopez, 2018; Widom et al., 2018).

It has been suggested that the cumulative effects of trauma increase children's and adolescents' risk for criminal careers, characterized by antisocial behavior, such as exploitation and coercion, and more chronic and severe violent offenses, which eventually warrant criminal charges and long-term incarceration as children and adolescents age out of juvenile justice systems (Pechorro et al., 2021; Pękala et al., 2021; Stensrud et al., 2019; Yohros, 2022). There are, however, several factors associated with career adaptability that moderate and mediate these outcomes and that have the potential to mitigate (or worsen) circumstances, including age, personality, cognitive capacities, self-esteem/efficacy, stress and coping, vocational identity, and interventions or responses to interventions related to career exploration, personal strengths and weaknesses, and decision-making (Keijzer et al., 2021; Longhi et al., 2021; Poole et al., 2017; Prescod & Zeligman, 2018; Rudolph et al., 2017).

The cumulative effects of ACEs, polyvictimization, and interpersonal trauma adversely affect adults with regard to career development, adjustment, satisfaction, and persistence (Davis et al., 2022; La Mott & Martin, 2019; Turner et al., 2017). As such, these individuals often experience depression, anxiety, and dissatisfaction with work, which undermine their ability to demonstrate their potential to supervisors and employers. This is often compounded by attachment disturbances, poor self-regulation, emotional reactivity in the workplace, and repeated disciplinary actions by administrators and human resource personnel, which cause individuals who have experienced (and re-experience) trauma to have poor job performance evaluations, appear unapproachable to others (because they experience heightened levels of physiological arousal, mood and behavior dysregulation, and/or behavioral avoidance) and, in turn, experience job instability (De Venter et al., 2020; Jahng, 2020; Kim & Wickrama, 2021).

Scholars have speculated that survivors of early trauma often display relational patterns corresponding to substantive behavioral and personality disturbances that intersect with workplace behaviors and employment outcomes (Baglivio et al., 2020; Fuchshuber et al., 2019; Richard-Lepouriel et al., 2019; Voestermans et al., 2021). Many adults affected by trauma develop long-lasting negative schemas about themselves and their ability to function and maintain long-term employment, including deep feelings of inferiority, fear, self-hatred, and distrust, all of which give rise to maladaptive personality styles and, in some cases, clinically significant characterological disturbances (DeCou et al., 2019; Jaffe et al., 2019). Some personality disturbances may appear more adaptive than others or are more likely to be positively reinforced by employers and organizations. Interpersonal traumas, such as violence, emotional and sexual abuse, and neglect, correlate with obsessive-compulsive personality disorder (OCPD), which can be characterized by workaholism, rigid control and orderliness, and low mental flexibility and openness (Kanehisa et al., 2017; Miller & Brock, 2017). These individuals are often highly productive and thriving in the workplace, partly because they overidentify with their vocational identity to cope with psychological distress, reconcile their unmet needs, or compensate for the loss of other salient identities and roles (e.g., caregiver, romantic partner, friend, uncle/aunt, spiritual or religious community member).

Adverse childhood experiences, polyvictimization, and developmental traumas have been shown to diminish an individual's educational and career development, exploration, and potential, including income potential/earnings. For example, a recent study found that higher ACEs positively correlated with high school non-completion, unemployment, and living in a household below the federal poverty level (Metzler et al., 2017). Failure to hold a job, being dismissed or fired, prematurely quitting a job (without financial preparations), and higher levels of financial problems, including Medicaid usage, financial debt, and referral to debt collection agencies, have all been linked to experiences of early trauma (Copeland et al., 2018; Zhao & Li, 2022).

A recent study by Lu and colleagues (2022) explores the work experiences of adults who have experienced early traumas. Respondents reported several ways in which psychological distress and trauma symptoms adversely affected their ability to function in the workplace. Responses included fear of interpersonal relationships, thought disturbances originating from the trauma, troublesome memories, dissociation, negative emotionality, insecure attachment, and physiological hypoarousal (i.e., fatigue). Trauma and insecure attachment have been linked to employee-reported intent to quit and relocate, low occupational or organizational commitment, and higher employee turnover rates (Kim et al., 2019; Steine et al., 2017; Weng et al., 2018).

Consider the following case of Kelly (Tarocchi et al., 2013) for illustration.

Kelly is a 37-year-old woman who sought psychological evaluation and treatment for psychological distress associated with complex trauma, anxiety/panic symptoms, and mood instability, which adversely affected her interpersonal relationships and ability to work effectively. According to the report, Kelly experienced sexual abuse, bullying, physical assaults at school, and domestic violence, which led her parents to divorce. She was devastated by their separation and recalled significant changes in her life. She developed a codependent relationship with her mother and had inconsistent contact with her father, which caused her to feel rejected and abandoned by him. At 14, Kelly ran away from home and developed an addiction to heroin to help her connect to others, including intimate relationships. At 17, Kelly became pregnant by an abusive partner. She eventually returned home to live with her mother as she became fearful of her boyfriend's violence and its potential effects on her baby. At age 30, Kelly moved out to gain independence, although she experienced fear and psychological distress, and difficulty maintaining relationships and employment. As such, she decided to send her son to live with his father while she reconciled her social and emotional needs and her son's safety and security.

In session, Kelly elaborated on her experiences and relationships. Regarding a recent breakup, she stated, "When we were together, I felt suffocated, and when we were apart, I was scared and lonely but free." Kelly elaborated more broadly on relationships, "I want to trust, but my experiences have taught me to maintain a certain reserve so I can remain more secure." Assessment results revealed that Kelly experiences social alienation, disorganized attachment, interpersonal betrayal trauma, and views herself negatively. Kelly improved self-regulation, coping, and interpersonal relationships in response to treatment. After experiencing a year of unemployment, she returned to work and reported feeling calm at work, less anxious, and connected to the workplace, including customers, coworkers, and her supervisor. She also received a positive performance evaluation. Unfortunately, Kelly lost her job after the company experienced financial strain in response to economic circumstances. However, she and several of her coworkers, who had also been affected by these circumstances, worked together to search for new job opportunities.

Kelly's experiences of trauma include sexual abuse, neglect and abandonment, exposure to interpersonal violence, and family instability. Disturbances in mood, behavior, and interpersonal relationships resulting from her traumatic experiences contributed to Kelly's challenges at work, including long-term unemployment. Kelly's response to treatment was positive and demonstrated her resilience, which is not uncommon for survivors of abuse and neglect, particularly when they are supported by healthcare providers, employers, family, and friends. At the same time, experiences of stress and strain at work, either from high demands, expectations, bottom-line performance metrics, or unhealthy interpersonal interactions with supervisors and coworkers undermine such opportunities and put individuals at high risk for underemployment, unemployment, and disability.

Workplace Stress

Some individuals within an organization, including management, leadership, staff, and customers/consumers/clients/patients, may also suffer from early traumas, which may be worsened by workplace stress. Workplace stress refers to the harmful physical and psychological responses to stress that occur when the requirements of a job do not align with an individual's capabilities, resources, or social and emotional needs (Hilton et al., 2021; Lockey et al., 2022). We may experience stress at work due to personal circumstances (e.g., food insecurity, financial stress, health problems), relationships (e.g., marital conflict, divorce, domestic violence), or workplace stressors (e.g., employee harassment, bullying, incivility, high demands or unrealistic expectations, low resources). Multiple stressors make it challenging for us to stay present for ourselves and our colleagues (Ham et al., 2022; Lagrosen & Lagrosen, 2022; Sun et al., 2021).

Researchers have demonstrated that chronic exposure to workplace stress positively predicts physical and mental health problems and potentiates cumulative physiological stress that leads to morbidity and mortality (Almroth et al., 2022; Attell et al., 2017; Li et al., 2021b; Niedhammer et al., 2021). Individuals adversely affected by trauma are particularly susceptible to workplace stress because they experience cumulative (toxic) stress, emotion and behavior disturbances, psychiatric comorbidities, and longstanding health problems. These individuals often experience persistent states of fear and anxiety at work, including recurring thoughts about being ostracized, neglected, or excluded by others. Consequently, adults who experience trauma are far more vulnerable to chronic and severe mental health problems because of workplace stress than adults who have not. These effects are likely to be more pervasive for individuals from marginalized communities, such as racial and sexual minorities, who sometimes experience discrimination in the workplace (Caceres et al., 2021; Holman, 2018; Wright & Chan, 2022).

Individuals who currently experience trauma or who experienced early trauma may have more difficulty setting boundaries between their personal life and work life. Increasing work demands and adverse experiences in the workplace often disrupt self-care, relational/marital satisfaction, and seeking social support, often because these individuals ruminate about work and become mentally and emotionally consumed by work-related stress. However, some workplaces are naturally more stressful than others, particularly those characterized as toxic workplace environments. A toxic workplace is characterized by chronic stress, anxiety, and physiological hyperarousal due to the fear of being criticized or ostracized by others (Brown et al., 2021; Rasool et al., 2021). As such, scholars have urged employers to refrain from labeling, stigmatizing, or disempowering any individual who has experienced trauma. Employers should realize that such individuals may be experiencing dysfunction in the workplace environment, such as unresponsive supervisors and administrators, who are charged with the responsibility of setting the tone for employees, modeling positive behaviors, providing employees with tools and resources, and protecting vulnerable employees in the workplace.

Maulik (2017) draws on the World Health Organization's conceptualization of workplace stress and toxic workplace practices, which states in part:

> Stress occurs in a wide range of work circumstances but is often made worse when employees feel they have little support from supervisors and

colleagues, as well as little control over work processes. Work-related stress can be caused by poor work organization (the way we design jobs and work systems, and the way we manage them), by poor work design (for example, lack of control over work processes), poor management, unsatisfactory working conditions and lack of support from colleagues and supervisors.

(World Health Organization, 2020)

Individuals who experience toxic workplaces commonly report fear, anxiety, perceived inadequacy, negative core beliefs, low self-esteem, and social avoidance (Chung, 2018; Wang et al., 2020). Scholars now conceptualize toxic workplace cultures as a behavioral vulnerability factor for developing psychological disorders. Interpersonally sensitive individuals experience long-standing, sometimes treatment-resistant depression and anxiety disorders as a result of toxic workplaces.

ACEs and polyvictimization trauma interact with toxic workplace environments in ways that increase an individual's risk for revictimization and psychological challenges (Cusack et al., 2021; Dash & Jena, 2020; Grundmann et al., 2018; Ørke et al., 2018; Walker et al., 2019, 2022). For example, exposure to workplace aggression and violence has been linked to a heightened risk of PTSD compared to nonexposed adults (Pihl-Thingvad et al., 2019). The cumulative effects of early abuse and neglect heighten responses to workplace problems (e.g., irritability, emotional numbing, dissociation, negative self-talk, and interpersonal conflicts; Caceres et al., 2021; Jaffe et al., 2019; Lahav et al., 2020; Shin et al., 2017).

Exposure to workplace stress may differentially affect individuals in particular professions (Aykanian & Mammah, 2022; Bryce et al., 2023; Grist & Caudle, 2021; Steen et al., 2021; Steinlin et al., 2017). Law enforcement personnel encounter stressful circumstances regularly, and early abuse and neglect worsen their psychological adjustment, physical health, and well-being. Studies have found that officers who experienced early abuse and neglect tend to have more difficulty regulating their emotions and behaviors and use harsher (and possibly abusive) police practices (DeVylder et al., 2019; McQuerrey Tuttle et al., 2022).

This heightened fear propensity disrupts self-awareness, interpersonal communication, and mastery of age-appropriate developmental competencies (e.g., establishing healthy relationship parameters, identifying and expressing feelings, and tolerating ambiguity). Unfortunately, most employers do not recognize DTD symptoms as such, and, regrettably, these individuals often do not receive the type of attention and treatment that they need to thrive. As a result, these individuals often experience disciplinary actions and other responses that can distract them from uncovering and responding appropriately to their early traumas and DTD challenges.

Trauma-Informed Care

DTD symptoms differ depending on the specific traumas experienced, the characteristics of the individuals involved, and the level of discordance between the individuals and their environments (person-environment fit theory suggests that people have an innate need to fit their environments and seek out environments that match their characteristics; Mackey et al., 2017; Van Vianen, 2018). Symptoms will also vary depending on each individual's degree of environmental support, perceived controllability of the stressful events, access to socioeconomic resources, and effective evaluations and treatments.

Organizations often have an employee code of conduct that describes standards of behavior and safeguards against inappropriate interactions between staff, such as those suggestive of bullying and intimidation. However, organizations may not have explicit policies, procedures, and supports for individuals with trauma (i.e., trauma-informed care for organizations). In addition, organizations may struggle to consistently enforce the employee code of conduct, which may cause employees who have experienced trauma to feel unsafe and possibly neglected by leadership. Because these individuals are in positions of power and individuals with early trauma often have had adverse experiences with caregivers, they may re-enact early traumas with managers when they feel abused or neglected.

Trauma-informed care (TIC) models have increased dramatically over the past two decades and have been shown to effectively apply to employment settings, organizations, and institutions. A trauma-informed workplace is characterized by a positive workplace culture and leadership practices that convey an understanding of the commonality and broad impact of ACEs and trauma on mood, cognition, interpersonal communication, and physiological health (Isobel et al., 2021; Koloroutis & Pole, 2021; Rodrigues et al., 2021). Trauma-informed workplaces respond to employees with empathy to minimize stigma, shame, and possible additional traumas deriving from workplace conflicts. Research suggests that trauma-informed practices in the workplace are often characterized by exemplary leaders who recognize the influence of organizational context and behavior in mitigating responses to trauma; demonstrate a commitment to trauma-informed training, education, and compliance; model appropriate behaviors; and treat employees with respect and dignity (Amateau et al., 2022; Bargeman et al., 2022; Kim et al., 2021; Levenson et al., 2021; Robey et al., 2021).

Contemporary research and trauma-informed workplace guidelines developed by the Substance Abuse and Mental Health Services Administration (2014) include the following:

- Develop a clear mission statement on trauma and trauma-informed care;
- Have delineated policies, procedures, and quality assurance measures in place;

- Assign coaches, advocates, or department leaders to facilitate trauma-informed interactions between employees, including helping to mitigate conflicts or crises and providing/soliciting immediate feedback to minimize poor self-regulation that may give rise to workplace hostility, aggression, and violence;
- Ensure transparency whenever possible, given that individuals with trauma may assume the worst possible outcome regardless of the circumstances and may respond inappropriately out of fear; and
- Provide regular and balanced feedback, including attention to positive behaviors and interactions, such as descriptive praise for effort, motivation, and accomplishments.

Drawing on trauma-informed principles has benefited organizations, employees, and the individuals they serve. Empowered leaders who consistently value and operationalize their stated policies and procedures can help employees focus on work and demonstrate their strengths, mainly because they are less focused on indications of fear and danger.

Concluding Thoughts

Individuals who have experienced early trauma face unique challenges in adulthood, including traumatic revictimization in the workplace (e.g., bullying, microaggressions, and feeling disempowered, marginalized, or distracted by possible signs of danger in the workplace). These experiences are particularly damaging to trauma survivors and can severely affect their ability to function, thrive, and demonstrate their strengths, talents, and skills. Stressful circumstances in the work environment often make it more difficult for employees to work and function properly, primarily when experiences of ACEs and early trauma are not recognized or understood by coworkers, employers, supervisors, or, more broadly, the overall workplace culture. Understanding power and the use and misuse of that power is vital to learning how to lead and support individuals who have experienced trauma, who inherently feel disempowered because they lost their power at a given point (or several points) in their lives. As such, employers must consider how to support these individuals effectively and develop people in the service of the organization, institution, or workplace without marginalizing their individual needs. Employers are encouraged to refrain from normalizing (and reinforcing) unhealthy practices, such as bullying, invalidation, exploitation, or labeling someone as challenging to work with, problematic, or annoying. Instead, cognitive reframing (emotion and behavior dysregulation as indicative of trauma-mediated fear, vulnerability, attachment insecurity, and helplessness) and focusing on safety, transparency, self-regulation, strengths, and resources will make all the difference in determining the success or repeated victimization of trauma survivors.

References

Abdinoor, N. M., & Ibrahim, M. B. (2019). Evaluating self-concept, career decision-making self-efficacy and parental support as predictors career maturity of senior secondary students from low income environment. *European Journal of Education Studies*, 6(7), 480–490. http://dx.doi.org/10.46827/ejes.v0i0.2703.

Ahn, J. S., Plamondon, A., & Ratelle, C. F. (2022). Different ways to support and thwart autonomy: Parenting profiles and adolescents' career decision-making. *Journal of Family Psychology*, 37(2), 161–172. https://doi.org/10.1037/fam0000982.

Akosah-Twumasi, P., Emeto, T. I., Lindsay, D., Tsey, K., & Malau-Aduli, B. S. (2018). A systematic review of factors that influence youths career choices – the role of culture. *Frontiers in Education*, 3, 58. https://doi.org/10.3389/feduc.2018.00058.

Almroth, M., Hemmingsson, T., Sörberg Wallin, A., Kjellberg, K., & Falkstedt, D. (2022). Psychosocial workplace factors and alcohol-related morbidity: A prospective study of 3 million Swedish workers. *European Journal of Public Health*, 32(3), 366–371. https://doi.org/10.1093/eurpub/ckac019.

Amateau, G., Gendron, T. L., & Rhodes, A. (2022). Stress, strength, and respect: Viewing direct care staff experiences through a trauma-informed lens. *Gerontology & Geriatrics Education*, 1–16. https://doi.org/10.1080/02701960.2022.2039132.

American Psychological Association. (2016). *Professional Practice Guidelines for Integrating the Role of Work and Career into Psychological Practice*. Retrieved from: http://www.apa.org/about/policy/work-career-practice.pdf.

Attell, B. K., Brown, K. K., & Treiber, L. A. (2017). Workplace bullying, perceived job stressors, and psychological distress: Gender and race differences in the stress process. *Social Science Research*, 65, 210–221. https://doi.org/10.1016/j.ssresearch.2017.02.001.

Aykanian, A., & Mammah, R. O. (2022). Prevalence of adverse childhood experiences among frontline homeless services workers in Texas. *Families in Society*, 103(4), 438–449. https://doi.org/10.1177/10443894211063579.

Baglivio, M. T., Wolff, K. T., DeLisi, M., & Jackowski, K. (2020). The role of adverse childhood experiences (ACEs) and psychopathic features on juvenile offending criminal careers to age 18. *Youth Violence and Juvenile Justice*, 18(4), 337–364. https://doi.org/10.1177/15412040209270.

Bargeman, M., Abelson, J., Mulvale, G., Niec, A., Theuer, A., & Moll, S. (2022). Understanding the conceptualization and operationalization of trauma-informed care within and across systems: A critical interpretive synthesis. *The Milbank Quarterly*, 100, 785–853https://doi.org/10.1111/1468-0009.12579.

Bocciardi, F., Caputo, A., Fregonese, C., Langher, V., & Sartori, R. (2017). Career adaptability as a strategic competence for career development: An exploratory study of its key predictors. *European Journal of Training and Development*, 41(1), 67–82. https://doi.org/10.1108/EJTD-07-2016-0049.

Bolat, N., & Odacı, H. (2017). High school final year students' career decision-making self-efficacy, attachment styles and gender role orientations. *Current Psychology*, 36(2), 252–259. https://doi.org/10.1007/s12144-016-9409-3.

Brown, A. O., Couser, G. P., Morrison III, D. E., & Agarwal, G. (2021). The stressful, hostile, and toxic workplace: An advanced understanding of a common clinical complaint. *Psychiatric Annals*, 51(2), 70–75. https://doi.org/10.3928/00485713-20210107-01.

Bryce, I., Pye, D., Beccaria, G., McIlveen, P., & Du Preez, J. (2023). A systematic literature review of the career choice of helping professionals who have experienced cumulative harm as a result of adverse childhood experiences. *Trauma, Violence, & Abuse*, 24(1), 72–85. https://doi.org/10.1177/15248380211016016.

Buckley, T. R. (2018). Black adolescent males: Intersections among their gender role identity and racial identity and associations with self-concept (global and school). *Child Development*, 89(4), e311–e322. https://doi.org/10.1111/cdev.12950.

Caceres, B. A., Wardecker, B. M., Anderson, J., & Hughes, T. L. (2021). Revictimization is associated with higher cardiometabolic risk in sexual minority women. *Women's Health Issues*, 31(4), 341–352. https://doi.org/10.1016/j.whi.2021.02.004.

Chung, M. C., AlQarni, N., Al Muhairi, S., & Mitchell, B. (2017). The relationship between trauma centrality, self-efficacy, posttraumatic stress and psychiatric co-morbidity among Syrian refugees: Is gender a moderator? *Journal of Psychiatric Research*, 94, 107–115. https://doi.org/10.1016/j.jpsychires.2017.07.001.

Chung, Y. W. (2018). Workplace ostracism and workplace behaviors: A moderated mediation model of perceived stress and psychological empowerment. *Anxiety, Stress, & Coping*, 31(3), 304–317. https://doi.org/10.1080/10615806.2018.1424835.

Copeland, W. E., Shanahan, L., Hinesley, J., Chan, R. F., Aberg, K. A., Fairbank, J. A., van den Oord, E., & Costello, E. J. (2018). Association of childhood trauma exposure with adult psychiatric disorders and functional outcomes. *JAMA Network Open*, 1(7), e184493. https://doi.org/10.1001/jamanetworkopen.2018.4493.

Cordeiro, P. M. G., Paixao, M. P., Lens, W., Lacante, M., & Luyckx, K. (2018). Parenting styles, identity development, and adjustment in career transitions: The mediating role of psychological needs. *Journal of Career Development*, 45(1), 83–97. https://doi.org/10.1177/08948453166727.

Creed, P. A., Kaya, M., & Hood, M. (2020). Vocational identity and career progress: The intervening variables of career calling and willingness to compromise. *Journal of Career Development*, 47(2), 131–145. https://doi.org/10.1177/08948453187949.

Cusack, S. E., Bourdon, J. L., Bountress, K., Saunders, T. R., Kendler, K. S., Dick, D. M., & Amstadter, A. B. (2021). Prospective predictors of sexual revictimization among college students. *Journal of Interpersonal Violence*, 36(17–18), 8494–8518. https://doi.org/10.1177/08862605198496.

Dash, S. S., & Jena, L. K. (2020). Self-deception, emotional neglect and workplace victimization: A conceptual analysis and ideas for research. *International Journal of Workplace Health Management*, 13(1), 81–94. https://doi.org/10.1108/IJWHM-03-2019-0036.

Davis, J. P., Tucker, J. S., Dunbar, M., Seelam, R., & D'Amico, E. J. (2022). Poly-victimization and opioid use during late adolescence and young adulthood: Health behavior disparities and protective factors. *Psychology of Addictive Behaviors*, 36(5), 440–451. https://doi.org/10.1037/adb0000770.

DeCou, C. R., Mahoney, C. T., Kaplan, S. P., & Lynch, S. M. (2019). Coping self-efficacy and trauma-related shame mediate the association between negative social reactions to sexual assault and PTSD symptoms. *Psychological Trauma: Theory, Research, Practice, and Policy*, 11(1), 51–54. https://doi.org/10.1037/tra0000379.

De Venter, M., Elzinga, B. M., Van Den Eede, F., Wouters, K., Van Hal, G. F., Veltman, D. J., Sabbe, B., & Penninx, B. (2020). The associations between childhood trauma and work functioning in adult workers with and without depressive and anxiety disorders. *European Psychiatry*, 63(1), e76. https://doi.org/10.1192/j.eurpsy.2020.70.

DeVylder, J., Lalane, M., & Fedina, L. (2019). The association between abusive policing and PTSD symptoms among U.S. police officers. *Journal of the Society for Social Work and Research*, 10(2), 261–273. https://doi.org/10.1086/703356.

Dray, K. K., Smith, V. R., Kostecki, T. P., Sabat, I. E., & Thomson, C. R. (2020). Moving beyond the gender binary: Examining workplace perceptions of nonbinary and transgender employees. *Gender, Work & Organization*, 27(6), 1181–1191. https://doi.org/10.1111/gwao.12455.

Fuchshuber, J., Hiebler-Ragger, M., Kresse, A., Kapfhammer, H. P., & Unterrainer, H. F. (2019). The influence of attachment styles and personality organization on emotional functioning after childhood trauma. *Frontiers in Psychiatry*, 10, 643. https://doi.org/10.3389/fpsyt.2019.00643.

Garriott, P. O., Raque-Bogdan, T. L., Zoma, L., Mackie-Hernandez, D., & Lavin, K. (2017). Social cognitive predictors of Mexican American high school students' math/science career goals. *Journal of Career Development*, 44(1), 77–90. https://doi.org/10.1177/0894845316633386.

Gbeleyi, O. A., Awaah, F., Okebukola, P. A., Shabani, J., & Potokri, O. C. (2022). Influence of students' career interests on perceived difficult concept in computer studies in Ghanaian and Nigerian secondary schools. *Humanities and Social Sciences Communications*, 9(1), 1–6. https://doi.org/10.1057/s41599-022-01215-3.

Green, Z. A. (2020). The mediating effect of well-being between generalized self-efficacy and vocational identity development. *International Journal for Educational and Vocational Guidance*, 20(2), 215–241. https://doi.org/10.1007/s10775-019-09401-7.

Grist, C. L., & Caudle, L. A. (2021). An examination of the relationships between adverse childhood experiences, personality traits, and job-related burnout in early childhood educators. *Teaching and Teacher Education*, 105, 103426. https://doi.org/10.1016/j.tate.2021.103426.

Grundmann, J., Lincoln, T. M., Lüdecke, D., Bong, S., Schulte, B., Verthein, U., & Schäfer, I. (2018). Traumatic experiences, revictimization and posttraumatic stress disorder in German inpatients treated for alcohol dependence. *Substance Use & Misuse*, 53(4), 677–685. https://doi.org/10.1080/10826084.2017.1361997.

Ham, E., Seto, M. C., Rodrigues, N. C., & Hilton, N. Z. (2022). Workplace stressors and PTSD among psychiatric workers: The mediating role of burnout. *International Journal of Mental Health Nursing*, 31(5), 1151–1163. https://doi.org/10.1111/inm.13015.

Hardcastle, K., Bellis, M. A., Ford, K., Hughes, K., Garner, J., & Ramos Rodriguez, G. (2018). Measuring the relationships between adverse childhood experiences and educational and employment success in England and Wales: findings from a retrospective study. *Public Health*, 165, 106–116. https://doi.org/10.1016/j.puhe.2018.09.014.

Hilton, N. Z., Ricciardelli, R., Shewmake, J., Rodrigues, N. C., Seto, M. C., & Ham, E. (2021). Perceptions of workplace violence and workplace stress: A mixed methods study of trauma among psychiatric workers. *Issues in Mental Health Nursing*, 42(9), 797–807. https://doi.org/10.1080/01612840.2021.1899350.

Holman, E. G. (2018). Theoretical extensions of minority stress theory for sexual minority individuals in the workplace: A cross-contextual understanding of minority stress processes. *Journal of Family Theory & Review*, 10(1), 165–180. https://doi.org/10.1111/jftr.12246.

Hou, C., Wu, Y., & Liu, Z. (2019). Career decision-making self-efficacy mediates the effect of social support on career adaptability: A longitudinal study. *Social Behavior and Personality: An International Journal*, 47(5), 1–13. https://doi.org/10.2224/sbp.8157.

Howard, K. A., & Ferrari, L. (2022). Social-emotional learning and career development in elementary settings. *British Journal of Guidance & Counselling*, 50(3), 371–385. https://doi.org/10.1080/03069885.2021.1959898.

Hu, S., Hood, M., Creed, P. A., & Shen, X. (2022). The relationship between family socioeconomic status and career outcomes: A life history perspective. *Journal of Career Development*, 49(3), 600–615. https://doi.org/10.1177/08948453209580.

Isobel, S., Wilson, A., Gill, K., Schelling, K., & Howe, D. (2021). What is needed for Trauma Informed Mental Health Services in Australia?: Perspectives of clinicians and managers. *International Journal of Mental Health Nursing*, 30(1), 72–82. https://doi.org/10.1111/inm.12811.

Jaffe, A. E., DiLillo, D., Gratz, K. L., & Messman-Moore, T. L. (2019). Risk for revictimization following interpersonal and noninterpersonal trauma: Clarifying the role of posttraumatic stress symptoms and trauma-related cognitions. *Journal of Traumatic Stress*, 32(1), 42–55. https://doi.org/10.1002/jts.22372.

Jahng, K. E. (2020). Narratives of working mothers experiencing workplace bullying: Trauma transferred to young children. *Family Relations*, 69(2), 320–334. https://doi.org/10.1111/fare.12402.

Jouriles, E. N., Choi, H. J., Rancher, C., & Temple, J. R. (2017). Teen dating violence victimization, trauma symptoms, and revictimization in early adulthood. *Journal of Adolescent Health*, 61(1), 115–119. https://doi.org/10.1016/j.jadohealth.2017.01.020.

Kanehisa, M., Kawashima, C., Nakanishi, M., Okamoto, K., Oshita, H., Masuda, K., Takita, F., Izumi, T., Inoue, A., Ishitobi, Y., Higuma, H., Ninomiya, T., & Akiyoshi, J. (2017). Gender differences in automatic thoughts and cortisol and alpha-amylase responses to acute psychosocial stress in patients with obsessive-compulsive personality disorder. *Journal of Affective Disorders*, 217, 1–7. https://doi.org/10.1016/j.jad.2017.03.057.

Keijzer, R., van der Rijst, R., van Schooten, E., & Admiraal, W. (2021). Individual differences among at-risk students changing the relationship between resilience and vocational identity. *International Journal of Educational Research*, 110, 101893. https://doi.org/10.1016/j.ijer.2021.101893.

Kim, J., Aggarwal, A., Maloney, S., & Tibbits, M. (2021). Organizational assessment to implement trauma-informed care for first responders, child welfare providers, and healthcare professionals. *Professional Psychology: Research and Practice*, 52(6), 569–578. https://doi.org/10.1037/pro0000408.

Kim, J., & Smith, C. K. (2021). Traumatic experiences and female university students' career adaptability. *The Career Development Quarterly*, 69(3), 263–277. https://doi.org/10.1002/cdq.12272.

Kim, J., & Wickrama, K. A. S. (2021). Early maternal employment status and attachment quality: An investigation of a conditional process model. *Journal of Family Issues*, 42(2), 395–421. https://doi.org/10.1177/0192513X20923704.

Kim, M. J., Bonn, M., Lee, C.-K., & Kim, J. S. (2019). Effects of employees' personality and attachment on job flow experience relevant to organizational commitment and consumer-oriented behavior. *Journal of Hospitality and Tourism Management*, 41, 156–170. https://doi-org.resources.njstatelib.org/10.1016/j.jhtm.2019.09.010.

Koçtürk, N., Ulaş, Ö., & Bilginer, Ç. (2019). Career development and educational status of the sexual abuse victims: The first data from Turkey. *School Mental Health*, 11(1), 179–190. https://doi.org/10.1007/s12310-018-9274-3.

Koloroutis, M., & Pole, M. (2021). Trauma-informed leadership and posttraumatic growth. *Nursing Management*, 52(12), 28–34. https://doi.org/10.1097/01.NUMA.0000800336.39811.a3.

Kvitkovičová, L., Umemura, T., & Macek, P. (2017). Roles of attachment relationships in emerging adults' career decision-making process: A two-year longitudinal research design. *Journal of Vocational Behavior*, 101, 119–132. https://doi.org/10.1016/j.jvb.2017.05.006.

Lagrosen, S., & Lagrosen, Y. (2022). Workplace stress and health – the connection to quality management. *Total Quality Management & Business Excellence*, 33(1–2), 113–126. https://doi.org/10.1080/14783363.2020.1807317.

Lahav, Y., Ginzburg, K., & Spiegel, D. (2020). Post-traumatic growth, dissociation, and sexual revictimization in female childhood sexual abuse survivors. *Child Maltreatment*, 25(1), 96–105. https://doi.org/10.1177/1077559519856.

La Mott, J., & Martin, L. A. (2019). Adverse childhood experiences, self-care, and compassion outcomes in mental health providers working with trauma. *Journal of Clinical Psychology*, 75(6), 1066–1083. https://doi.org/10.1002/jclp.22752.

Lee, Y., & Lee, J. Y. (2018). A multilevel analysis of individual and organizational factors that influence the relationship between career development and job-performance improvement. *European Journal of Training and Development*, 42(5/6), 286–304. https://doi.org/10.1108/EJTD-11-2017-0097.

Lent, R. W., Morris, T. R., Penn, L. T., & Ireland, G. W. (2019). Social-cognitive predictors of career exploration and decision-making: Longitudinal test of the career self-management model. *Journal of Counseling Psychology*, 66(2), 184–194. https://doi.org/10.1037/cou0000307.

Levenson, J. S., Craig, S. L., & Austin, A. (2021). Trauma-informed and affirmative mental health practices with LGBTQ+ clients. *Psychological Services*, 20(Suppl 1), 134–144. https://doi.org/10.1037/ser0000540.

Lewis, J. A., Raque-Bogdan, T. L., Lee, S., & Rao, M. A. (2018). Examining the role of ethnic identity and meaning in life on career decision-making self-efficacy. *Journal of Career Development*, 45(1), 68–82. https://doi.org/10.1177/08948453176968.

Li, F., Jiao, R., Yin, H., & Liu, D. (2021a). A moderated mediation model of trait gratitude and career calling in Chinese undergraduates: Life meaning as mediator and moral elevation as moderator. *Current Psychology: A Journal for Diverse Perspectives on Diverse Psychological Issues*. Advance online publication. https://doi.org/10.1007/s12144-021-01455-7.

Li, J., Atasoy, S., Fang, X., Angerer, P., & Ladwig, K. H. (2021b). Combined effect of work stress and impaired sleep on coronary and cardiovascular mortality in hypertensive workers: The MONICA/KORA cohort study. *European Journal of Preventive Cardiology*, 28(2), 220–226. https://doi.org/10.1177/2047487319839183.

Li, T., Tien, H. L. S., Gu, J., & Wang, J. (2022). The relationship between social support and career adaptability: the chain mediating role of perceived career barriers and career maturity. *International Journal for Educational and Vocational Guidance*, 1–18. https://doi.org/10.1007/s10775-021-09515-x.

Lim, S. A., & You, S. (2019). Long-term effect of parents' support on adolescents' career maturity. *Journal of Career Development*, 46(1), 48–61. https://doi.org/10.1177/089484531773186.

Lin, W. H., & Chiao, C. (2022). The relationship between adverse childhood experience and heavy smoking in emerging adulthood: The role of not in education, employment, or training status. *The Journal of Adolescent Health*, 70(1), 155–162. https://doi.org/10.1016/j.jadohealth.2021.07.022.

Lockey, S., Graham, L., Zheng, Y., Hesketh, I., Plater, M., & Gracey, S. (2022). The impact of workplace stressors on exhaustion and work engagement in policing. *The Police Journal*, 95(1), 190–206. https://doi.org/10.1177/0032258X2110165.

Longhi, D., Brown, M., & Fromm Reed, S. (2021). Community-wide resilience mitigates adverse childhood experiences on adult and youth health, school/work, and
problem behaviors. *The American Psychologist*, 76(2), 216–229. https://doi.org/10.
1037/amp0000773.

Lu, W., Bates, F. M., Waynor, W. R., Bazan, C., Gao, C. E., & Yanos, P. T. (2022). I
feel frozen: Client perceptions of how posttraumatic stress disorder impacts employment. *Psychiatric Rehabilitation Journal*, 45(2), 136–143. https://doi.org/10.1037/p
rj0000477.

Macia, K. S., Blonigen, D. M., Shaffer, P. M., Cloitre, M., & Smelson, D. A. (2021).
Trauma-related differences in socio-emotional functioning predict housing and
employment outcomes in homeless veterans. *Social Science & Medicine*, 281, 114096.
https://doi.org/10.1016/j.socscimed.2021.114096.

Mackey, J. D., Perrewé, P. L., & McAllister, C. P. (2017). Do I fit in?: Perceptions of
organizational fit as a resource in the workplace stress process. *Group & Organization
Management*, 42(4), 455–486. https://doi.org/10.1177/105960111562515.

Maulik, P. K. (2017). Workplace stress: A neglected aspect of mental health wellbeing.
The Indian Journal of Medical Research, 146(4), 441–444. https://doi.org/10.4103/ijmr.
IJMR_1298_17.

McQuerrey Tuttle, B., Cho, Y., & Waldrop, T. C. (2022). Pre-career exposure to violence as a predictor of emotional distress among police recruits. *The Police Journal*. https://
doi.org/10.1177/0032258X211064712.

McWhirter, E. H., Garcia, E. A., & Bines, D. (2018). Discrimination and other education barriers, school connectedness, and thoughts of dropping out among Latina/o
students. *Journal of Career Development*, 45(4), 330–344. https://doi.org/10.1177/
08948453176968.

Metzler, M., Merrick, M. T., Klevens, J., Ports, K. A., & Ford, D. C. (2017). Adverse
childhood experiences and life opportunities: Shifting the narrative. *Children and Youth
Services Review*, 72, 141–149. https://doi.org/10.1016/j.childyouth.2016.10.021.

Miller, M. L., & Brock, R. L. (2017). The effect of trauma on the severity of obsessive-
compulsive spectrum symptoms: A meta-analysis. *Journal of Anxiety Disorders*, 47, 29–44.
https://doi.org/10.1016/j.janxdis.2017.02.005.

Negru-Subtirica, O., & Pop, E. I. (2018). Reciprocal associations between educational
identity and vocational identity in adolescence: A three-wave longitudinal investigation. *Journal of Youth and Adolescence*, 47(4), 703–716. https://doi.org/10.1007/
s10964-017-0789-y.

Niedhammer, I., Bertrais, S., & Witt, K. (2021). Psychosocial work exposures and health
outcomes: A meta-review of 72 literature reviews with meta-analysis. *Scandinavian Journal
of Work, Environment & Health*, 47(7), 489–508. https://doi.org/10.5271/sjweh.3968.

Ørke, E. C., Vatnar, S. K. B., & Bjørkly, S. (2018). Risk for revictimization of intimate
partner violence by multiple partners: A systematic review. *Journal of Family Violence*,
33(5), 325–339. https://doi.org/10.1007/s10896-018-9952-9.

Parola, A., & Marcionetti, J. (2022). Career decision-making difficulties and life satisfaction: The role of career-related parental behaviors and career adaptability. *Journal of
Career Development*, 49(4), 831–845. https://doi.org/10.1177/0894845321995.

Pechorro, P., DeLisi, M., Abrunhosa Gonçalves, R., & Pedro Oliveira, J. (2021). The
role of low self-control as a mediator between trauma and antisociality/criminality in
youth. *International Journal of Environmental Research and Public Health*, 18(2), 567. https://
doi.org/10.3390/ijerph18020567.

Peila-Shuster, J. J. (2018). Fostering hope and career adaptability in children's career development. *Early Child Development and Care*, 188(4), 452–462. https://doi.org/10. 1080/03004430.2017.1385610.

Pękala, K., Kacprzak, A., Pękala-Wojciechowska, A., Chomczyński, P., Olszewski, M., Marczak, M., Kozłowski, R., Timler, D., Zakonnik, Ł., Sienkiewicz, K., Kozłowska, E., & Rasmus, P. (2021). Risk factors of early adolescence in the criminal career of polish offenders in the light of life course theory. *International Journal of Environmental Research and Public Health*, 18(12), 6583. https://doi.org/10.3390/ijerph18126583.

Pihl-Thingvad, J., Andersen, L. L., Brandt, L. P. A., & Elklit, A. (2019). Are frequency and severity of workplace violence etiologic factors of posttraumatic stress disorder?: A 1-year prospective study of 1,763 social educators. *Journal of Occupational Health Psychology*, 24(5), 543–555. https://doi.org/10.1037/ocp0000148.

Poole, J. C., Dobson, K. S., & Pusch, D. (2017). Childhood adversity and adult depression: The protective role of psychological resilience. *Child Abuse & Neglect*, 64, 89–100. https://doi.org/10.1016/j.chiabu.2016.12.012.

Prescod, D. J., & Zeligman, M. (2018). Career adaptability of trauma survivors: The moderating role of posttraumatic growth. *The Career Development Quarterly*, 66(2), 107–120. https://doi.org/10.1002/cdq.12126.

Pulliam, N., & Bartek, S. (2018). College and career readiness in elementary schools. *International Electronic Journal of Elementary Education*, 10(3), 355–360. https://doi.org/ 10.26822/iejee.2018336193.

Ramos, K., & Lopez, F. G. (2018). Attachment security and career adaptability as predictors of subjective well-being among career transitioners. *Journal of Vocational Behavior*, 104, 72–85. https://doi.org/10.1016/j.jvb.2017.10.004.

Rasool, S. F., Wang, M., Tang, M., Saeed, A., & Iqbal, J. (2021). How toxic workplace environment effects the employee engagement: The mediating role of organizational support and employee wellbeing. *International Journal of Environmental Research and Public Health*, 18(5), 2294. https://doi.org/10.3390/ijerph18052294.

Richard-Lepouriel, H., Kung, A. L., Hasler, R., Bellivier, F., Prada, P., Gard, S., Ardu, S., Kahn, J. P., Dayer, A., Henry, C., Aubry, J. M., Leboyer, M., Perroud, N., & Etain, B. (2019). Impulsivity and its association with childhood trauma experiences across bipolar disorder, attention deficit hyperactivity disorder and borderline personality disorder. *Journal of Affective Disorders*, 244, 33–41. https://doi.org/10.1016/j.jad. 2018.07.060.

Robey, N., Margolies, S., Sutherland, L., Rupp, C., Black, C., Hill, T., & Baker, C. N. (2021). Understanding staff- and system-level contextual factors relevant to trauma-informed care implementation. *Psychological Trauma: Theory, Research, Practice, and Policy*, 13(2), 249–257. https://doi.org/10.1037/tra0000948.

Robson, D. A., Allen, M. S., & Howard, S. J. (2020). Self-regulation in childhood as a predictor of future outcomes: A meta-analytic review. *Psychological Bulletin*, 146(4), 324–354. https://doi.org/10.1037/bul0000227.

Rodrigues, N. C., Ham, E., Kirsh, B., Seto, M. C., & Hilton, N. Z. (2021). Mental health workers' experiences of support and help-seeking following workplace violence: A qualitative study. *Nursing & Health Sciences*, 23(2), 381–388. https://doi.org/ 10.1111/nhs.12816.

Rogers, M. E., Creed, P. A., & Praskova, A. (2018). Parent and adolescent perceptions of adolescent career development tasks and vocational identity. *Journal of Career Development*, 45(1), 34–49. https://doi.org/10.1177/0894845316667.

Rudolph, C. W., Lavigne, K. N., & Zacher, H. (2017). Career adaptability: A meta-analysis of relationships with measures of adaptivity, adapting responses, and adaptation results. *Journal of Vocational Behavior*, 98, 17–34. https://doi.org/10.1016/j.jvb.2016.09.002.

Samuelson, K. W., Bartel, A., Valadez, R., & Jordan, J. T. (2017). PTSD symptoms and perception of cognitive problems: The roles of posttraumatic cognitions and trauma coping self-efficacy. *Psychological Trauma: Theory, Research, Practice, and Policy*, 9(5), 537–544. https://doi.org/10.1037/tra0000210.

Sawitri, D. R., & Creed, P. A. (2017). Collectivism and perceived congruence with parents as antecedents to career aspirations: A social cognitive perspective. *Journal of Career Development*, 44(6), 530–543. https://doi.org/10.1177/0894845316666857.

Shin, K. M., Chung, Y. K., Shin, Y. J., Kim, M., Kim, N. H., Kim, K. A., Lee, H., & Chang, H. Y. (2017). Post-traumatic cognition mediates the relationship between a history of sexual abuse and the post-traumatic stress symptoms in sexual assault victims. *Journal of Korean Medical Science*, 32(10), 1680–1686. https://doi.org/10.3346/jkms.2017.32.10.1680.

Steen, J. T., Straussner, S. L. A., & Senreich, E. (2021). Adverse childhood experiences and career-related issues among licensed social workers: A qualitative study. *Smith College Studies in Social Work*, 91(3), 216–233. https://doi.org/10.1080/00377317.2021.1887790.

Steine, I. M., Winje, D., Krystal, J. H., Bjorvatn, B., Milde, A. M., Grønli, J., Nordhus, I. H., & Pallesen, S. (2017). Cumulative childhood maltreatment and its dose-response relation with adult symptomatology: Findings in a sample of adult survivors of sexual abuse. *Child Abuse & Neglect*, 65, 99–111. https://doi.org/10.1016/j.chiabu.2017.01.008.

Steinlin, C., Dölitzsch, C., Kind, N., Fischer, S., Schmeck, K., Fegert, J. M., & Schmid, M. (2017). The influence of sense of coherence, self-care and work satisfaction on secondary traumatic stress and burnout among child and youth residential care workers in Switzerland . *Child & Youth Services*, 38(2), 159–175. https://doi.org/10.1080/0145935X.2017.1297225.

Stensrud, R. H., Gilbride, D. D., & Bruinekool, R. M. (2019). The childhood to prison pipeline: Early childhood trauma as reported by a prison population. *Rehabilitation Counseling Bulletin*, 62(4), 195–208. https://doi.org/10.1177/00343552187748.

Substance Abuse and Mental Health Services Administration. (2014). *Trauma-Informed Care in Behavioral Health Services*. Treatment Improvement Protocol (TIP) Series 57. HHS Publication No. (SMA) 13–4801. Rockville, MD: Substance Abuse and Mental Health Services Administration.

Sun, X., Qiao, M., Deng, J., Zhang, J., Pan, J., Zhang, X., & Liu, D. (2021). Mediating effect of work stress on the associations between psychological job demands, social approval, and workplace violence among health care workers in Sichuan province of China. *Frontiers in Public Health*, 9, 743626. https://doi.org/10.3389/fpubh.2021.743626.

Super, D. E. (1980). A life-span, life-space approach to career development. *Journal of Vocational Behavior*, 16(3), 282–298. https://doi.org/10.1016/0001-8791(80)90056–90051.

Super, D. E. (1990). A life-span, life-space approach to career development. In D. Brown & L. Brooks (Eds.), *Career choice and development: Applying contemporary theories to practice* (pp. 197–261). San Francisco, CA: Jossey-Bass.

Šverko, I., & Babarović, T. (2019). Applying career construction model of adaptation to career transition in adolescence: A two-study paper. *Journal of Vocational Behavior*, 111, 59–73. https://doi.org/10.1016/j.jvb.2018.10.011.

Tarocchi, A., Aschieri, F., Fantini, F., & Smith, J. D. (2013). Therapeutic assessment of complex trauma: A single-case time-series study. *Clinical Case Studies*, 12(3), 228–245. https://doi.org/10.1177/1534650113479442.

Turner, H. A., Shattuck, A., Finkelhor, D., & Hamby, S. (2017). Effects of poly-victimization on adolescent social support, self-concept, and psychological distress. *Journal of Interpersonal Violence*, 32(5), 755–780. https://doi.org/10.1177/0886260515558637.

Ulusoy, F., & Akcan, A. (2022). Comparison of adverse childhood experiences of working and nonworking adolescents. *Journal of Child and Adolescent Psychiatric Nursing*, 35(3), 277–284. https://doi.org/10.1111/jcap.12375.

van der Kolk, B., Pynoos, R., Cicchetti, D., Cloitre, M., D'Andrea, W., Ford, J., & Teicher, M. (2009). Proposal to include a developmental trauma disorder diagnosis for children and adolescents in DSM-V. http://www.traumacenter.org/announcements/dtd_papers_oct_09.pdf.

Van Vianen, A. E. (2018). Person–environment fit: A review of its basic tenets. *Annual Review of Organizational Psychology and Organizational Behavior*, 5, 75–101. https://doi.org/10.1146/annurev-orgpsych-032117-104702.

Voestermans, D., Eikelenboom, M., Rullmann, J., Wolters-Geerdink, M., Draijer, N., Smit, J. H., Thomaes, K., & van Marle, H. (2021). The association between childhood trauma and attachment functioning in patients with personality disorders. *Journal of Personality Disorders*, 35(4), 554–572. https://doi.org/10.1521/pedi_2020_34_474.

Walker, H. E., Freud, J. S., Ellis, R. A., Fraine, S. M., & Wilson, L. C. (2019). The prevalence of sexual revictimization: A meta-analytic review. *Trauma, Violence, & Abuse*, 20(1), 67–80. https://doi.org/10.1177/15248380176923.

Walker, H. E., & Wamser-Nanney, R. (2022). Revictimization risk factors following childhood maltreatment: A literature review. *Trauma, Violence, & Abuse*, 15248380221093692. https://doi.org/10.1177/15248380221093692.

Wang, Z., Zaman, S., Rasool, S. F., Zaman, Q. U., & Amin, A. (2020). Exploring the relationships between a toxic workplace environment, workplace stress, and project success with the moderating effect of organizational support: Empirical evidence from Pakistan. *Risk Management and Healthcare Policy*, 13, 1055–1067. https://doi.org/10.2147/RMHP.S256155.

Watson, M., & McMahon, M. (2022). Critical perspectives on childhood career development learning: expanding horizons. *British Journal of Guidance & Counselling*, 50(3), 474–480. https://doi.org/10.1080/03069885.2022.2063255.

Weisgram, E. S., & Bruun, S. T. (2018). Predictors of gender-typed toy purchases by prospective parents and mothers: The roles of childhood experiences and gender attitudes. *Sex Roles*, 79(5), 342–357. https://doi.org/10.1007/s11199-018-0928-2.

Weng, Q., Wu, S., McElroy, J. C., & Chen, L. (2018). Place attachment, intent to relocate and intent to quit: The moderating role of occupational commitment. *Journal of Vocational Behavior*, 108, 78–91. https://doi.org/10.1016/j.jvb.2018.06.002.

Widom, C. S., Fisher, J. H., Nagin, D. S., & Piquero, A. R. (2018). A prospective examination of criminal career trajectories in abused and neglected males and females followed up into middle adulthood. *Journal of Quantitative Criminology*, 34(3), 831–852. https://doi.org/10.1007/s10940-017-9356-7.

World Health Organization. (2020, October 19). Occupational health: Stress in the workplace. *World Health Organization.* https://www.who.int/news-room/questions-and-answers/item/ccupational-health-stress-at-the-workplace.

Wright, G. G., & Chan, C. D. (2022). Integrating trauma-informed care into career counseling: A response to COVID-19 job loss for Black, indigenous, and people of color. *Journal of Employment Counseling,* 59(2), 91–99. https://doi.org/10.1002/joec.12186.

Xu, H. (2021). Childhood environmental adversity and career decision-making difficulty: A life history theory perspective. *Journal of Career Assessment,* 29(2), 221–238. https://doi.org/10.1177/1069072720940978.

Yohros, A. (2022). Examining the relationship between adverse childhood experiences and juvenile recidivism: A systematic review and meta-analysis. *Trauma, Violence & Abuse,* 15248380211073846. Advance online publication. https://doi.org/10.1177/15248380211073846.

Zacher, H., Rudolph, C. W., Todorovic, T., & Ammann, D. (2019). Academic career development: A review and research agenda. *Journal of Vocational Behavior,* 110, 357–373. https://doi.org/10.1016/j.jvb.2018.08.006.

Zhao, C., & Li, X. (2022). Living under the shadow: Adverse childhood experiences and entrepreneurial behaviors in Chinese adults. *Journal of Business Research,* 138, 239–255. https://doi.org/10.1016/j.jbusres.2021.09.016.

Zheng, X., Fang, Z., Shangguan, S., & Fang, X. (2022). Associations between childhood maltreatment and educational, health and economic outcomes among middle-aged Chinese: The moderating role of relative poverty. *Child Abuse & Neglect,* 130(Pt 4), 105162. https://doi.org/10.1016/j.chiabu.2021.105162.

9

DEVELOPMENTAL TRAUMA AND HEALTH

Behavioral Medicine and Primary Care Psychology

> Traumatized people chronically feel unsafe inside their bodies: The past is alive in the form of gnawing interior discomfort. Their bodies are constantly bombarded by visceral warning signs, and, in an attempt to control these processes, they often become expert at ignoring their gut feelings and in numbing awareness of what is played out inside. They learn to hide from their selves.
>
> *(van der Kolk, 2014, p. 97)*

Over the last several decades, researchers and practitioners have recognized the devastation caused by cumulative stress and polyvictimization, including the extensive physiological disturbances that compromise health, social and occupational functioning, and mental and spiritual well-being (Brindle et al., 2018; Chang et al., 2019; Crouch et al., 2018; Janusek et al., 2017; Mikhail et al., 2018; Li et al., 2017; Ridout et al., 2018). Broad debilitating medical conditions, such as migraine headaches, chronic heart and kidney disease, and cancer, are linked to ACEs and early interpersonal trauma (Downey et al., 2017; Garrido et al., 2018; Llabre et al., 2017; López-Martínez et al., 2018; Sonu et al., 2019; Wiss & Brewerton, 2020). Trauma is associated with poor treatment adherence and, at the same time, high-risk behaviors, such as heavy smoking, alcohol and illicit drug abuse, and sexual promiscuity and sexually transmitted infections (Cuca et al., 2019; Haller et al., 2022; London et al., 2017). The combination of behavioral risks and comorbid medical disorders often results in a poor quality of life and higher rates of functional impairments and disability, particularly in the absence of prevention efforts and trauma-informed interventions. Trauma-informed care approaches are necessarily patient-centered, often requiring multiple visits and collaborative patient-provider interactions, including sharing the role of the expert with patients in ways that empower them to advocate for their needs and preferences in treatment and medical

DOI: 10.4324/9781003304715-9

decision-making (Cuevas et al., 2018; Kia-Keating et al., 2019). In doing so, providers must be prepared to discuss and address trauma's impact on health and well-being.

Research suggests that patients benefit from discussing experiences of ACEs and trauma, including regular screening and evaluation by healthcare providers (Goldstein et al., 2017). Regrettably, patients also often report that such discussions are rare and often omitted from their primary care visits (Purkey et al., 2018). Thus, understanding and appreciating trauma in evaluation and treatment, including associated health-risk behaviors and medical comorbidities, are highly consequential to healthcare providers' understanding and treatment of individuals who experienced early repeated abuse, neglect, violence, and traumatic loss. In fact, we now understand that trauma symptoms can manifest as exclusively physical symptoms and disorders, giving rise to broad multisystem (e.g., nervous, respiratory) health problems and more severe functional impairments. In this final chapter, I want to devote space to discussing trauma and health more carefully, including functional medical syndromes associated with trauma, the patient-provider relationship, and the use of evidence-based, culturally congruent, trauma-informed care practices.

Trauma and Physical Health

Physiological stress among individuals affected by trauma is particularly damaging because their bodies tend to frequently mobilize high levels of stress hormones, metabolic resources (e.g., glucose), and neurotransmitters to prepare them for imminent danger, which can cause issues such as sleep disturbances, eating disorders, and alcohol and drug abuse (Clemens et al., 2018). Trauma survivors may also have learned to suppress or repress their feelings, including experiences of depression, anxiety, guilt, and shame, which have additive adverse effects on their health and well-being, including compromising adaptive immunity and their ability to prevent and recover from acute and chronic illnesses. For example, metabolic disturbances, such as obesity, cardiovascular disease, and diabetes mellitus, are associated with trauma, and trauma precipitates early-onset disease and comorbidities (Jaworska-Andryszewska & Rybakowski, 2019; Kuras et al., 2017; Lee et al., 2018; Nelson et al., 2020). Regrettably, children, adolescents, and adults adversely affected by traumas often spend their lives protecting themselves, including their bodies, and they may avoid healthcare providers (because of attachment disturbances, dissociative responses to stress, or fear of being revictimized by authority figures) or, by comparison, become highly dependent (or codependent) on them.

Social isolation, fear of vulnerability and rejection, distrust of institutions and healthcare providers, and socio-economic adversity increase the risk for repeated hospitalizations, incomplete or ineffective treatments, and high medical expenditures from reliance on emergency medical services. Studies suggest that individuals who have experienced early trauma often rely on emergency medical services to cope with depression, anxiety, and loneliness or because mainstream healthcare services have failed to adequately address their psychological and medical needs (Vandyk et al., 2019). Their reasons for seeking medical treatment may be clear and specific (e.g., to address common problems, such as a cold) or complex, multifaceted, and related to the physiological disturbances of toxic stress, ACEs, and trauma (e.g., functional neurological disorders, gastrointestinal complaints, mental health problems). Further, patients may have difficulty communicating their needs effectively, trusting primary care providers, and maintaining high levels of treatment adherence.

Some individuals may become over-reliant on healthcare providers in response to psychological and somatic distress, heightened pain sensitivity, or to reconcile attachment disturbances (e.g., developing a codependent relationship with healthcare providers to cope with social isolation, anxiety, depression, and sleep disturbances). Consequently, under- and overutilization of healthcare services at the extremes of the continuum are likely to develop as individuals impacted by trauma cope with fear, anger/resentment, dissociation, and physiological distress (Hargreaves et al., 2019; Purkey et al., 2018).

Trauma and Somatic Symptoms of Distress

Heightened physical sensitivity and body awareness/preoccupation often causes DTD patients to experience somatic stress, stress-related symptoms, and functional medical disorders. Some individuals who have experienced developmental trauma will develop symptoms corresponding to somatic symptom disorders (SSDs). SSDs, as defined by DSM-5 criteria, are characterized by a preoccupation with health and a propensity to (mis)interpret bodily sensations as indications of severe illness and disease, which give rise to psychological distress, anxious rumination, and, in some circumstances, severe functional impairments.

The APA's conceptualization of somatic stress syndromes considers various contributing factors, diagnostic symptoms, and medical and psychiatric comorbidities. For example, healthcare providers often explore the possibility that mood and personality disorders may contribute to somatic distress or that psychological symptoms expressed through medical problems may result from obsessive-compulsive disorders, such as illness anxiety disorder (illness anxiety is marked by a pervasive fear of illness and a propensity to generalize physical and psychological distress symptoms as indications of chronic, severe and possibly disabling irreversible conditions; Lebel et al., 2020; Newby et al., 2017). Conversely, providers must also maintain objectivity throughout the evaluation process and consider the possibility that patients may need long-term care because of the incapacitating distress caused by trauma-mediated medical problems. Providers must also consider whether patients are amplifying their symptoms (i.e., feigning) for some secondary gain (i.e., malingering). We see these types of responses among individuals experiencing alcohol and drug addiction, personality disorders (antisocial and histrionic), or social and economic adversities (low-income incarcerated individuals).

Systemic Inflammation

In addition to the well-documented somatic expression of stress and disruptions to neurotransmitters and stress hormones linked to toxic stress, trauma has also been associated with high circulating inflammatory markers known to cause health problems and chronic diseases, such as c-reactive protein (CRP), which is produced by the liver to help individuals respond to acute stress, injury, and infection (Elliot et al., 2017; Friend et al., 2022). Trauma contributes to longstanding multisystem inflammation that disrupts normal immunity, compromises physical and mental health, and leads to auto-immune disorders (Speer et al., 2018).

Several neuropsychiatric disorders have been linked to early trauma and inflammation, including autism spectrum disorders (ASD), anxiety, depression, and schizophrenia. Scholars speculate that maternal stress and trauma cause heightened proinflammatory cytokine activity and infections that, in turn, adversely affect children's immune responses and nervous system development. The maternal immune activation hypothesis suggests that physiological stress and illness, repeated infection, injuries, and sleep disturbances during pregnancy compromise children's adaptive immunity and increase their risk for birth complications and medical, psychiatric, and developmental disturbances across the lifespan. As a further illustration, consider that a broad range of physiological conditions, such as chronic pain and peripheral (nervous system) neuropathies, are linked to systemic inflammation and toxic stress and trauma.

Systemic Inflammation and Neurological Disturbances

Bell's Palsy (BP) and Peripheral Neuropathy

One such condition is Bell's palsy (BP), which is characterized by unilateral (one side) facial paralysis. Research suggests that BP is often caused by poor immunity, stress and sleep deprivation, and vulnerability to infections, which are linked to oxidative stress and systemic inflammation (i.e., cytotoxic immunity; Burke et al., 2017; Davies et al., 2020; Demir et al., 2018; Kınar et al., 2021; Nelson et al., 2017; Terzi et al., 2017; You et al., 2019). Research also suggests that individuals who experience high-risk pregnancies and trauma-mediated obesity, hypertension, diabetes, and migraines are also at high risk for BP and tend to be less responsive to treatment (Kim et al., 2019, 2020; Psillas et al., 2021; Zhao et al., 2017). Individuals who experience BP also often experience general and social anxiety as well as depression, partly because of facial disfigurement and poor motor control (Díaz-Aristizabal et al., 2019; Lee et al., 2019; Pouwels et al., 2021; Siemann et al., 2022; Tseng et al., 2017).

Trauma and Dementia

Trauma has also been linked to a high risk of developing neurological and functional neurological disturbances, including fibromyalgia, dementia, and Alzheimer's disease (Hellou et al., 2017; Karatzias et al., 2017; Kienle et al., 2017; Ludwig et al., 2018; Spagnolo et al., 2020; Williams et al., 2019). Dementia is a neurological disorder that causes a progressive deterioration of the nervous system and measurable disturbances in memory, personality, and executive functioning. Dementia includes Alzheimer's disease and pseudodementia, which refers to cognitive disturbances that mirror dementia and originate from psychological causes, including depression and psychological trauma. Experiences of early abuse and neglect have been shown to increase the risk of developing dementia and pseudodementia, including early onset (Desmarais et al., 2020; Donley et al., 2018; Radford et al., 2017; Roberts et al., 2022; Tanaka et al., 2021), and these risks are compounded by alcohol use, poverty and food insecurity, history of stroke, head injury with loss of consciousness, and epilepsy. Scholars speculate that the link between trauma and dementia stems from trauma-mediated neuroinflammation (dementias are linked to disturbances in cellular and intracellular communication, such as amyloid β plaques and neurofibrillary tangles, and these circumstances are worsened by systemic inflammation, which further compromises immune responses; Hoeijmakers et al., 2017; Kinney et al., 2018).

Traumatic Brain Injury (TBI)

Traumatic Brain Injury (TBI) is a medical condition healthcare providers should be aware of that might signal the presence of DTD in children, adolescents, and adults, especially those who present with recurrent injuries and hospital visits. Physically abused children can sustain head injuries due to direct contact with caregivers, accidental injuries due to lack of caregiver attention and supervision, or physical assaults at school or in their communities (Guinn et al., 2019; Song et al., 2018). It has been suggested that early abuse is associated with TBIs and TBIs heighten the risk of behavioral disturbances and psychological disorders, including anxiety, traumatic stress, and antisocial behavior leading to criminal records and recidivism (Kaplan et al., 2018; O'Rourke et al., 2018; Rosen & Ayers, 2020; Schofield et al., 2019). TBI and DTD both cause traumatic amnesia, disrupted attention, mood and behavior disturbances, headaches, as well as overlapping physiological disturbances of the nervous system (e.g., asymmetrical white matter tract abnormalities and gray matter changes in the basolateral amygdala, hippocampus, and prefrontal cortex; Kaplan et al., 2018).

Epilepsy and Seizure Disorders

TBIs and trauma are also linked to epilepsy, a neurological disorder characterized by repeated seizures. Seizures are characterized by sudden, uncontrolled physiological disturbances in the nervous system that adversely affect an individual's cognitive and behavioral capacities (e.g., motor deficits, confusion, memory disturbances). Seizure disorders linked to trauma include psychogenic nonepileptic seizures (PNES) (Perez et al., 2017). PNES are seizure episodes caused by psychological distress that lack measurable physiological changes (by conventional measurement standards) of a seizure. PNES has been linked to psychiatric disorders, including trauma, cognitive dissociation, and attachment disturbances (Baroni et al., 2018; Labudda et al., 2017, 2018; Lloyd et al., 2022). Research suggests that other factors also correlate with PNES. For example, higher levels of anticipatory anxiety of repeated seizures, social anxiety and avoidance, somatization, and a poorer quality of life differentiate individuals with PNES from those with other seizure disorders (Ertan et al., 2021; Myers et al., 2019).

Consider the following recent report by Yrondi et al. (2020), who describe a patient who experienced severe seizures requiring surgical intervention and who disclosed early abuse and neglect one month after surgery was completed.

PA is a 41-year-old male suffering from temporal lobe epilepsy, which began at age 9. Seizures were associated with loss of consciousness, sensory and motor disturbances, amnesia, and epigastric pain. He had been on oxcarbazepine, an anticonvulsant medication that regulates physiological activity in the nervous system. The treatment helped to control the frequency and intensity of seizures. Regrettably, his seizures worsened (became more frequent and severe) in 2016, and conventional treatments were no longer effective in mitigating seizure activity. In 2017, PA underwent surgery, specifically partial removal of the amygdala, hippocampus, and temporal lobe. The surgery dramatically improved his seizures. However, PA experienced psychological trauma symptoms, which had previously been underappreciated by PA (and his providers), who avoided discussions of his experiences of early abuse and neglect. PA experienced severe depression, physiologic fatigue, anxiety, and PTSD, including intrusive thoughts related to early abuse by a family member, sleep disturbances, irritability, and physiological hyperarousal. Standardized assessment revealed clinically significant symptoms of emotional and physical abuse and emotional neglect. PA was treated with antidepressant medication (sertraline) and trauma-focused CBT, which mitigated psychological distress and improved his ability to cope and recover from his traumas.

PA's case demonstrates the complexity of evaluating and treating individuals with comorbid medical and psychiatric health problems effectively, particularly when medical problems overshadow psychological needs and mental health disturbances. In addition, early trauma often happens when individuals are helpless, unable to defend themselves, or feel unsafe physically and psychologically. The needs of individuals affected by trauma are diverse partly because they differ in their trauma experiences, awareness of the impact of those experiences on their physical health, as well as their healthcare needs, psychological and social capital, and ability to prioritize their health effectively. Trauma survivors often experience guilt and shame, including in prioritizing their needs over the needs of others.

Trauma and attachment disturbances originating from repeated abuse and neglect are likely to make it challenging for these individuals to seek medical treatment and disclose their psychological and emotional suffering to healthcare providers. This is especially true when individuals use dissociation to cope, which can increase an individual's felt level of vulnerability. Disclosing traumatic experiences to healthcare providers in a position of authority can be especially challenging and stigmatizing and, if unexplored in treatment, can give rise to behavioral disturbances and traumatic reenactments (e.g., arguing with medical staff and rejecting treatment recommendations).

Trauma-Informed Medical Care

Research suggests that trauma-informed care helps systems, providers, and the individuals they support in diverse ways. Studies have demonstrated several benefits to implementing and maintaining trauma-informed care practices across multiple medical settings, including maternal-fetal medicine, intensive care units, and emergency departments (Ashana et al., 2020; Sanders & Hall, 2018). TIC has been shown to improve retention rates, self-efficacy, emotion regulation, and attitudes and beliefs, as well as underscore the dynamic relationships between individuals and the social, cultural, and systems/institutions that support them (Hales et al., 2017, 2019; Sundborg, 2019).

Understanding trauma-informed principles and the effects of trauma on the provider-patient relationship also requires social, cultural, and systems-level support, such as establishing trauma-informed institutional norms and values; collaborations with interdisciplinary professionals; trauma-informed policies and procedures, including by health maintenance organizations; and ongoing medical education, training, and supervision/mentoring (Brown et al., 2022; Grossman et al., 2021; McClinton & Laurencin, 2020; Roberts et al., 2019).

Patient-Provider Interactions

Healthcare providers that are culturally competent, empathic, and relationally focused are likely to help trauma survivors recover from their traumas more effectively (Goldstein et al., 2020; Loria et al., 2021; Meredith et al., 2022; Tomaz & Castro-Vale, 2020). Competency in addressing a combination of early experiences of abuse, attachment trauma, and revictimization, including by healthcare providers, must also be considered more broadly in patient-physician interactions and healthcare systems of care. Individuals with symptoms characteristic of DTD often face social adversities that contribute to their poor health, including relational, financial, occupational, and legal problems, which often intersect with multiple minority stressors, including racial, sexual, and religious minority discrimination (Craig et al., 2020; Stolbach & Anam, 2017; DiGuiseppi et al. 2022). Thus, understanding and appreciating the extensive cognitive, behavioral, and interpersonal disturbances linked to trauma, including attention, mood and self-awareness, executive functioning (i.e., prioritizing needs, keeping up with appointments), and interpersonal communication, can mitigate (or worsen) these outcomes.

Given that DTD stems from early interpersonal trauma, positive patient-physician interactions can mitigate the effects of trauma and promote resiliency, often overshadowed by an exclusive focus on cognitive and behavioral disturbances, illness, and disease. Research suggests that respectful non-reactive (mindful) interactions with patients experiencing trauma are vital to their capacity to self-regulate, cope, care for themselves and others, and recover from the damaging effects of early stress and trauma (Robertshaw et al., 2017). Providers must reconcile the natural tendency to personalize and react negatively to an individual's reactions, respond with compassion and appreciation for traumatic origins of mood and behavior disturbances, and avoid revictimization. Escalating levels of psychological distress and crisis are fight-flight-freeze reactions to fear, helplessness, and perceptions of vulnerability or neglect by healthcare providers, who may be unaware of the individual's needs and coping strategies. Increasing levels of behavioral, physiological, cognitive, and emotional dysregulation are likely to worsen when patients are forced to wait for extended periods and feel rushed, invalidated, and stigmatized by staff and healthcare providers.

Trauma-Informed Assessment

Trauma-informed care calls for a change in standard healthcare practice models, and it underscores multicultural and systems models of care and evidence-based, person-centered approaches. Although mainstream healthcare traditionally emphasizes authority and expertise (on behalf of the healthcare provider) and a focus on clearly delineated signs, symptoms, and diagnostic criteria, practitioners must also recognize the diverse responses to trauma associated with DTD and the need for flexibility, collaboration, and individualized care to respond to these adaptations effectively.

Biopsychosocial approaches and integrative healthcare models consider biological, psychological, social, and cultural symptoms and illness, and they encourage healthcare providers to broaden their practices to include multidimensional assessments and treatments (Brown et al., 2017; Achenbach et al.,

2017; Longenecker et al., 2020). Evaluators must carefully consider neurodevelopmental, medical, and psychological disorders and comorbidities, including autism, ADHD, learning disorders, anxiety/panic, depression, psychosis, and the broad range of physiological, neuropsychiatric, and functional medical disorders discussed in this chapter.

Standardized interviews as well as person-centered evaluation and psychometric instruments specifically designed to assess for trauma symptoms, comorbidities, and stress-mediated psychological, relational, and physiological disturbances have been developed for this purpose. One of the most widely used measures of trauma and DTD is the Developmental Trauma Disorder Semi-structured Interview (DTD-SI), a clinician-administered measure for trauma in children, adolescents, and adults (Ford et al., 2018, 2022). The DTD-SI is a valid, reliable, and culturally informed measure of trauma that assesses for emotional and behavioral disturbances, psychological and somatic distress, disruptions in attention and self-awareness, insecure attachment and relationship conflicts, and personality disturbances associated with early repeated traumas (Spinazzola et al., 2018; van der Kolk et al., 2019). Likewise, the ICD-11 Trauma Questionnaire (ICD-TQ) is a screening measure for complex trauma and polyvictimization (Cloitre et al., 2018, 2021). PTSD and complex PTSD (c-PTSD) symptoms assessed by the ICD-TQ include re-experiencing, avoidance, perceived threat, emotion dysregulation, insecure attachment, and negative core beliefs (i.e., disturbances in self-organization [DSO]; Haselgruber et al., 2020; Redican et al., 2021; Rocha et al., 2020). Empirical research and systematic reviews of assessment tools and evaluation procedures designed to assess for ACEs, trauma, and developmental trauma are increasingly being reported in research (e.g., Trauma Symptom Checklist, UCLA PTSD Reaction Index, Childhood Trauma Questionnaire; Charak, et al., 2017; Denton et al., 2017; Jardin et al., 2017; Kaplow et al., 2020; Schmidt et al., 2020).

Treatment

In addition to TF-CBT therapies discussed in previous chapters, studies have also provided support for several other therapies, including eye movement desensitization and reprocessing (EMDR) and EEG neurofeedback (Askovic et al., 2017; Rogel et al., 2020; Schlumpf et al., 2019). EMDR is a psychological treatment for trauma and complex developmental traumas that involves processing traumatic experiences through mental imagery (of the traumatic events) and reprocessing those experiences in a safe and measured way to the images, self-thoughts, emotions, and body sensations associated with early abuse and neglect. Likewise, neurofeedback is a physiological therapy designed to help patients, including those affected by trauma, regulate their thoughts, feelings, and nervous system functioning. More specifically, scholars have linked physiological activity to differentiated states of mood, cognition, and behavior, including attention and distraction, auditory and visual processing, anxiety and homeostasis, on the hypoarousal-hyperarousal continuum (scholars measure and describe this process using terms like *alpha, beta, delta, gamma,* and *theta,* and they use this information to help individuals self-regulate, cope, problem solve, and manage their physical and emotional health more effectively).

In addition to psychotherapies, individuals with indications of complex developmental trauma often require medication to regulate their mood and behavior. Research suggests that several medications effectively reduce trauma symptoms and improve psychological and behavioral functioning, including antidepressants (e.g., mirtazapine, sertraline) and anti-inflammatory medication (e.g., prazosin; Bennett et al., 2022; Edelsohn et al., 2021; Coventry et al., 2020). Alternative treatments for trauma and PTSD, such as psychedelic drugs, are currently being explored in randomized clinical trials (Healy et al., 2021; Luoma et al., 2020; Siegel et al., 2021).

Concluding Thoughts

Throughout this chapter and across all chapters in this book, I have highlighted the pernicious outcomes associated with early stress and trauma, including the lack of secure attachment that could have helped individuals with DTD cope more effectively. Adequate training in trauma-informed care can help healthcare providers address the extensive needs of individuals affected by interpersonal trauma and polyvictimization, including physical and mental health disorders, comorbidities, social and economic adversities (poverty, unemployment, discrimination, incarceration, and recidivism), and functional impairments often requiring disability. Avoiding discussions related to ACEs and trauma, or minimizing the impact of these experiences on an individual's health and well-being, is likely to reinforce avoidance coping, shame, and stigma as well as continue to cause or worsen health problems, including chronic diseases linked to social determinants of health and health disparities. These individuals often suffer in silence or are misunderstood when conveying a need for help, regardless of their behavioral disturbances. They may vacillate between avoidance, anger and aggression, dissociation/confusion, and codependency, likely mirroring the chaos of early (repeated) abuse and neglect, and revictimization as adolescents and adults.

A trauma-informed approach can help practitioners understand and respond to their needs effectively, such as the tendency to express psychological distress through physical (somatic) symptoms. These expressions may also intersect with cultural norms and beliefs and thus necessitate careful evaluation, including how individuals and providers describe and conceptualize physical and psychological stress and illness.

As definitions and conceptualizations of trauma have changed over the years and continue to change in response to emerging research, health maintenance organizations must contend with mounting empirical evidence advancing diverse responses to trauma, including psychiatric and medical disorders that may not be described in mainstream diagnostic frameworks (ICD and DSM disorder taxonomies). We must also consider that healthcare systems and health maintenance organizations often focus on the extent to which psychological and medical problems adversely affect functioning, which effectively penalizes those who have less access to resources or who can (barely) function at school and work but are afraid to ask for help, admit vulnerability, and depend on others when others have let them down for the vast majority of their life. The DTD framework also underscores strength-based resources that may mitigate toxic stress and promote wellness and resilience under the same conditions, such as spirituality, mindfulness/meditation, and stress-related growth.

The implications of ACEs, trauma, complex developmental trauma, and trauma-informed practices are far-reaching in that these conditions affect (and are influenced by) biological risks (prenatal environment, early exposure to toxic stress and systemic inflammation), social circumstances (school and work, relationships, incarceration, and recidivism), psychological factors (diverse psychiatric symptoms and disorders, negative core beliefs, high-risk behavior), and cultural contexts (shame and stigma, gender norms and pressures to conform to those norms, racism, and discrimination). Coordinated research, practice, and policy-development efforts are needed to effectively address the cumulative effects of trauma at the individual level and, more broadly, on the societal level.

Studies are needed to reconcile several unanswered questions. Developmental trauma is associated with insecure attachment; however, studies on other underlying causes and contributing factors (independent of and in addition to the insecure attachment), such as negative core beliefs, reward and reinforcement value and saliency, executive dysfunction, and moral and spiritual development, are needed.

The extent to which ACEs precipitate trauma is also an area that needs further research. ACEs encompass a broad range of possibly traumatic experiences, including parental divorce and exposure to violence; however, increasingly, scholars have cautioned against the specific use of ACE scores, given that ACEs are common and experiencing these events does not necessarily equate to trauma, PTSD, and DTD. Nevertheless, ACEs continue to be vital to understanding the risk factors associated with trauma, and, for DTD in particular, the health needs and outcomes that might otherwise remain underappreciated and undertreated by healthcare providers (DTD is associated with broad physical and psychological disorders, and mainstream evaluation practices, such as screening for PTSD, may undermine traumatic adaptations commonly associated with developmental traumas). In this regard, a shift from patient-focused evaluation and treatment to a focus on social systems, organizations, and institutions is particularly vital given that responses to stress and trauma are likely to be worsened by environments that are invalidating, neglectful, and possibly abusive or mitigated by circumstances that are safe, supportive, respectful, and predictable. In other words, trauma-informed care is the responsibility of the individual as well as social systems and institutions. As such, individuals in positions of power are urged to consider their contributions to the behavioral and interpersonal responses to trauma linked to DTD and to acknowledge and accept that they play a role in the recovery process and in helping victims of trauma realize their potential, find value in trusting others, and learn that recovery is inextricably linked to interpersonal relationships and their ability to forgive and love themselves regardless of the circumstances.

References

Achenbach, T. M., Ivanova, M. Y., & Rescorla, L. A. (2017). Empirically based assessment and taxonomy of psychopathology for ages 1½–90+ years: Developmental, multi-informant, and multicultural findings. *Comprehensive Psychiatry*, 79, 4–18. http s://doi.org/10.1016/j.comppsych.2017.03.006.

Ashana, D. C., Lewis, C., & Hart, J. L. (2020). Dealing with "difficult" patients and families: Making a case for trauma-informed care in the intensive care unit. *Annals of the American Thoracic Society*, 17(5), 541–544. https://doi.org/10.1513/AnnalsATS. 201909-700IP.

Askovic, M., Watters, A. J., Aroche, J., & Harris, A. W. (2017). Neurofeedback as an adjunct therapy for treatment of chronic posttraumatic stress disorder related to refugee trauma and torture experiences: Two case studies. *Australasian Psychiatry*, 25(4), 358–363. https://doi.org/10.1177/1039856217715988.

Baroni, G., Martins, W. A., Piccinini, V., da Rosa, M. P., de Paola, L., Paglioli, E., Margis, R., & Palmini, A. (2018). Neuropsychiatric features of the coexistence of epilepsy and psychogenic nonepileptic seizures. *Journal of Psychosomatic Research*, 111, 83–88. https://doi.org/10.1016/j.jpsychores.2018.05.014.

Bennett, A., Crosse, K., Ku, M., Edgar, N. E., Hodgson, A., & Hatcher, S. (2022). Interventions to treat post-traumatic stress disorder (PTSD) in vulnerably housed populations and trauma-informed care: A scoping review. *BMJ open*, 12(3), e051079. https://doi.org/10.1136/bmjopen-2021-051079.

Brindle, R. C., Cribbet, M. R., Samuelsson, L. B., Gao, C., Frank, E., Krafty, R. T., Thayer, J. F., Buysse, D. J., & Hall, M. H. (2018). The relationship between childhood trauma and poor sleep health in adulthood. *Psychosomatic Medicine*, 80(2), 200–207. https://doi.org/10.1097/PSY.0000000000000542.

Brown, T., Ashworth, H., Bass, M., Rittenberg, E., Levy-Carrick, N., Grossman, S., Lewis-O'Connor, A., & Stoklosa, H. (2022). Trauma-informed care interventions in emergency medicine: A systematic review. *The Western Journal of Emergency Medicine*, 23(3), 334–344. https://doi.org/10.5811/westjem.2022.1.53674.

Brown, T. A., Berner, L. A., Jones, M. D., Reilly, E. E., Cusack, A., Anderson, L. K., ..., & Wierenga, C. E. (2017). Psychometric evaluation and norms for the Multidimensional Assessment of Interoceptive Awareness (MAIA) in a clinical eating disorders sample. *European Eating Disorders Review*, 25(5), 411–416. https://doi.org/10. 1002/erv.2532.

Burke, N. N., Finn, D. P., McGuire, B. E., & Roche, M. (2017). Psychological stress in early life as a predisposing factor for the development of chronic pain: Clinical and preclinical evidence and neurobiological mechanisms. *Journal of Neuroscience Research*, 95(6), 1257–1270. https://doi.org/10.1002/jnr.23802.

Chang, X., Jiang, X., Mkandarwire, T., & Shen, M. (2019). Associations between adverse childhood experiences and health outcomes in adults aged 18–59 years. *PloS One*, 14(2), e0211850. https://doi.org/10.1371/journal.pone.0211850.

Charak, R., De Jong, J. T. V. M., Berckmoes, L. H., Ndayisaba, H., & Reis, R. (2017). Assessing the factor structure of the childhood trauma questionnaire, and cumulative effect of abuse and neglect on mental health among adolescents in conflict-affected Burundi. *Child Abuse & Neglect*, 72, 383–392. https://doi.org/10.1016/j.chiabu.2017.09.009.

Clemens, V., Huber-Lang, M., Plener, P. L., Brähler, E., Brown, R. C., & Fegert, J. M. (2018). Association of child maltreatment subtypes and long-term physical health in a German representative sample. *European Journal of Psychotraumatology*, 9(1), 1510278. https://doi.org/10.1080/20008198.2018.1510278.

Cloitre, M., Hyland, P., Prins, A., & Shevlin, M. (2021). The international trauma questionnaire (ITQ) measures reliable and clinically significant treatment-related change in PTSD and complex PTSD. *European Journal of Psychotraumatology*, 12(1), 1930961. https://doi.org/10.1080/20008198.2021.1930961.

Cloitre, M., Shevlin, M., Brewin, C. R., Bisson, J. I., Roberts, N., Maercker, A., Karatzias, T., & Hyland, P. (2018). The international trauma questionnaire: Development of a self-report measure of ICD-11 PTSD and complex PTSD. *Acta Psychiatrica Scandinavica*, 138(6), 536–546. https://doi.org/10.1111/acps.12956.

Coventry, P. A., Meader, N., Melton, H., Temple, M., Dale, H., Wright, K., Cloitre, M., Karatzias, T., Bisson, J., Roberts, N. P., Brown, J., Barbui, C., Churchill, R., Lovell, K., McMillan, D., & Gilbody, S. (2020). Psychological and pharmacological interventions for posttraumatic stress disorder and comorbid mental health problems following complex traumatic events: Systematic review and component network meta-analysis. *PLoS Medicine*, 17(8), e1003262. https://doi.org/10.1371/journal.pmed.1003262.

Craig, S. L., Austin, A., Levenson, J., Leung, V., Eaton, A. D., & D'Souza, S. A. (2020). Frequencies and patterns of adverse childhood events in LGBTQ+ youth. *Child Abuse & Neglect*, 107, 104623. https://doi.org/10.1016/j.chiabu.2020.104623.

Crouch, E., Radcliff, E., Strompolis, M., & Srivastav, A. (2018). Safe, stable, and nurtured: Protective factors against poor physical and mental health outcomes following exposure to adverse childhood experiences (ACEs). *Journal of Child & Adolescent Trauma*, 12(2), 165–173. https://doi.org/10.1007/s40653-018-0217-9.

Cuca, Y. P., Shumway, M., Machtinger, E. L., Davis, K., Khanna, N., Cocohoba, J., & Dawson-Rose, C. (2019). The association of trauma with the physical, behavioral, and social health of women living with HIV: Pathways to guide trauma-informed health care interventions. *Women's Health Issues*, 29(5), 376–384. https://doi.org/10.1016/j.whi.2019.06.001.

Cuevas, K., Balbo, J., Duval, K., & Beverly, E. (2018). Neurobiology of sexual assault and osteopathic considerations for trauma-informed care and practice. *Journal of Osteopathic Medicine*, 118(2), e2–e10. https://doi.org/10.7556/jaoa.2018.018.

Davies, A. J., Rinaldi, S., Costigan, M., & Oh, S. B. (2020). Cytotoxic immunity in peripheral nerve injury and pain. *Frontiers in Neuroscience*, 14, 142. https://doi.org/10.3389/fnins.2020.00142.

Demir, C. Y., Bozan, N., Kocak, O. F., Cokluk, E., Sultanoglu, Y., & Ersoz, M. E. (2018). Thiol/Disulphide homeostasis and oxidative stress in patients with peripheral facial paralysis. *Eastern Journal of Medicine*, 23(3), 206. https://doi.org/10.5505/ejm. 2018.62533.

Denton, R., Frogley, C., Jackson, S., John, M., & Querstret, D. (2017). The assessment of developmental trauma in children and adolescents: A systematic review. *Clinical Child Psychology and Psychiatry*, 22(2), 260–287. https://doi.org/10.1177/ 1359104516631607.

Desmarais, P., Weidman, D., Wassef, A., Bruneau, M. A., Friedland, J., Bajsarowicz, P., Thibodeau, M. P., Herrmann, N., & Nguyen, Q. D. (2020). The interplay between post-traumatic stress disorder and dementia: A systematic review. *The American Journal of Geriatric Psychiatry*, 28(1), 48–60. https://doi.org/10.1016/j.jagp.2019.08.006.

Díaz-Aristizabal, U., Valdés-Vilches, M., Fernández-Ferreras, T. R., Calero-Muñoz, E., Bienzobas-Allué, E., & Moracén-Naranjo, T. (2019). Correlations between impairment, psychological distress, disability, and quality of life in peripheral facial palsy. *Neurologia (Barcelona, Spain)*, 34(7), 423–428. https://doi.org/10.1016/j.nrl. 2017.03.004.

DiGuiseppi, G. T., Davis, J. P., Srivastava, A., Layland, E. K., Pham, D., & Kipke, M. D. (2022). Multiple minority stress and behavioral health among young Black and Latino sexual minority men. *LGBT Health*, 9(2), 114–121. https://doi.org/10.1089/ lgbt.2021.0230.

Donley, G., Lönnroos, E., Tuomainen, T. P., & Kauhanen, J. (2018). Association of childhood stress with late-life dementia and Alzheimer's disease: The KIHD study. *European Journal of Public Health*, 28(6), 1069–1073. https://doi.org/10.1093/eurpub/ cky134.

Downey, J. C., Gudmunson, C. G., Pang, Y. C., & Lee, K. (2017). Adverse childhood experiences affect health risk behaviors and chronic health of Iowans. *Journal of Family Violence*, 32(6), 557–564. https://doi.org/10.1007/s10896-017-9909-4.

Edelsohn, G. A., Eren, K., Parthasarathy, M., Ryan, N. D., & Herschell, A. (2021). Inter-class concomitant pharmacotherapy in Medicaid-insured youth receiving psychiatric residential treatment. *Frontiers in Psychiatry*, 12, 658283. https://doi.org/10. 3389/fpsyt.2021.658283.

Elliot, A. J., Mooney, C. J., Infurna, F. J., & Chapman, B. P. (2017). Associations of lifetime trauma and chronic stress with C-reactive protein in adults ages 50 years and older: Examining the moderating role of perceived control. *Psychosomatic Medicine*, 79 (6), 622–630. https://doi.org/10.1097/PSY.0000000000000476.

Ertan, D., Hubert-Jacquot, C., Maillard, L., Sanchez, S., Jansen, C., Fracomme, L., Schwan, R., Hopes, L., Javelot, H., Tyvaert, L., Vignal, J. P., El-Hage, W., & Hingray, C. (2021). Anticipatory anxiety of epileptic seizures: An overlooked dimension linked to trauma history. *Seizure*, 85, 64–69. https://doi.org/10.1016/j.seizure.2020. 12.006.

Ford, J. D., Spinazzola, J., van der Kolk, B., & Chan, G. (2022). Toward an empirically based Developmental Trauma Disorder diagnosis and semi-structured interview for children: The DTD field trial replication. *Acta Psychiatrica Scandinavica*, 145(6), 628–639. https://doi.org/10.1111/acps.13424.

Ford, J. D., Spinazzola, J., van der Kolk, B., & Grasso, D. J. (2018). Toward an empirically based Developmental Trauma Disorder diagnosis for children: Factor structure, item characteristics, reliability, and validity of the developmental trauma disorder semi-structured interview. *The Journal of Clinical Psychiatry*, 79(5), 17m11675. https://doi.org/10.4088/JCP.17m11675.

Friend, S. F., Nachnani, R., Powell, S. B., & Risbrough, V. B. (2022). C-Reactive Protein: Marker of risk for post-traumatic stress disorder and its potential for a mechanistic role in trauma response and recovery. *The European Journal of Neuroscience*, 55(9–10), 2297–2310. https://doi.org/10.1111/ejn.15031.

Garrido, E. F., Weiler, L. M., & Taussig, H. N. (2018). Adverse childhood experiences and health-risk behaviors in vulnerable early adolescents. *The Journal of Early Adolescence*, 38(5), 661–680. https://doi.org/10.1177/0272431616687671.

Goldstein, E., Athale, N., Sciolla, A. F., & Catz, S. L. (2017). Patient preferences for discussing childhood trauma in primary care. *The Permanente Journal*, 21, 16-055. https://doi.org/10.7812/TPP/16-055.

Goldstein, E., Benton, S. F., & Barrett, B. (2020). Health risk behaviors and resilience among low-income, black primary care patients: Qualitative findings from a trauma-informed primary care intervention study. *Family & Community Health*, 43(3), 187–199. https://doi.org/10.1097/FCH.0000000000000260.

Grossman, S., Cooper, Z., Buxton, H., Hendrickson, S., Lewis-O'Connor, A., Stevens, J., Wong, L. Y., & Bonne, S. (2021). Trauma-informed care: Recognizing and resisting re-traumatization in health care. *Trauma Surgery & Acute Care Open*, 6(1), e000815. https://doi.org/10.1136/tsaco-2021-000815.

Guinn, A. S., Ports, K. A., Ford, D. C., Breiding, M., & Merrick, M. T. (2019). Associations between adverse childhood experiences and acquired brain injury, including traumatic brain injuries, among adults: 2014 BRFSS North Carolina. *Injury Prevention*, 25(6), 514–520. https://doi.org/10.1136/injuryprev-2018-042927.

Hales, T., Kusmaul, N., & Nochajski, T. (2017). Exploring the dimensionality of trauma-informed care: Implications for theory and practice. *Human Service Organizations: Management, Leadership & Governance*, 41(3), 317–325. https://doi.org/10.1080/23303131.2016.1268988.

Hales, T. W., Green, S. A., Bissonette, S., Warden, A., Diebold, J., Koury, S. P., & Nochajski, T. H. (2019). Trauma-informed care outcome study. *Research on Social Work Practice*, 29(5), 529–539. https://doi.org/10.1177/1049731518766618.

Haller, K., Fritzsche, S., Kruse, I., O'Malley, G., Ehrenthal, J. C., & Stamm, T. (2022). Associations between personality functioning, childhood trauma and non-adherence in cardiovascular disease: A psychodynamically-informed cross-sectional study. *Frontiers in Psychology*, 13, 913081. https://doi.org/10.3389/fpsyg.2022.913081.

Hargreaves, M. K., Mouton, C. P., Liu, J., Zhou, Y. E., & Blot, W. J. (2019). Adverse childhood experiences and health care utilization in a low-income population. *Journal of Health Care for the Poor and Underserved*, 30(2), 749–767. https://doi.org/10.1353/hpu.2019.0054.

Haselgruber, A., Sölva, K., & Lueger-Schuster, B. (2020). Validation of ICD-11 PTSD and complex PTSD in foster children using the International Trauma Questionnaire. *Acta Psychiatrica Scandinavica*, 141(1), 60–73. https://doi.org/10.1111/acps.13100.

Healy, C. J., Lee, K. A., & D'Andrea, W. (2021). Using psychedelics with therapeutic intent is associated with lower shame and complex trauma symptoms in adults with histories of child maltreatment. *Chronic Stress*, 5, 24705470211029881. https://doi.org/10.1177/24705470211029881.

Hellou, R., Häuser, W., Brenner, I., Buskila, D., Jacob, G., Elkayam, O., Aloush, V., & Ablin, J. N. (2017). Self-reported childhood maltreatment and traumatic events among Israeli patients suffering from fibromyalgia and rheumatoid arthritis. *Pain Research & Management*, 3865249. https://doi.org/10.1155/2017/3865249.

Hoeijmakers, L., Ruigrok, S. R., Amelianchik, A., Ivan, D., van Dam, A. M., Lucassen, P. J., & Korosi, A. (2017). Early-life stress lastingly alters the neuroinflammatory response to amyloid pathology in an Alzheimer's disease mouse model. *Brain, Behavior, and Immunity*, 63, 160–175. https://doi.org/10.1016/j.bbi.2016.12.023.

Janusek, L. W., Tell, D., Gaylord-Harden, N., & Mathews, H. L. (2017). Relationship of childhood adversity and neighborhood violence to a proinflammatory phenotype in emerging adult African American men: An epigenetic link. *Brain, Behavior, and Immunity*, 60, 126–135. https://doi.org/10.1016/j.bbi.2016.10.006.

Jardin, C., Venta, A., Newlin, E., Ibarra, S., & Sharp, C. (2017). Secure attachment moderates the relation of sexual trauma with trauma symptoms among adolescents from an inpatient psychiatric facility. *Journal of interpersonal violence*, 32(10), 1565–1585. https://doi.org/10.1177/0886260515589928.

Jaworska-Andryszewska, P., & Rybakowski, J. K. (2019). Childhood trauma in mood disorders: Neurobiological mechanisms and implications for treatment. *Pharmacological Reports*, 71(1), 112–120. https://doi.org/10.1016/j.pharep.2018.10.004.

Kaplan, G. B., Leite-Morris, K. A., Wang, L., Rumbika, K. K., Heinrichs, S. C., Zeng, X., Wu, L., Arena, D. T., & Teng, Y. D. (2018). Pathophysiological bases of comorbidity: Traumatic brain injury and post-traumatic stress disorder. *Journal of Neurotrauma*, 35(2), 210–225. https://doi.org/10.1089/neu.2016.4953.

Kaplow, J. B., Rolon-Arroyo, B., Layne, C. M., Rooney, E., Oosterhoff, B., Hill, R., Steinberg, A. M., Lotterman, J., Gallagher, K. A. S., & Pynoos, R. S. (2020). Validation of the UCLA PTSD reaction index for DSM-5: A developmentally informed assessment tool for youth. *Journal of the American Academy of Child and Adolescent Psychiatry*, 59(1), 186–194. https://doi.org/10.1016/j.jaac.2018.10.019.

Karatzias, T., Howard, R., Power, K., Socherel, F., Heath, C., & Livingstone, A. (2017). Organic vs. functional neurological disorders: The role of childhood psychological trauma. *Child Abuse & Neglect*, 63, 1–6. https://doi.org/10.1016/j.chiabu.2016.11.011.

Kia-Keating, M., Barnett, M. L., Liu, S. R., Sims, G. M., & Ruth, A. B. (2019). Trauma-responsive care in a pediatric setting: Feasibility and acceptability of screening for adverse childhood experiences. *American Journal of Community Psychology*, 64(3–4), 286–297. https://doi.org/10.1002/ajcp.12366.

Kienle, J., Rockstroh, B., Bohus, M., Fiess, J., Huffziger, S., & Steffen-Klatt, A. (2017). Somatoform dissociation and posttraumatic stress syndrome – two sides of the same medal?: A comparison of symptom profiles, trauma history and altered affect regulation between patients with functional neurological symptoms and patients with PTSD. *BMC Psychiatry*, 17(1), 248. https://doi.org/10.1186/s12888-017-1414-z.

Kim, S. Y., Lee, C. H., Lim, J. S., Kong, I. G., Sim, S., & Choi, H. G. (2019). Increased risk of Bell palsy in patient with migraine: A longitudinal follow-up study. *Medicine*, 98(21), e15764. https://doi.org/10.1097/MD.0000000000015764.

Kim, S. Y., Oh, D. J., Park, B., & Choi, H. G. (2020). Bell's palsy and obesity, alcohol consumption and smoking: A nested case-control study using a national health screening cohort. *Scientific Reports*, 10(1), 4248. https://doi.org/10.1038/s41598-020-61240-7.

Kınar, A., Ulu, Ş., Bucak, A., & Kazan, E. (2021). Can systemic immune-inflammation index (SII) be a prognostic factor of Bell's palsy patients? *Neurological Sciences*, 42(8), 3197–3201. https://doi.org/10.1007/s10072-020-04921-5.

Kinney, J. W., Bemiller, S. M., Murtishaw, A. S., Leisgang, A. M., Salazar, A. M., & Lamb, B. T. (2018). Inflammation as a central mechanism in Alzheimer's disease.

Alzheimer's & Dementia (New York), 4, 575–590. https://doi.org/10.1016/j.trci.2018. 06.014.

Kuras, Y. I., McInnis, C. M., Thoma, M. V., Chen, X., Hanlin, L., Gianferante, D., & Rohleder, N. (2017). Increased alpha-amylase response to an acute psychosocial stress challenge in healthy adults with childhood adversity. *Developmental Psychobiology*, 59(1), 91–98. https://doi.org/10.1002/dev.21470.

Labudda, K., Frauenheim, M., Illies, D., Miller, I., Schrecke, M., Vietmeier, N., Brandt, C., & Bien, C. G. (2018). Psychiatric disorders and trauma history in patients with pure PNES and patients with PNES and coexisting epilepsy. *Epilepsy & Behavior*, 88, 41–48. https://doi.org/10.1016/j.yebeh.2018.08.027.

Labudda, K., Illies, D., Herzig, C., Schröder, K., Bien, C. G., & Neuner, F. (2017). Current psychiatric disorders in patients with epilepsy are predicted by maltreatment experiences during childhood. *Epilepsy Research*, 135, 43–49. https://doi.org/10. 1016/j.eplepsyres.2017.06.005.

Lebel, S., Mutsaers, B., Tomei, C., Leclair, C. S., Jones, G., Petricone-Westwood, D., Rutkowski, N., Ta, V., Trudel, G., Laflamme, S. Z., Lavigne, A.-A., & Dinkell, A. (2020). Health anxiety and illness-related fears across diverse chronic illnesses: A systematic review on conceptualization, measurement, prevalence, course, and correlates. *PLoS One*, 15(7), e0234124. https://doi.org/10.1371/journal.pone.0234124.

Lee, E. E., Martin, A. S., Tu, X., Palmer, B. W., & Jeste, D. V. (2018). Childhood adversity and schizophrenia: The protective role of resilience in mental and physical health and metabolic markers. *The Journal of Clinical Psychiatry*, 79(3), 17m11776. https://doi.org/10.4088/JCP.17m11776.

Lee, S. Y., Kong, I. G., Oh, D. J., & Choi, H. G. (2019). Increased risk of depression in Bell's palsy: Two longitudinal follow-up studies using a national sample cohort. *Journal of Affective Disorders*, 251, 256–262. https://doi.org/10.1016/j.jad.2019.03.059.

Li, Z., He, Y., Wang, D., Tang, J., & Chen, X. (2017). Association between childhood trauma and accelerated telomere erosion in adulthood: A meta-analytic study. *Journal of Psychiatric Research*, 93, 64–71. https://doi.org/10.1016/j.jpsychires.2017.06.002.

Llabre, M. M., Schneiderman, N., Gallo, L. C., Arguelles, W., Daviglus, M. L., Gonzalez, F., 2nd, Isasi, C. R., Perreira, K. M., & Penedo, F. J. (2017). Childhood trauma and adult risk factors and disease in Hispanics/Latinos in the US: Results from the Hispanic community health study/study of Latinos (HCHS/SOL) sociocultural ancillary study. *Psychosomatic Medicine*, 79(2), 172–180. https://doi.org/10.1097/PSY. 0000000000000394.

Lloyd, M., Winton-Brown, T. T., Hew, A., Rayner, G., Foster, E., Rychkova, M., Ali, R., Velakoulis, D., O'Brien, T. J., Kwan, P., & Malpas, C. B. (2022). Multi-dimensional psychopathological profile differences between patients with psychogenic nonepileptic seizures and epileptic seizure disorders. *Epilepsy & Behavior*, 135, 108878. https://doi.org/10.1016/j.yebeh.2022.108878.

London, S., Quinn, K., Scheidell, J. D., Frueh, B. C., & Khan, M. R. (2017). Adverse experiences in childhood and sexually transmitted infection risk from adolescence into adulthood. *Sexually Transmitted Diseases*, 44(9), 524–532. https://doi.org/10.1097/ OLQ.0000000000000640.

Longenecker, J. M., Krueger, R. F., & Sponheim, S. R. (2020). Personality traits across the psychosis spectrum: A hierarchical taxonomy of psychopathology conceptualization of clinical symptomatology. *Personality and Mental Health*, 14(1), 88–105. https:// doi.org/10.1002/pmh.1448.

López-Martínez, A. E., Serrano-Ibáñez, E. R., Ruiz-Párraga, G. T., Gómez-Pérez, L., Ramírez-Maestre, C., & Esteve, R. (2018). Physical health consequences of interpersonal trauma: A systematic review of the role of psychological variables. *Trauma, Violence & Abuse*, 19(3), 305–322. https://doi.org/10.1177/1524838016659488.

Loria, H., McLeigh, J., Craker, K., & Bird, S. (2021). Trauma-informed, integrated primary care: A medical home model for children with prenatal drug exposure who enter foster care. *Children and Youth Services Review*, 127, 106089. https://doi.org/10.1016/j.childyouth.2021.106089.

Ludwig, L., Pasman, J. A., Nicholson, T., Aybek, S., David, A. S., Tuck, S., Kanaan, R. A., Roelofs, K., Carson, A., & Stone, J. (2018). Stressful life events and maltreatment in conversion (functional neurological) disorder: Systematic review and meta-analysis of case-control studies. *The Lancet: Psychiatry*, 5(4), 307–320. https://doi.org/10.1016/S2215-0366(18)30051–30058.

Luoma, J. B., Chwyl, C., Bathje, G. J., Davis, A. K., & Lancelotta, R. (2020). A meta-analysis of placebo-controlled trials of psychedelic-assisted therapy. *Journal of Psychoactive Drugs*, 52(4), 289–299. https://doi.org/10.1080/02791072.2020.1769878.

McClinton, A., & Laurencin, C. T. (2020). Just in TIME: Trauma-Informed Medical Education. *Journal of Racial and Ethnic Health Disparities*, 7(6), 1046–1052. https://doi.org/10.1007/s40615-020-00881-w.

Meredith, L. S., Wong, E., Osilla, K. C., Sanders, M., Tebeka, M. G., Han, B., Williamson, S. L., & Carton, T. W. (2022). Trauma-informed collaborative care for African American primary care patients in federally qualified health centers: A pilot randomized trial. *Medical Care*, 60(3), 232–239. https://doi.org/10.1097/MLR.0000000000001681.

Mikhail, J. N., Nemeth, L. S., Mueller, M., Pope, C., & NeSmith, E. G. (2018). The social determinants of trauma: A trauma disparities scoping review and framework. *Journal of Trauma Nursing*, 25(5), 266–281. https://doi.org/10.1097/JTN.0000000000000388.

Myers, L., Trobliger, R., Bortnik, K., Zeng, R., Saal, E., & Lancman, M. (2019). Psychological trauma, somatization, dissociation, and psychiatric comorbidities in patients with psychogenic nonepileptic seizures compared with those in patients with intractable partial epilepsy. *Epilepsy & Behavior*, 92, 108–113. https://doi.org/10.1016/j.yebeh.2018.12.027.

Nelson, C. A., Scott, R. D., Bhutta, Z. A., Harris, N. B., Danese, A., & Samara, M. (2020). Adversity in childhood is linked to mental and physical health throughout life. *BMJ (Clinical research ed.)*, 371, m3048. https://doi.org/10.1136/bmj.m3048.

Nelson, S. M., Cunningham, N. R., & Kashikar-Zuck, S. (2017). A conceptual framework for understanding the role of adverse childhood experiences in pediatric chronic pain. *The Clinical Journal of Pain*, 33(3), 264–270. https://doi.org/10.1097/AJP.0000000000000397.

Newby, J. M., Hobbs, M. J., Mahoney, A. E., Wong, S. K., & Andrews, G. (2017). DSM-5 illness anxiety disorder and somatic symptom disorder: Comorbidity, correlates, and overlap with DSM-IV hypochondriasis. *Journal of Psychosomatic Research*, 101, 31–37. https://doi.org/10.1016/j.jpsychores.2017.07.010.

O'Rourke, C., Linden, M. A., & Lohan, M. (2018). Traumatic brain injury and abuse among female offenders compared to non-incarcerated controls. *Brain Injury*, 32(13–14), 1787–1794. https://doi.org/10.1080/02699052.2018.1539872.

Perez, D. L., Matin, N., Barsky, A., Costumero-Ramos, V., Makaretz, S. J., Young, S. S., Sepulcre, J., LaFrance Jr, W. C., Keshavan, M. S., & Dickerson, B. C. (2017).

Cingulo-insular structural alterations associated with psychogenic symptoms, childhood abuse and PTSD in functional neurological disorders. *Journal of Neurology, Neurosurgery, and Psychiatry,* 88(6), 491–497. https://doi.org/10.1136/jnnp-2016-314998.

Pouwels, S., Sanches, E. E., Chaiet, S. R., de Jongh, F. W., Beurskens, C., Monstrey, S. J., Luijmes, R. E., Siemann, I., Ramnarain, D., Marres, H., & Ingels, K. (2021). Association between duration of peripheral facial palsy, severity, and age of the patient, and psychological distress. *Journal of Plastic, Reconstructive & Aesthetic Surgery,* 74 (11), 3048–3054. https://doi.org/10.1016/j.bjps.2021.03.092.

Psillas, G., Dimas, G. G., Sarafidou, A., Didangelos, T., Perifanis, V., Kaiafa, G., Mirkopoulou, D., Tegos, T., Savopoulos, C., & Constantinidis, J. (2021). Evaluation of effects of diabetes mellitus, hypercholesterolemia and hypertension on Bell's palsy. *Journal of Clinical Medicine,* 10(11), 2357. https://doi.org/10.3390/jcm10112357.

Purkey, E., Patel, R., Beckett, T., & Mathieu, F. (2018). Primary care experiences of women with a history of childhood trauma and chronic disease: Trauma-informed care approach. *Canadian Family Physician,* 64(3), 204–211. https://www.cfp.ca/content/cfp/64/3/204.full.pdf.

Radford, K., Delbaere, K., Draper, B., Mack, H. A., Daylight, G., Cumming, R., Chalkley, S., Minogue, C., & Broe, G. A. (2017). Childhood stress and adversity is associated with late-life dementia in aboriginal Australians. *The American Journal of Geriatric Psychiatry,* 25(10), 1097–1106. https://doi.org/10.1016/j.jagp.2017.05.008.

Redican, E., Nolan, E., Hyland, P., Cloitre, M., McBride, O., Karatzias, T., Murphy, J., & Shevlin, M. (2021). A systematic literature review of factor analytic and mixture models of ICD-11 PTSD and CPTSD using the International Trauma Questionnaire. *Journal of Anxiety Disorders,* 79, 102381. https://doi.org/10.1016/j.janxdis.2021.102381.

Ridout, K. K., Khan, M., & Ridout, S. J. (2018). Adverse childhood experiences run deep: Toxic early life stress, telomeres, and mitochondrial DNA copy number, the biological markers of cumulative stress. *Bioessays: News and Reviews in Molecular, Cellular and Developmental Biology,* 40(9), e1800077. https://doi.org/10.1002/bies.201800077.

Roberts, A. L., Zafonte, R., Chibnik, L. B., Baggish, A., Taylor, H., Baker, J., Whittington, A. J., & Weisskopf, M. G. (2022). Association of adverse childhood experiences with poor neuropsychiatric health and dementia among former professional US football players. *JAMA Network Open,* 5(3), e223299. https://doi.org/10.1001/jamanetworkopen.2022.3299.

Roberts, S. J., Chandler, G. E., & Kalmakis, K. (2019). A model for trauma-informed primary care. *Journal of the American Association of Nurse Practitioners,* 31(2), 139–144. https://doi.org/10.1097/JXX.0000000000000116.

Robertshaw, L., Dhesi, S., & Jones, L. L. (2017). Challenges and facilitators for health professionals providing primary healthcare for refugees and asylum seekers in high-income countries: A systematic review and thematic synthesis of qualitative research. *BMJ Open,* 7(8), e015981. https://doi.org/10.1136/bmjopen-2017-015981.

Rocha, J., Rodrigues, V., Santos, E., Azevedo, I., Machado, S., Almeida, V., Silva, C., Almeida, J., & Cloitre, M. (2020). The first instrument for complex PTSD assessment: Psychometric properties of the ICD-11 Trauma Questionnaire. *Revista Brasileira de Psiquiatria,* 42(2), 185–189. https://doi.org/10.1590/1516-4446-2018-0272.

Rogel, A., Loomis, A. M., Hamlin, E. D., Hodgdon, H., Spinazzola, J., & van der Kolk, B. (2020). The impact of neurofeedback training on children with developmental trauma: A randomized controlled study. *Psychological Trauma: Theory, Research, Practice, and Policy,* 12(8), 918. https://doi.org/10.1037/tra0000648.

Rosen, V., & Ayers, G. (2020). An update on the complexity and importance of accurately diagnosing post-traumatic stress disorder and comorbid traumatic brain injury. *Neuroscience Insights,* 15, 2633105520907895. https://doi.org/10.1177/2633105520907895.

Sanders, M. R., & Hall, S. L. (2018). Trauma-informed care in the newborn intensive care unit: Promoting safety, security and connectedness. *Journal of Perinatology,* 38(1), 3–10. https://doi.org/10.1038/jp.2017.124.

Schlumpf, Y. R., Nijenhuis, E. R., Klein, C., Jäncke, L., & Bachmann, S. (2019). Functional reorganization of neural networks involved in emotion regulation following trauma therapy for complex trauma disorders. *Neuroimage: Clinical,* 23, 101807. https://doi.org/10.1016/j.nicl.2019.101807.

Schmidt, M. R., Narayan, A. J., Atzl, V. M., Rivera, L. M., & Lieberman, A. F. (2020). Childhood maltreatment on the Adverse Childhood Experiences (ACEs) scale versus the Childhood Trauma Questionnaire (CTQ) in a perinatal sample. *Journal of Aggression, Maltreatment & Trauma,* 29(1), 38–56. https://doi.org/10.1080/10926771.2018.1524806.

Schofield, P. W., Mason, R., Nelson, P. K., Kenny, D., & Butler, T. (2019). Traumatic brain injury is highly associated with self-reported childhood trauma within a juvenile offender cohort. *Brain Injury,* 33(4), 412–418. https://doi.org/10.1080/02699052.2018.1552020.

Siegel, A. N., Meshkat, S., Benitah, K., Lipsitz, O., Gill, H., Lui, L. M., …, & Rosenblat, J. D. (2021). Registered clinical studies investigating psychedelic drugs for psychiatric disorders. *Journal of Psychiatric Research,* 139, 71–81. https://doi.org/10.1016/j.jpsychires.2021.05.019.

Siemann, I., Sanches, E. E., de Jongh, F. W., Luijmes, R., Ingels, K., Beurskens, C., Monstrey, S. J., Ramnarain, D., Marres, H., & Pouwels, S. (2022). Psychological counselling in patients with a peripheral facial palsy: Initial experience from an expert centre. *Journal of Plastic, Reconstructive & Aesthetic Surgery,* 75(5), 1639–1643. https://doi.org/10.1016/j.bjps.2021.11.079.

Song, M. J., Nikoo, M., Choi, F., Schütz, C. G., Jang, K., & Krausz, R. M. (2018). Childhood trauma and lifetime traumatic brain injury among individuals who are homeless. *The Journal of Head Trauma Rehabilitation,* 33(3), 185–190. https://doi.org/10.1097/HTR.0000000000000310.

Sonu, S., Post, S., & Feinglass, J. (2019). Adverse childhood experiences and the onset of chronic disease in young adulthood. *Preventive Medicine,* 123, 163–170. https://doi.org/10.1016/j.ypmed.2019.03.032.

Spagnolo, P. A., Norato, G., Maurer, C. W., Goldman, D., Hodgkinson, C., Horovitz, S., & Hallett, M. (2020). Effects of TPH2 gene variation and childhood trauma on the clinical and circuit-level phenotype of functional movement disorders. *Journal of Neurology, Neurosurgery, and Psychiatry,* 91(8), 814–821. https://doi.org/10.1136/jnnp-2019-322636.

Speer, K., Upton, D., Semple, S., & McKune, A. (2018). Systemic low-grade inflammation in post-traumatic stress disorder: A systematic review. *Journal of Inflammation Research,* 11, 111–121. https://doi.org/10.2147/JIR.S155903.

Spinazzola, J., van der Kolk, B., & Ford, J. D. (2018). When nowhere is safe: Interpersonal trauma and attachment adversity as antecedents of posttraumatic stress disorder and developmental trauma disorder. *Journal of Traumatic Stress,* 31(5), 631–642. https://doi.org/10.1002/jts.22320.

Stolbach, B. C., & Anam, S. (2017). Racial and ethnic health disparities and trauma-informed care for children exposed to community violence. *Pediatric Annals*, 46(10), e377–e381. https://doi.org/10.3928/19382359-20170920-01.

Sundborg, S. A. (2019). Knowledge, principal support, self-efficacy, and beliefs predict commitment to trauma-informed care. *Psychological Trauma: Theory, Research, Practice, and Policy*, 11(2), 224–231. https://doi.org/10.1037/tra0000411.

Tanaka, T., Hirai, S., Hosokawa, M., Saito, T., Sakuma, H., Saido, T., Hasegawa, M., & Okado, H. (2021). Early-life stress induces the development of Alzheimer's disease pathology via angiopathy. *Experimental Neurology*, 337, 113552. https://doi.org/10.1016/j.expneurol.2020.113552.

Terzi, S., Dursun, E., Yılmaz, A., Özergin Coşkun, Z., Özgür, A., Çeliker, M., & Demirci, M. (2017). Oxidative stress and antioxidant status in patients with Bell's palsy. *Journal of Medical Biochemistry*, 36(1), 18–22. https://doi.org/10.1515/jomb-2016-0033.

Tomaz, T., & Castro-Vale, I. (2020). Trauma-informed care in primary health settings – which is even more needed in times of COVID-19. *Healthcare (Basel, Switzerland)*, 8 (3), 340. https://doi.org/10.3390/healthcare8030340.

Tseng, C. C., Hu, L. Y., Liu, M. E., Yang, A. C., Shen, C. C., & Tsai, S. J. (2017). Bidirectional association between Bell's palsy and anxiety disorders: A nationwide population-based retrospective cohort study. *Journal of Affective Disorders*, 215, 269–273. https://doi.org/10.1016/j.jad.2017.03.051.

van der Kolk, B., Ford, J. D., & Spinazzola, J. (2019). Comorbidity of developmental trauma disorder (DTD) and post-traumatic stress disorder: Findings from the DTD field trial. *European Journal of Psychotraumatology*, 10(1), 1562841. https://doi.org/10.1080/20008198.2018.1562841.

van der Kolk, B. A. (2014). *The body keeps the score: Brain, mind, and body in the healing of trauma*. New York: Penguin Books.

Vandyk, A., Bentz, A., Bissonette, S., & Cater, C. (2019). Why go to the emergency department? Perspectives from persons with borderline personality disorder. *International Journal of Mental Health Nursing*, 28(3), 757–765. https://doi.org/10.1111/inm.12580.

Williams, B., Ospina, J. P., Jalilianhasanpour, R., Fricchione, G. L., & Perez, D. L. (2019). Fearful attachment linked to childhood abuse, alexithymia, and depression in motor functional neurological disorders. *The Journal of Neuropsychiatry and Clinical Neurosciences*, 31(1), 65–69. https://doi.org/10.1176/appi.neuropsych.18040095.

Wiss, D. A., & Brewerton, T. D. (2020). Adverse childhood experiences and adult obesity: A systematic review of plausible mechanisms and meta-analysis of cross-sectional studies. *Physiology & Behavior*, 223, 112964. https://doi.org/10.1016/j.physbeh.2020.112964.

You, D. S., Albu, S., Lisenbardt, H., & Meagher, M. W. (2019). Cumulative childhood adversity as a risk factor for common chronic pain conditions in young adults. *Pain Medicine*, 20(3), 486–494. https://doi.org/10.1093/pm/pny106.

Yrondi, A., Valton, L., Bouilleret, V., Aghakhani, N., Curot, J., & Birmes, P. J. (2020). Post-traumatic stress disorder with flashbacks of an old childhood memory triggered by right temporal lobe epilepsy surgery in adulthood. *Frontiers in Psychiatry*, 11, 351. https://doi.org/10.3389/fpsyt.2020.00351.

Zhao, H., Zhang, X., Tang, Y. D., Zhu, J., Wang, X. H., & Li, S. T. (2017). Bell's palsy: Clinical analysis of 372 cases and review of related literature. *European Neurology*, 77(3–4), 168–172. https://doi.org/10.1159/000455073.

INDEX

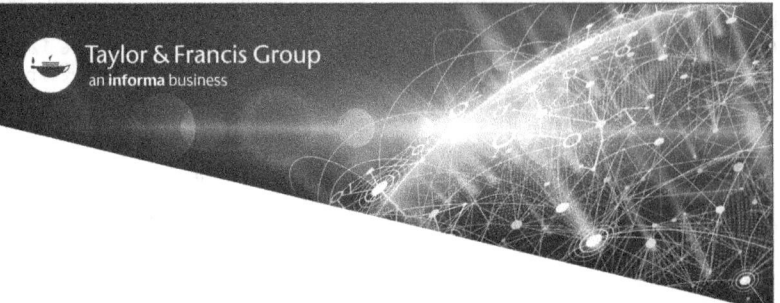
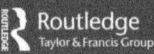
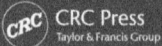